Joseph Paul Hardy III
6/17/83

Pathophysiology and Techniques of Cardiopulmonary Bypass

Volume I

This volume is one of the Cardiothoracic Surgery Series,
Edited by Joe R. Utley

Pathophysiology and Techniques of Cardiopulmonary Bypass

Volume I

Editor

Joe R. Utley, M.D.
Professor of Surgery
University of California
San Diego

Editorial Associate

E. Alexandra Ashleigh, B.A.

SANS TACHE
WILLIAMS & WILKINS
Baltimore/London

Made in the United States of America

Library of Congress Cataloging in Publication Data

Main entry under title:

Pathophysiology and techniques of cardiopulmonary bypass.

(Cardiothoracic surgery series)
Includes index.
1. Cardiopulmonary bypass. I. Utley, Joe R. II. Ashleigh, E. Alexandra (Elizabeth Alexandra) III. Series. [DNLM: 1. Aortocoronary bypass. 2. Postoperative complications. WG 169 P297] RD598.P37 617'.412 81-13044
ISBN 0-683-08501-8 AACR2

Composed and printed at the
Waverly Press, Inc.
Mt. Royal and Guilford Aves.
Baltimore, MD 21202, U.S.A.

Series Editor's Foreword

The goal of the cardiothoracic surgery series is to bring together new information in the basic, clinical, and applied sciences, which are important to the work of cardiothoracic surgeons. With this series we hope to increase the communication between surgeons, other physicians, and health professionals who are actively involved in the care of the cardiothoracic surgery patient. The complexity of care in cardiothoracic surgery involves not only the surgeon, but also the cardiologist, pulmonologist, internist, anesthesiologist, perfusionist, intensive care nurse, and operating room nurse, as well as many other health professionals. The body of knowledge used daily by these professionals includes not only knowledge from the surgical disciplines, but also knowledge from the basic sciences of chemistry, physics, biology, engineering, and physiology. It is hoped that this series will "enrich the flavor of the intellectual stew," and not only add to the reader's knowledge but also stimulate his critical thinking regarding problems related to the care of his patients. The reader may find more questions than answers in some of the material.

Summarized in the first volume are many of the organ system complications related to cardiopulmonary bypass as well as chapters related to specific clinical techniques and problems. Other chapters are related to basic science with specific relevance to cardiopulmonary bypass. The subject of each monograph will be selected according to the emergence of new developments in this specialty and the desire to relate knowledge gained in many disciplines to the current problems in cardiothoracic surgery.

—Joe R. Utley, M.D.

Preface

Cardiopulmonary bypass is used in the treatment of patients with heart disease over 100,000 times each year in the United States. The current safety of cardiopulmonary bypass is evidenced by the low mortality rates for aortocoronary bypass procedures. Nonetheless, cardiopulmonary bypass constitutes a major intervention with potential complications that can adversely affect virtually any organ system. The current safety of cardiopulmonary bypass is due to many years of concerted effort by surgeons, physiologists, biochemists, engineers, anesthesiologists, perfusionists, and the medical device industry to improve the quality of instrumentation used in cardiopulmonary bypass and to better understand the effects of cardiopulmonary bypass. In this monograph we have attempted to bring together widely diversified material related to cardiopulmonary bypass and to state the current understanding of the physiologic effects of cardiopulmonary bypass and its effect on various organ systems, and to discuss some of the current controversies regarding cardiopulmonary bypass. The monograph should prove useful to cardiac surgeons, cardiac surgery residents and trainees, anesthesiologists, intensivists, cardiologists, perfusionists, and persons working in the medical device industry.

—Joe R. Utley, M.D.

Acknowledgments

Numerous people's efforts have contributed to the production of this monograph. The editor wishes to acknowledge the support of the faculty in the Division of Cardiothoracic Surgery at the University of California at San Diego, many of whom are contributors to this volume. The work of editing and manuscript preparation has been greatly aided by the very careful work of Elizabeth Ashleigh, Judith Bohannan, Cleonice Gordon, and Linny Sarnecki.

Contributors

V. Paul Addonizio, Jr., M.D., Resident of Surgery, University of Pennsylvania, Philadelphia.

John P. Connors, M.D., Associate Professor of Surgery, Washington University, St. Louis.

Walter P. Dembitsky, M.D., Assistant Clinical Professor of Surgery, University of California, San Diego.

L. Henry Edmunds, Jr., M.D., Professor of Surgery, University of Pennsylvania, Philadelphia.

Robert J. Ellis, M.D., Associate Professor of Surgery, University of California, San Diego.

Mary Hartley-Winkler, R.N., C.C.P. University of California, San Diego.

Leland B. Housman, M.D., Clinical Instructor of Surgery, University of California, San Diego.

John J. Lamberti, M.D., Associate Clinical Professor of Surgery, University of California, San Diego.

David M. Long, M.D., Ph.D., Associate Clinical Professor of Surgery, University of California, San Diego.

William Y. Moores, M.D., Assistant Professor of Surgery, University of California, San Diego.

Diane J. Sansonetti, M.D., Resident in Surgery, University of California, San Diego.

Julie A. Swain, M.D., Assistant Professor of Surgery, University of California, San Diego.

Edward P. Todd, M.D., Ph.D., Professor of Surgery, University of Kentucky, Lexington.

Daniel J. Ullyot, M.D., Associate Professor of Surgery, University of California, San Francisco.

Joe R. Utley, M.D., Professor of Surgery, University of California, San Diego.

J. Deane Waldman, M.D., Associate Clinical Professor of Pediatrics, University of California, San Diego.

Jordan Waldman, M.D., Associate Clinical Professor of Anesthesiology, University of California, San Diego.

Fred N. White, Ph.D., Professor of Medicine (Physiology), Director, Physiological Research Laboratory, Scripps Institution of Oceanography, University of California, San Diego.

John A. Young, M.D., Assistant Professor of Surgery, University of California, San Diego.

Barry L. Zimmerman, M.D., Assistant Clinical Professor of Anesthesia, University of California, San Diego.

Contents

CHAPTER 1

OXYGEN DELIVERY DURING CARDIOPULMONARY BYPASS

WILLIAM Y. MOORES, M.D.

MYOCARDIAL OXYGEN DELIVERY

The cardiac output depends upon continuous oxygen delivery through the coronary circulation. Myocardial function is immediately impaired with decreased coronary flow. Studies have shown that decrease in coronary flow is followed by a proportionate decrease in myocardial function.[1] Myocardial oxygen demand must be met by adequate oxygen supply delivered to the myocardial cell. Delivery to the cell depends upon anatomic integrity of the coronary vessels, oxygen-carrying capacity of the blood, and release of oxygen to the myocardium.

Interventions during cardiopulmonary bypass can significantly effect the myocardial oxygen demands. With anesthesia induction, there are variations in myocardial oxygen demands. Arterial hypertension during anesthesia induction increases oxygen demands and may produce myocardial ischemia, especially in patients with coronary disease. The interaction of hypertension and anesthetic agents may significantly effect myocardial oxygen consumption. Wilkinson and his associates,[2] in a canine study, showed that hypertension during halothane anesthesia caused a decrease in myocardial performance which was not accompanied by decreased oxygen consumption. We compared myocardial performance under halothane and morphine sulfate anesthesia in our laboratory. During normoxia halothane significantly decreased myocardial performance which was matched by a proportionate decrease in myocardial oxygen consumption. Morphine sulfate anesthesia decreased neither myocardial performance nor oxygen consumption. When these swine were subjected to hypoxia (PO_2 40 torr), stroke volume at a given end diastolic pressure decreased with both anesthetic agents. The depression with halothane was greater than with morphine and, furthermore, this reduction in stroke volume was not accompanied by a proportionate fall in myocardial oxygen consumption.[3, 4] We concluded from these studies that halothane is not an appropriate anesthetic agent during bypass.

Shifts of the oxyhemoglobin dissociation curve to the right or left may affect myocardial oxygen consumption. The ability of hemoglobin (Hgb) to release oxygen over a specific arterial to coronary sinus pO_2 gradient may be affected by drugs or changes in pH that shift the oxyhemoglobin dissociation curve to the right or left.

During cardiopulmonary bypass when the circulation is being sustained by the heart-lung machine, the myocardial oxygen needs are reduced. Hypothermia decreases the myocardial oxygen demand. Hypothermia decreases the oxygen availability by increasing oxygen-hemoglobin affinity with a shift in the oxygen-hemoglobin dissociation curve to the left. During rewarming these changes in oxygen availability reverse, but at different rates. Many factors may affect the myocardial supply/demand ratio during cardiopulmonary bypass. These include the myocardial oxygen consumption, the partial pressure of oxygen in blood, the blood temperature, the blood pressure and coronary flow, the hemoglobin content of blood, and the oxygen-hemoglobin dissociation curve. Progressive hemodilution, changes in the oxygen-hemoglobin dissociation curve, and utilization of stroma free hemoglobin during cardiopulmonary bypass will be presented in this chapter.

Hemodilution during Cardiopulmonary Bypass

The use of a nonblood prime is advantageous for blood conservation with cardiopulmonary bypass. Tissue perfusion is improved as well. The safety of hemodilution during cardiopulmonary bypass was noted in 1965 by several investigators.[5–7] Subsequent reports documented increased edema and decreased left ventricular[8–11] function with hemodilution employing crystalloid solutions. Other studies compared crystalloid and colloid primes.[12, 13] Hemodilution using crystalloid primes to a hematocrit of 20% appears to be safe during cardiopulmonary bypass. Experimental studies show no change in oxygen consumption or venous pO_2 levels in dogs on cardiopulmonary bypass at a hematocrit level of 20%.[14]

Studies of hemodilution without cardiopulmonary bypass do not directly apply to the cardiopulmonary bypass situation, but do offer some information regarding an appropriate level of hemodilution that is tolerated by various organ systems. These studies have generally examined a sequential decrease in hematocrit with bleeding and volume replacements. One of these studies sequentially reduced the hematocrit value to 10% in dogs without effecting changes in baseline oxygen consumption at this low hematocrit value.[15] Another study looking at sequential decreases in hematocrit values in baboons found irreversible damage to the neurologic tissue with hematocrits in the 10–15% range.[16] One investigator noted no change in left ventricular function with a hematocrit 20%.[5] In spite of the preservation of myocardial function, this study documented a decrease in myocardial compliance accompanied by an increased myocardial oxygen consumption and a decreased coronary sinus oxygen tension. Coronary perfusion pressure was also noted to be a more significant determinant of myocardial performance at this low hematocrit level. As might be expected, a decrease in the hematocrit value has been associated with an increase in coronary blood flow[17] and heart rate.[18] If the period of hemodilution is prolonged, one may find an increase in the myocardial arteriovenous oxygen difference, as shown by Hagl and his coworkers[19] when they examined prolonged hemodilution at a hematocrit 20%.

Unpublished studies from our own laboratory examining severe hemodilution in swine have shown relatively normal preservation of left ventricular function in swine with a hematocrit of 15%. We also noted near normal preservation of myocardial performance in a single animal with a hematocrit 7%. All of these studies were done in normal animals where the changes in coronary blood flow, heart rate, arteriovenous oxygen difference, and tissue edema were frequently not reflected in performance changes. Unfortunately, these findings may have limited application for the patient with an abnormal myocardium, which is compirsed of coronary disease. It would seem obvious that hemodilution requiring an increase in coronary blood flow and heart rate may lead to further myocardial damage in patients with fixed coronary stenoses.

The combination of hemodilution and hypothermia during cardiopulmonary bypass has the benefit of decreasing oxygen consumption and lowering blood viscosity and improving tissue perfusion.[11, 20] In one study, Laver and his associates examined hemodilution and hypothermia in 17 patients who required cardiopulmonary bypass and circulatory arrest for congenital or acquired heart disease. The hematocrit values at the time of circulatory arrest varied from 5–17%. Although several of the patients died from their complex lesions, they were unable to attribute any deaths to the effect of hemidilution. The lower limit of hematocrit necessary to support organ function is not precisely known. Baboons have been exchanged transfused to a hematocrit of 10% before manifesting a precipitous drop in pH, oxygen consumption, and cardiac output.[21] These animals were sequentially hemodiluted to 10% hematocrit and showed an increase in cardiac output during progressive hemodilution prior to reaching the critical level of 10%.

Most applications of hemodilution during cardiopulmonary bypass deal with nonworking myocardium, and the safe level of hemodilution for the nonworking myocardium during bypass and subsequently for the working myocardium recovering from bypass has not been well worked out. As mentioned before, the preliminary data from our laboratory seems to support the concept that hemodilution to a hematocrit value of 15% is acceptable for the working myocardium immediately following cardiopulmonary bypass.

THE OXYGEN HEMOGLOBIN DISSOCIATION CURVE

The relationship between oxygen content and the partial pressure of oxygen in the blood is described by a sigmoid-shaped oxygen-hemoglobin dissociation curve (Fig. 1.1). The sigmoidal shape allows hemoglobin to remain highly saturated at a pO_2 value of 100 torr, and to release a large amount of oxygen with small drops in pO_2. Without this unique hemoglobin-oxygen relationship, oxygen would only be present in solution, and release would be a linear function related only to pO_2. The shape and position of this sigmoid oxygen-hemoglobin dissociation curve can vary. This variation can result in an alteration in the oxygen that is delivered over the same range of pO_2 values. Variation in the oxyhemoglobin dissociation curve is most frequently described as a change in the P-50 of the hemoglobin. The P-50 is defined as the oxygen tension present when the hemoglobin is 50% saturated. An increase in the hemoglobin-oxygen affinity is associated with a decrease in the P-50 value since the stronger attachment of the oxygen to the hemoglobin means that the partial pressure exerted by the oxygen is less when the Hgb is 50% saturated. Another term used to describe the oxyhemoglobin dissociation curve relationship is the Hill coefficient or the slope of the log plot of the dissociation curve. The P50 may remain stationary while a change in the slope occurs. The resultant release of O_2 over an arterial-venous PO_2 difference changes. A steeper slope means that more O_2 can be released over a smaller O_2 tension difference. Shifts in the oxygen-hemoglobin dissociation curve may be encountered with changes in the pH, pCO_2 and temperature.[22-25] The effects of these variations are described in Figure 1.1.

Variations during Cardiopulmonary Bypass

The oxygen-hemoglobin dissociation curve is altered by conditions encountered during cardiopulmonary bypass. These alterations include an increase in the oxygen-hemoglobin affinity, resulting in decreased oxygen delivery over a normal arterial and venous pO_2 range if a decrease in temperature, an increase in pH, or a decrease in hemoglobin concentration occurs. The substrate 2,3-diphosphoglycerate (2,3-DPG) has been closely linked to variation in the oxygen-hemoglobin dissociation curve.[26, 27] This organic phosphate, whose concentration rapidly decreases in aged blood, is required for blood to maintain a normal oxygen-hemoglobin dissociation relationship with the curve adequately positioned to the right. Low levels of 2,3-diphosphoglycerate results in a curve that is significantly shifted to the left, with a resultant decrease in oxygen delivery over a normal arterial-venous pO_2 range.

Variations in P-50

Many investigators have attempted to relate the oxygen-hemoglobin dissociation curve to myocardial performance. Most studies in animals have documented decreased myocardial performance when low P-50 blood was used. These studies have documented lowered venous pO_2 when blood with greater oxygen-hemoglobin affinity was used. Valeri and associates[28] have studied changes in postoperative myocardial performance with transfusion of blood enriched with 2,3-diphosphoglycerate. They found that replacement with 2,3-DPG-enriched blood increased cardiac index immediately following cardiopulmonary bypass.

In our own laboratory we have studied the importance of 2,3-DPG-enriched blood using a right heart bypass swine myocardial model. Animals are transfused with swine blood en-

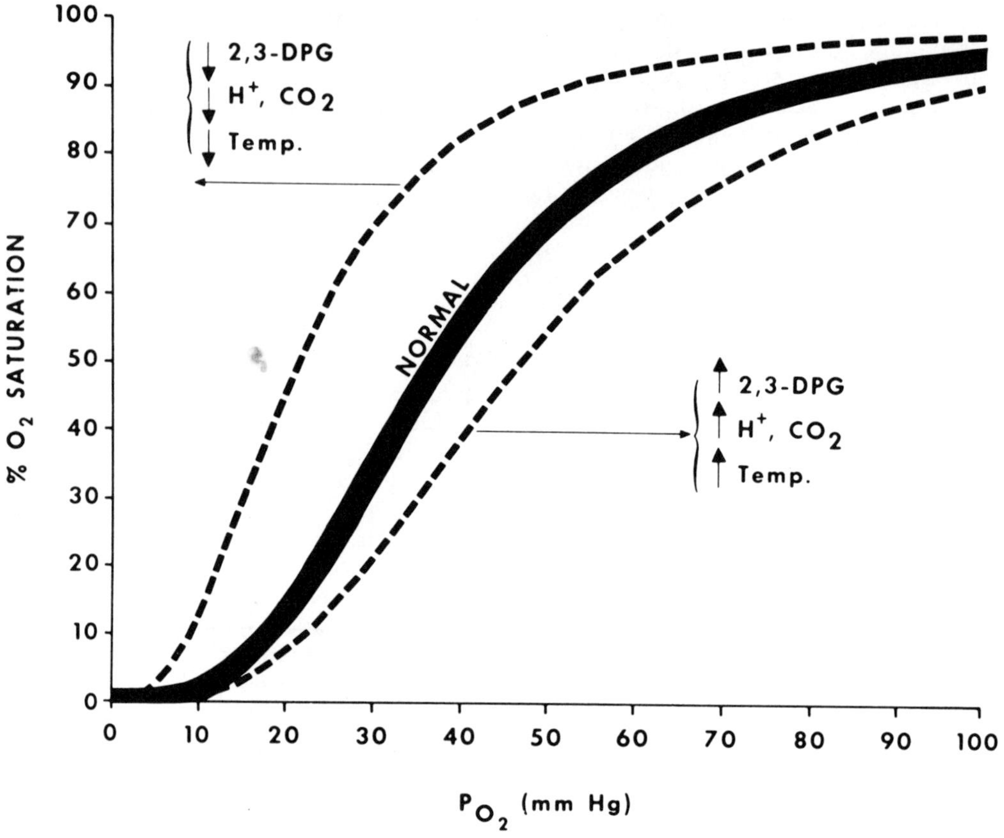

Figure 1.1. A schematic representation of the oxyhemoglobin dissociation curve showing the effect of 2,3-diphosphoglycerate hydrogen ion concentration, CO_2 concentration, and temperature on the position of the curve

riched with 2,3-DPG and increased P-50 or blood having depleted of 2,3-DPG and decreased P-50 value. The surgical preparation is seen in Figure 1.2. The results are summarized in Table 1.1 In this study we shifted the P-50 value from normal of 35 torr to an elevated value of 40 torr or a depressed value of 25 torr. This change in the P-50 was accompanied by changes in the concentration of 2,3-DPG. We did not document an increased stroke volume with the low hemoglobin-oxygen affinity blood having an increased P-50; however, we show a decrease in cardiac performance when the swine were exchange transfused with blood having an increased hemoglobin-oxygen affinity. This decrease in myocardial performance was matched by a decrease in the arterial-coronary sinus oxygen content difference as well as an increase in coronary blood flow. The coronary sinus pO_2 value was abnormally elevated in those animals perfused with high P-50 blood. Our conclusion was that an increase in the P-50 did not result in enhanced myocardial performance, and depression in the P-50 did result in decrements in stroke volume and the arterial coronary sinus oxygen content difference.

Examples of Multiple Factors

As previously stated, the clinical and experimental evidence associates increased myocardial performance with a normal or right-shifted oxygen-hemoglobin dissociation curve. When arterial and venous pO_2 values are normal, oxygen delivery is increased with a right shift of the curve. The curve is not linear, and oxygen delivery may

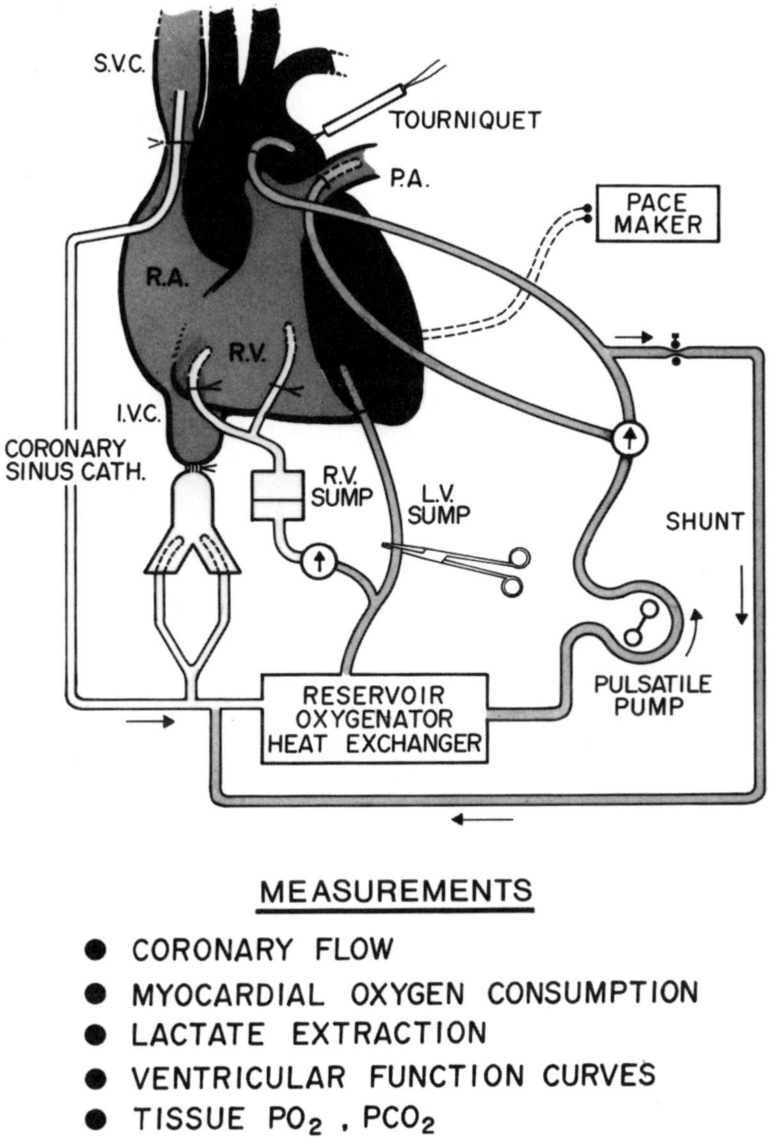

Figure 1.2. Right heart bypass preparation in swine. This diagram illustrates the pump circuit and resultant measurements from this preparation. *SVC*, superior vena cava; *IVC*, inferior vena cava; *RA*, right atrium; *LV*, left ventricle; *RV*, right ventricle; *PA*, pulmonary artery.

not be increased with right shift in the curve and low pO_2 values. The shape of the curve and the Hill coefficient (n) determines the oxygen delivered over a given pO_2 difference. The delivered oxygen can be determined over an arterial venous pO_2 difference with variations in P-50 and Hill coefficient (n). The influence of n and P-50 on oxygen delivery is in normoxia is shown in Figure 1.3. The oxygen tension goes from 90 torr in the arteries to 30 torr in the veins. Oxygen delivery is increased as the P-50 is elevated, although the increase in oxygen delivery tends to level off at a P-50 of 50 torr. Oxygen delivery is

Table 1.1
Importance of 2,3-DPG-enriched Blood in Cardiopulmonary Bypass Surgery

	Low HOA		High HOA	
	Control	Test	Control	Test
P-50 (torr)	35.8 ± 0.6	39.8 ± 1.0*	34.2 ± 1.1	25.6 ± 0.8*
2,3-DPG (μmoles/g Hgb)	25 ± 6	33 ± 6*	20 ± 2	9 ± 2*
Stroke volume (ml)	20 ± 2	19 ± 1	18 ± 1	14 ± 2*
A-CSO₂Δ (vol %)	8.7 ± 0.5	7.6 ± 0.9	8.1 ± 0.7	6.0 ± 0.3*
Coronary blood flow (ml/100 g heart)	104 ± 19	157 ± 19	122 ± 18	188 ± 19*
Coronary sinus PO_2	28 ± 1	35 ± 2*	28 ± 3	31 ± 3

* $P < 0.05$, test vs. control.
† P-50, PO_2 at 50% saturation; Hgb, hemoglobin; 2,3-DPG, 2,3-diphosphoglycerate; ml, milliliters; A-$CSO_2\Delta$, arterial-coronary sinus oxygen difference; HOA, hemoglobin-oxygen affinity.

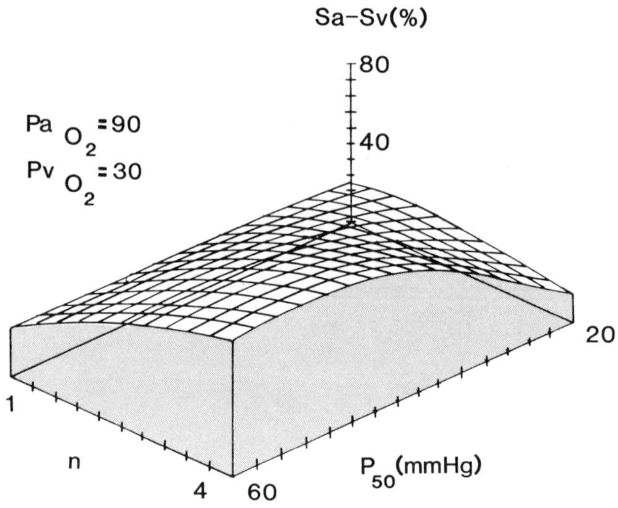

Figure 1.3. Three-dimensional representation of the amount of oxygen delivered (height of roof) when the P50 value and/or the end value are varied in an animal having an arterial oxygen tension of 90 torr and a venous oxygen tension of 30 torr. Sa-Sv, arteriovenous oxygen difference.

also increased as the n value increases from 1 to 4. In hypoxic situations with arterial pO_2 of 40 torr and a venous pO_2 of 20 torr is illustrated in Figure 1.4. In this situation, oxygen delivery increases as P-50 increases to 30 torr; however, oxygen delivery is decreased as the P-50 value increases to a value of 60 torr. In this situation the Hill slope value appears to have no real effect at a P-50 value of 60; however, there is a marked effect of the Hill slope if the P-50 value is maintained at around 30 torr. Therefore, a high Hill coefficient is disadvantageous only when both arterial and venous saturation differences are at the extreme of the oxygen dissociation curve.

Since the optimum position of the oxygen-hemoglobin dissociation curve depends on the arterial and venous pO_2 values, it is possible to construct an equation which will determine the optimum P-50 value that is appropriate for a given set of arterial and venous pO_2 values.[29] The optimum P-50 value can be determined by taking the square root of the product of the arterial and venous pO_2 values. A graphic representation of the optimal P-50 is seen in Figure 1.5 where the hemoglobin saturation is related to changes in P-50 at a venous oxygen tension of 30 and an arterial oxygen tension of 90 torr. It can be seen from this graph that the optimal P-50 is slightly in excess of 50 torr. A P-50 that is

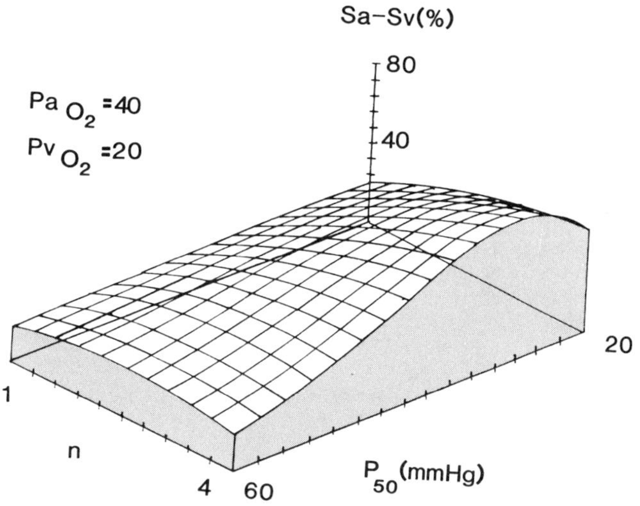

Figure 1.4. A three-dimensional representation illustrating the amount of oxygen delivered (height of roof) when the P50 value and/or the end value are varied in an animal with an arterial oxygen tension of 40 torr and a venous oxygen tension of 20 torr.

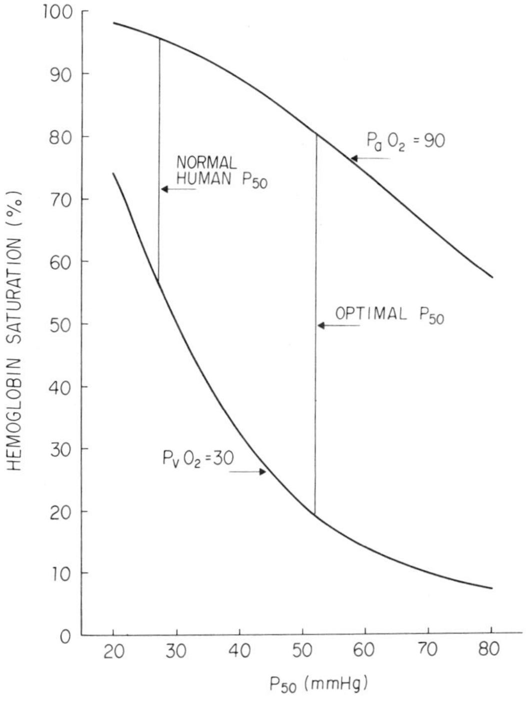

Figure 1.5. Diagram showing the hemoglobin saturation and percent at an arterial oxygen tension of 90 and a venous oxygen of 30 as the P50 is varied from 0 to 80. The normal P50 range is given at a P50 of 27; the optimal P50 which maximizes the saturation difference at these oxygen tensions is given at 52 torr.

in excess of that value will allow more oxygen to be removed from the venous blood at a pO_2 of 30, but the benefits of that increased removal will be more than compensated for by the decreased oxygen present at an arterial pO_2 of 90 at the higher P-50 values. Figure 1.6 shows the variation in cardiac output required if a given quantity of oxygen is to be delivered when the arterial oxygen tension and venous oxygen tension are 90 torr and 30 torr, respectively. If 6 liters of cardiac output are required to deliver a given amount of oxygen at these arterial and venous oxygen tensions at a normal P-50 of 27, then an output of something less than 4 liters per minute would be required to deliver the same amount of oxygen over the same arterial and venous oxygen tensions at an optimal P-50 of 52 torr.

ARTIFICIAL PERFUSION SOLUTIONS

If the limits of hemodilution are to be extended with an increased saving of blood during bypass, then some type of oxygen-carrying blood substitute is probably required. Additional oxygen may be placed into simple solution with an increase in the pO_2 value above 100 torr, and with a decrease in the temperature of the perfusate. Stroma free hemoglobin solution is such a blood substitute. This solution is not available for clinical usage.

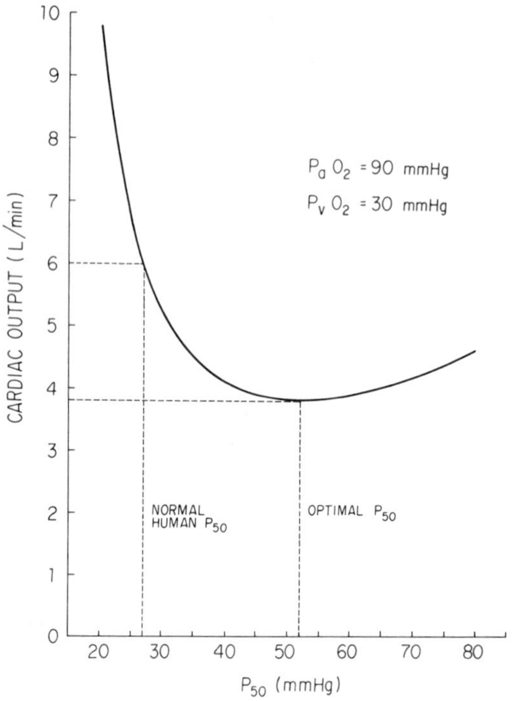

Figure 1.6. Diagram depicting the amount of cardiac output required to deliver a given amount of oxygen at an arterial oxygen tension of 90 and a venous oxygen tension of 30. Note the approximately 6 liters of cardiac output that are required to deliver the same amount of oxygen that could be delivered with slightly less than 4 liters per minute at the optimal P50.

Stroma Free Hemoglobin Solution

The search for a cell-free blood substitute has spanned many years. A crude hemoglobin solution was used experimentally by Amberson prior to 1934.[30] In more recent times, stroma free hemoglobin solutions have not possessed the kidney damaging characteristics of the initially evaluated crude solutions.[31, 32] At present, stroma free hemoglobin solution may have most of the desirable characteristics of a truly effective artificial blood. These major advantages include: its existence as a naturally occurring protein; its oxygen transporting characteristics[21, 33, 34]; its oncotic activity[30, 35] and its low viscosity.[36] Furthermore, it does not require typing or cross matching, does not cause microaggregation,[37, 38] and has not been found to cause any significant allergic problems.[39, 40]

Solutions now being investigated have virtually no nephrotoxicity, coagulation-anticoagulation properties, antigenicity, and methemoglobin conversion problems. These adverse properties of the initial hemoglobin solutions were reported by many investigators,[41–44] but their association with stromal components have meant their disappearance with true stroma free hemoglobin solutions. These solutions are prepared by high speed centrifugation and micropore filtration. Investigators have refined their techniques to solve the problems of vascular retention and oxygen off-loading.[45, 46]

The ability of these solutions to maintain life in totally exchanged dogs and baboons has been demonstrated with most solutions.[21, 32, 34, 47] The usefulness of stroma free hemoglobin solution as a resuscitation solution has been examined.[48–51] Many authors demonstrated increased effectiveness with stroma free hemoglobin solution over other crystalline resuscitation fluids. They have shown that such parameters as acid-base status, mitochondrial function, survival, and renal function return more closely to normal with stroma free hemoglobin solutions than with a nonhemoglobin-containing solutions. The major theoretical advantage of stroma free hemoglobin solution over other oncotically active proteins is the ability of stroma-free hemoglobin solution to transport oxygen.

The problem of the high hemoglobin-oxygen affinity (low P50) of these solutions, as well as the short *in vivo* biologic disappearance time, have recently been studied.[45, 52, 53] Although the short biological life of these solutions poses special problems regarding the use of stroma free hemoglobin solutions as a long-term blood replacement following major blood loss and during cardiopulmonary bypass, it is the high oxygen affinity that may limit the usefulness of the solution for both acute and chronic maintenance of oxygen transport in a patient being perfused with a low level of circulating erythrocytes.

Stroma free hemoglobin solution is essentially free of the organic phosphate 2,3-diphosphoglycerate (2,3-DPG), and this absence of 2,3-DPG has been felt to correlate

Table 1.2
Value of Stroma Free Hemoglobin Solution as a Perfusion Prime

	I. Stroma Free Hemoglobin Solution (Hct = 5%)		II. Albumin Solution (Hct = 5%)		III. Albumin Solution (Hct = 10%)	
	Control	Test	Control	Test	Control	Test
SV	20 ± 3†	10 ± 4	23 ± 5	0	21 ± 4	4 ± 3
Hct	26 ± 2	5 ± 1	30 ± 3	4 ± 1	31 ± 3	10 ± 0.6
Hgb	8.7 ± 0.7	5.4 ± 0.3	10.2 ± 0.8	1.5 ± 0.2	10.4 ± 1	3.4 ± 0.2

* SV, stroke volume at left ventricular end diastolic pressure (LVEDP) of 14 torr; Hct, hematocrit (vol %); Hgb, hemoglobin concentration (g/deciliter).
† Values are means ± SE.

with a low P50 seen in stroma free hemoglobin solutions. Recent studies describe a chemically modified stroma-free hemoglobin solution that has been manufactured by adding pyridoxal-5-phosphate (PLP) to the basic hemoglobin solution. Others have investigated solutions with improved oxygen off-loading.[54] Studies using nonaltered stroma free hemoglobin solution have shown a normal oxygen consumption in baboons maintained at 0 hematocrit.[21] Other investigators have observed significant fall in the tissue pO_2 values of abdominal viscera of animals transfused with stroma free hemoglobin solutions to a hematocrit value of 10%.[55] This tissue hypoxia was accompanied by an increase in oxygen-hemoglobin affinity of the animal's circulating hemoglobin (erythrocytic and stroma free hemoglobin combined) as the hematocrit value was decreased.

We attempted to determine the value of stroma free hemoglobin solution as a perfusion prime in a swine study that employed a surgical model identical to that described earlier in this chapter. The animal preparation and the measurements were those listed in Figure 1.2. An initial study[56] examined hemodilution on cardiopulmonary bypass to a hematocrit level of 5% with either stroma free hemoglobin solution or an equivalent oncotically active albumin solution. The data from this study, as well as data for animals supported at hematocrit level of 10% with albumin solution, are presented in Table 1.2. This study showed that no significant stroke volume could be maintained with albumin solution at hematocrit values of 5 or 10%, but if the perfusion solutions contained stroma free hemoglobin solution at a hematocrit value of 5%, then stroke volume could be maintained, although at a significantly decreased value. The findings from this study, as well as the studies enumerated above, lend support to the concept that stroma free hemoglobin solution may be a very appropriate artificial blood substitute for use during cardiopulmonary bypass.[57, 58] Some of its present disadvantages, such as a short *in vivo* retention time, may be advantageous when the solution is used as an extracorporeal circulation prime where one would want excretion of the prime solution following discontinuation of cardiopulmonary bypass.

CONCLUSION

The problem of supplying adequate oxygen to the myocardium and other organ systems during and following cardiopulmonary bypass is a complex one involving many factors. These factors may oppose each other in providing adequate oxygen to the body and the myocardium, and it is only by increasing our understanding of the dynamics of oxygen delivery with artificial perfusion that we can design perfusion that adequately provides for oxygen needs.

References

1. Stowe DF, Mathey DG, Moores WY, Glantz SA, Townsend RM, Kabra P, Chatterjee K, Parmley WW, Tyberg JV: Segment stroke work and metabolism depend on coronary blood flow in the pig. Am J Phys 234:H597, 1978.
2. Wilkinson PL, Tyberg JV, Moyers JR, White AE: Changes in myocardial oxygen consumption, efficiency and haemodynamics when systemic pressure is increased during morphine and added halothane anaesthesia in dogs. Can Anaesth Soc J 27:230, 1980.

3. Moores WY, Weiskopf RB, Dembitsky WP, Utley JR: Comparative effects of halothane and morphine anesthesia on myocardial function and metabolism during cyanosis in swine. Surg Forum 30:221, 1979.
4. Weiskopf RB, Moores WY, Riordan KK, Townsley MI, Crum JD, Willford DC, Dembitsky WP: Left ventricular dynamics: A comparison of morphine and halothane during normoxia. Proceedings of the Annual Meeting of the American Society of Anesthetists. Chicago, Illinois, 1978.
5. Litwak RS, Gadboys HL, Kahn M, Wisoff BG: High flow total body perfusion utilizing diluted perfusate in a large prime system. J Thorac Cardiovasc Surg 49:74, 1965.
6. Neville WE, Scicchitano L, Maben H, Banuchi F, Peacock H: Cardiopulmonary bypass with large volume nonblood perfusate. Experimental and clinical observations. Circulation 31(Suppl 1):130, 1965.
7. Roe BB, Hutchinson JC, Swenson EE: High-flow body perfusion with calculated hemodilution. Ann Thorac Surg 1:581, 1965.
8. Buckberg GD, Towers B, Paglia DE, Mulder DG, Maloney JV: Subendocardial ischemia after cardiopulmonary bypass. J Thoracic Cardiovasc Surg 64: 669, 1972.
9. Morales AR, Fine G, Taber RE: Cardiac surgery and myocardial necrosis. Arch Pathol 83:71, 1967.
10. Foglia RP, Lazar HL, Steed DL, Follette DM, Manganaro AJ, Deland E, Buckberg GD: Iatrogenic myocardial edema with crystalloid primes: Effect on left ventricular compliance, performance and perfusion. Surg Forum 29:312, 1978.
11. Utley JR, Todd EP, Wachtel CC, Cain RB, Collins JC: Effects of hypothermia, hemodilution and pump oxygenation on organ water content and blood flow. Surg Forum 27:217, 1976.
12. Hallowell P, Bland JHL, Dalton BC, Erdmann AJ III, Lappas DG, Laver MB, Philbin D, Thomas S, Lowenstein E: The effect of hemodilution with albumen on Ringer's lactate on water balance and blood use in open-heart surgery. Ann Thorac Surg 25:22, 1978.
13. Laks H, Standeven J, Blair O, Hahn J, Jellinek M, Willman VL: The effects of cardiopulmonary bypass with crystalloid and colloid hemodilution on myocardial extravascular water. J Thoracic Cardiovasc Surg 73:129, 1977.
14. Kawashima Y, Yamamoto Z, Manabe H: Safe limits of hemodilution in cardiopulmonary bypass. Surgery 76:391, 1974.
15. Wright CJ: The effects of severe progressive hemodilution on regional blood flow and oxyen consumption. Surgery 79:299, 1976.
16. Nagao S, Roccaforte P, Moody RA: The effects of isovolemic hemodilution and reinfusion of packed erythrocytes on somatosensory and visual evoked potentials. J Surg Res 25:530, 1978.
17. Murray JF, Rapaport E: Coronary blood flow and myocardial metabolism in acute experimental anaemia. Cardiovasc Res 6:360–367, 1972.
18. Buckberg G, Brazier J: Coronary blood flow and cardiac function during hemodilution. Bibl. Haematol., No. 41, p. 173, 1975.
19. Hagl S, Bornikoel K, Mayr N, Messmer K, Sebening F: Cardiac performance during limited hemodilution. No. 41, p. 152, 1975.
20. Laver MB, Buckley MJ, Austen WG: Extreme hemodilution with profound hypothermia and circulatory arrest. Bibl. Haematol, No. 41, p. 152, 1975.
21. Moss GS, DeWoskin R, Rosen AL, Levine H, Palani CK: Transport of oxygen and carbon dioxide by hemoglobin-saline solution in the red cell-free primate. Surg. Gynecol Obstet. 12:357, 1976.
22. Bohr C, Hasselbalch K, Krogh A: Ueber einen in biologischer beziehung wichtigen einfluss, den die kohlensaurespannung des blutes auf dessen sauerstoffbindung übt. Skand Arch Physiol 16:402, 1904.
23. German B, Wyman J Jr: The titration curves of oxygenated and reduced hemoglobin. J Biol Chem 117:533, 1937.
24. Astrup P, Engel K, Severinghaus JW, Munson E: The influence of temperature and pH on the dissociation curve of oxyhemoglobin of human blood. Scand J Clin Lab Invest 17:515, 1965.
25. Severinghaus JW: Respiration and hypothermia. Ann NY Acad Sci 80:384, 1959.
26. Chanutin A, Curnish RR: Effects of organic and inorganic phosphates on the oxygen equilibrium of human erythrocytes. Arch Biochem Biophys 121:96, 1967.
27. Benesch R, Benesch RE: The effect of organic phosphates from the human erythrocyte on the allosteric properties of hemoglobin. Biochem Biophys Res Commun 26:162, 1967.
28. Dennis RC, Hechtman HB, Berger RL, Vito L, Weisel RD, Valeri CR: Transfusion of 2,3 DPG-enriched red blood cells to improve cardiac function. Ann Thorac Surg 26:17, 1978.
29. Willford DC, Hill EP, Moores WY: Theoretical analysis of optimal P50. Submitted to J Appl Physiol, 1980.
30. Amberson WR, Flexner J, Steggerda FR, Mulder AG, Tendler MJ, Pankratz DS, Lang EP: On the use of Ringer-Locke solutions containing hemoglobin as a substitute for normal blood in mammals. J Cell Comp Physiol 5:359, 1934.
31. Rabiner SF, Helbert JR, Lopas H, Friedman LH: Evaluation of a stroma-free hemoglobin solution for use as a plasma expander. J Exp Med 126:1127, 1967.
32. Peskin GW, O'Brien K, Rabiner SF: Stroma-free hemoglobin solution: The "ideal" blood substitute? Surgery 66:185, 1969.
33. Bonhard K: Acute oxygen supply by infusion of hemoglobin solutions. Fed Proc 34:1466, 1975.
34. De Venuto F, Moores WY, Zegna AI, Zuck TF: Total and partial blood exchange in the rat with hemoglobin prepared by crystallization. Transfusion 17:555, 1977.
35. DeVenuto F, Zegna AI: Plasma oncotic pressure during and after blood exchange with crystalline hemoglobin solution. Surg Gynecol Obstet, 147:379, 1978.
36. Usami S, Chien S, Gregersen MI: Hemoglobin solution as a plasma expander: Effects on blood viscosity. Proc Soc Exp Biol Med 136:1232, 1971.
37. Hamilton PB, Farr LE, Hiller A, Van Slyke DD: Preparation of hemoglobin solution for intravenous

infusion. J Exp Med 86:455, 1947.
38. DeVenuto F: Stability of crystalline hemoglobin solution during extended storage. J Lab Clin Med, in press, 1981.
39. Cochin A, Das Gupta TK, DeWoskin R, Moss GS: Immunogenic properties of stroma *vs.* stroma-free hemoglobin solution. Surg Forum 23:19, 1972.
40. Sasazuki T: Studies on haptoglobin. Immunochemical properties of haptoglobin and antihemoglobin antibody. Proc Jap Acad 46:820, 1970.
41. Hamilton PB, Hiller A, Van Slyke DD: Renal effects of hemoglobin infusions in dogs in hemorrhagic shock. J Exp Med 86:477, 1947.
42. Baker SB de C, Dawes RLF: Experimental hemoglobinuric nephrosis. J Pathol Bacteriol 87:49, 1964.
43. Jaenike JR: The renal lesion associated with hemoglobinemia. I. Its production and functional evolution in the rat. J Exp Med 123:523, 1966.
44. Rabiner SF, Friedman LH: The role of intravascular hemolysis and the reticuloendothelial system in the production of a hypercoagulable state. Br J Haematol 14:105, 1968.
45. Greenburg AG, Schooley M, Peskin GW: Improved retention of stroma-free hemoglobin solution by chemical modification. J Trauma 17:501, 1977.
46. Greenburg AG, Elia C, Levine B, Belsha J, Peskin GW: Hemoglobin solution and the oxyhemoglobin dissociation curve. J Trauma 15:943, 1975.
47. Palani CK, DeWaskin, Michuda M, Rosen AL, Moss GS: *In vivo* oxygen transport with a stroma-free hemoglobin solution in primates. Surg Forum 25: 199, 1974.
48. Elia C, Sternberge HJ, Greenburg AG, Peskin GW: Stroma-free hemoglobin in the resuscitation of hemorrhagic shock. Surg Forum 25:201, 1974.
49. Collins JA, Braitberg A, Butcher HR Jr: A direct comparison of various fluid regimens in the resuscitation of rates following hemorrhage. In: Acute Fluid Replacement in the Therapy of Shock, Chap 22, edited by Malinin TI, Zeppa R, Drucker WR, and Callahan AB, New York, Stratton Intercontinental Medical Book Corp., 1974, p. 169.
50. Relihan M, Litwin MS: Clearance rate and renal effects of stroma-free hemoglobin on acidotic dogs. Surg Gynecol Obstet 137:73, 1973.
51. Jesch F, Endrich B, Pfieffer R, Messmer K: Resuscitation from acute blood loss with use of stroma-free hemoglobin solution. Eur Surg Res 8(Suppl. 2):168, 1976.
52. Messmer K, Jesch F, Schaff J, Schonberg M, Pielsticker K, Bonhard K: Oxygen supply by stroma free hemoglobin. In: Blood Substitutes and Plasma Expanders. Alan R. Liss, New York, 1978, pp. 175 and 190.
53. Greenburg AG, Pearl J, Belsha J, Peskin GW: An improved stroma-free hemoglobin solution. Surg Forum 26:53, 1975.
54. Moss GW: Personal communication.
55. Sunder-Plassman L, Sinagowitz, Rink R, Dieterle R, Messmer K, Kessler M: The local oxygen supply in tissue of abdominal viscera and of skeletal muscle in extreme hemodilution with stroma free hemoglobin solution. Adv Exp Med Biol 37A:395–400, 1973.
56. Moores WY, De Venuto F, Heydorn WH, Weiskopf RB, Baysinger M, Greenburg AG, Utley JR: Extending the limits of hemodilution on cardiopulmonary bypass using stroma-free hemoglobin solution. J Thorac Cardiovasc Surg 81:155, 1981.
57. Glogar DH, Clark LC Jr, Kloner RA, DeBoer LMV, Muller J, Braunwald E: Fluorocarbons—Synthetic oxygen carrying compounds which reduce myocardial ischemia. Circulation 62(Supp III):144, 1980.
58. Engelman RM, Rousou JH, Dobbs WA: Fluosol-DA, and artificial blood for total cardiopulmonary bypass. Program abstract, Society for Thoracic Surgery, 1981.

CHAPTER 2

FLUOROCARBONS AND SYNTHETIC BLOODS: CAPABILITIES AND FUTURE USES

DAVID M. LONG, M.D., Ph.D.

Synthetic blood is a product of work done by Dr. Leland C. Clark, Jr., a chemist whose many technologic contributions have had an enormous impact on the conduct of cadiopulmonary bypass (CPB). Dr. Clark invented the telethermometer. The next discovery of Dr. Clark's was that of the use of silicone antifoam for bubble oxygenators. Prior to the use of this agent, debubbling was performed by inefficient, traumatic mechanical devices. The oxygen electrode has been called the "Clark" electrode. Oxygen levels were monitored by the color of the blood during the initial years of open heart surgery since it took a long time to get the results of oxygen content measurements determined with the Van Slyke apparatus. Synthetic blood may be the most important discovery that Clark has made.

The unique properties of perfluorocarbon liquids were discovered while Clark and his colleagues[1] were screening a large number of compounds to increase diffusivity of oxygen from the blood to the sensing mechanism of the oxygen electrode. The properties of high O_2 solubility and chemical inertness were then tested in fluid ventilation studies by Clark and Gollan.[1] After this experiment, Gollan and Clark[2] tested the material as an organ perfusate. Sloviter and Kaminoto[3] made flurocarbon emulsions with albumin and found they could maintain the metabolic demands of the isolated perfused brain with fluorochemicals quite as well as with whole blood. Geyer et al. exchange transfused rats with fluorocarbon emulsions and had survival with erythrocyte concentrations of 0.5%. The enthusiasm generated by these initial studies was soon blunted by the realization that certain fluorochemicals, such as the perfluorotributylamine used by Geyer,[5] was eliminated from the body at an extremely slow and unacceptable rate. Since that time there has been a search for new fluorocarbons and emulsifying agents in order to obtain that combination that will make the ideal erythrocyte substitute.

CHEMICAL AND PHYSICAL PROPERTIES

As a result of 16 years of experiments, it is now possible to focus on six properties of the fluorocarbons:

1. Oxygen solubility
2. Chemical reactivity
3. Biological reactivity
4. Vapor pressure
5. Emulsion stability
6. Critical solution temperature and transpiration rate.

The initial experiments with fluid ventilation were performed with perfluorobutyltetrahyrdrofuran. (The 3M Company code for this compound was FX80, later changed to FC-75.) FC-75 was also used by Golland and Clark[2] to perfuse the heart for short periods. Sloviter and Kaminoto[3] made emulsions of this compound with bovine albumin as the emulsifying agent and perfused the isolated brain successfully, but when emulsions of FC-75 were adminstered intravenously to animals, they died in several hours with hyperinflated lungs. As was learned later, the vapor pressure of this compound is 51 torr, which is too high and promotes intravascular vaporization of fluorocarbons. Perfluorotributylamine (code names FC-43 and FC-47) was used by Geyer et al.,[4, 5] who also used Pluronic F-68 as the emulsifying agent. FC-47 has a very low vapor pressure of 2.5 torr and also makes a very stable emulsion of small particle size. With this preparation, Geyer was able to exchange transfuse rats to an erythrocyte hematocrit of 0.5% with permanent survival. The rats were placed in an oxygen-enriched atmosphere initially, and as they produced red blood cells to replace the fluorocarbon emulsion, the oxygen concentration of the atmosphere was gradually reduced. White blood cells, antibodies, and coagulation factors were not replaced by the fluorocarbon infusion, but the rats did not develop infections or bleed from the puncture sites used for the exchange transfusions. The perfluorotributylamine was "scrubbed" from the circulation by the phagocytic cells of the reticuloendothelial system. Elimination of fluorocarbons occurs as a vapor that escapes through the lungs and skin in much the same manner as an inert gas is eliminated. Because the vapor pressure of FC-47 is so low, the half-life is 895 days, and the FC-47 is stored in the body of the animals for virtually their entire life span. This long dwell time has not caused death or serious side effects other than massive organomegaly of the liver and spleen. Nevertheless, such a long dwell time is unacceptable for human use from a medicolegal point of view. FC-47 has been abandoned from consideration as a synthetic blood, except for laboratory usage in organ perfusion.

Perfluorodecalin was used by Clark et al. and Naito and his colleagues[7] because of its lower vapor pressure (12.7 torr). Perfluorodecalin has a more acceptable half-life of about 7 days. The disadvantage with perfluorodecalin is that it is difficult to make stable emulsions with this compound. Naito et al.[7] and his collaborators at Green Cross Corporation have used seven parts of perfluorodecalin in three parts of perfluorotripropylamine to prepare stable fine emulsions. This preparation is known commercially as Fluosol DA and has Pluronic F-68 as well as yolk phospholipid as emulsifying agents.[8] The half-life of perfluorotripropylamine is 63 days. Fluosol DA has been used successfully in human volunteers and more than 200 patients.

Oxygen Solubility Property

The oxygen solubility of perfluorocarbons varies from compound to compound. Ghosh et al.[9] reviewed some of the problems associated with measuring the oxygen solubility of perfluorocarbons. A list of the oxygen solubilities and vapor pressures of six perfluorochemicals of interest as synthetic bloods is given in Table 2.1. It is important to note that these O_2 solubilities are given for neat fluorocarbon liquids. The synthetic bloods are emulsions containing anywhere from 10% to 50% of perfluorocarbon. The O_2 content of the emulsions is directly related to the concentration of the emulsion and O_2 solubility of the particular fluorochemical. In Figure 2.1, we have compared the oxyhemoglobin dissociation curve for whole blood and the oxygen content of plasma with the oxygen content of fluorochemical emulsions of different concentrations at different partial pressures of oxygen. An oxygen solubility of 50 ml/100 ml of perfluorocarbon was used in plotting these graphs since this is the approximate oxygen solubility of perfluorocytlbromide (PFOB), the fluorochemical used in our laboratories.

The comparisons illustrated in Figure 2.1 may be helpful in understanding some of the phenomena observed when using synthetic bloods. It can be seen that the oxygen content is high with PFOB concentrations of 10% or more, but only with high partial pressures of oxygen. When mixtures of fluorochemical emulsions and whole blood are present, the

Table 2.1
Oxygen Solubilities and Vapor Pressures of Six Perfluorochemicals Used as Synthetic Bloods

	Oxygen Solubility (ml/100 ml, 25°C)	Vapor Pressure (mm Hg, 37.5°C)
1. Perfluoroctylbromide	52.7*	14
2. Perfluoroheptobromide	51.4	40
3. FC-75	52.2	51
4. Perfluorodimethyladamantane	39.4	—
5. Perfluorodecalin	40.3	13.6
6. FC-47	38.4	2.5

* This data was obtained from Wesseler et al.[32] and from specifications supplied by the manufacturers of the fluorochemicals.

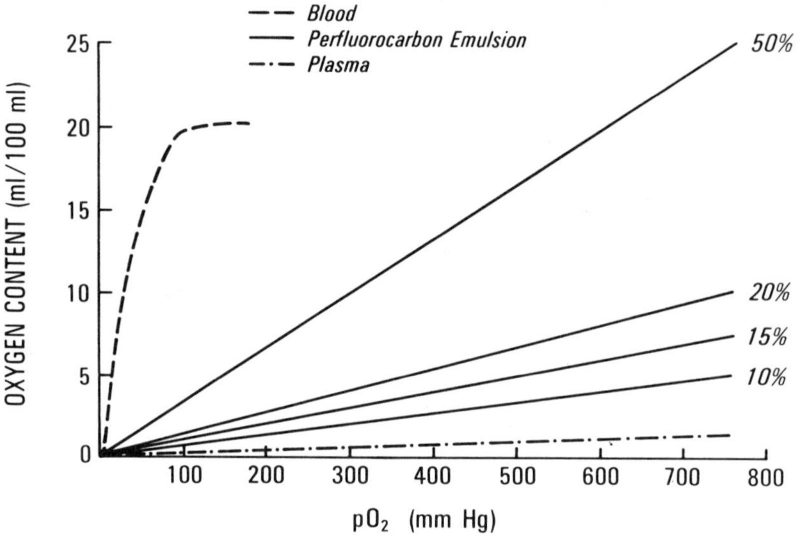

Figure 2.1. The oxygen content of perfluoroctylbromide emulsions of concentrations 10, 15, 20, and 50% is compared with the oxygen solubility of plasma and the normal oxyhemoglobin dissociation curve. Note that the oxygen solubility of perfluorocarbon and plasma obeys Henry's law and has a linear relationship with partial pressure of oxygen in contrast to the sigmoidal pattern of the oxyhemoglobin dissociation curve of whole blood.

dissolved oxygen is released before hemoglobin releases oxygen as long as the partial pressure of O_2 is high. In most of the animal experiments reported thus far, the fluorochemical concentration was at least 10%, and the animals were breathing 95 to 100% O_2. Under these circumstances, the venous pO_2 and the tissue pO_2 have been between 200 and 400 mm Hg, and all of the oxygen delivered was from the fluorochemical emulsions.

Tremper et al.[10] performed detailed hemodynamic studies on a patient whose hemoglobin concentration had decreased to 3.5 g/dl as a result of hemorrhage. This patient was given 1000 ml of Fluosol DA 20% prior to hysterectomy. The concentration of Fluosol DA in the blood increased to a maximum of 2.7%. With the patient breathing an FIO_2 of 1.0, the arterial O_2 concentration was 8.1 ml/dl, and the venous partial pressure of O_2 was 90 torr. The oxygen consumption of the patient remained the same before and after

Fluosol DA, but the cardiac index decreased from 7.2 to 5.9 liters/minute/M^2. Tremper estimated that 27% of the O_2 delivery was by Fluosol DA. The hemodynamic studies reported in this single case presentation are illustrative of the types of information that are needed to make critical decisions on the value of synthetic bloods.

Carbon dioxide solubility is as important as O_2 solubility since CO_2 metabolism is directly associated with and influences O_2 metabolism. The solubility of CO_2 in perfluorocarbons is many times greater than the O_2 solubility. CO_2 transport is not impaired by fluorochemicals, and partial pressures of CO_2 are either normal or decreased.

RATES OF ELIMINATION

As mentioned above, the slow rate of elimination from the body was a critical factor in eliminating FC-47 as an erythrocyte substitute for use in humans. Yokayama et al.[8] found the half-lives for perfluorodecalin and perfluorotripropylamine were 7 and 63 days, respectively. The elimination rate for perfluorocytlbromide is about the same as that for perfluorodecalin according to Clark. Clark et al.[11] have done the most extensive studies of the elimination rates of different fluorochemicals and have found vapor pressure as well as chemical structure to be important factors in the rate of elimination. Critical solution temperature and transpiration rates are used by Clark to evaluate the rate of elimination of fluorocarbons from the body. Although there has been great emphasis placed on the rate of elimination from the body, there is no evidence to point to any particular time factor as being ideal or acceptable. It is generally assumed that the longer a substance stays in the body and the higher the concentration, the greater the opportunity for producing adverse effects. This hypothesis has a number of exceptions that are noteworthy. Cardiovascular surgeons have developed many different types of materials and compounds that have been implanted permanently with no significant side effects. Nevertheless, carcinogenic compounds usually exert their adverse effects by virtue of long dwell time, high concentration, or repeated exposure, so there is reason to develop fluorochemicals with the shortest dwell time feasible. Medicolegal considerations and anxiety over litigation are sometimes given significant priority when one is making decisions about commercial development.

Intravascular elimination rates are of prime consideration in selecting materials for synthetic blood. Coarse emulsions are eliminated from the blood stream rapidly and produce reticuloendothelial blockade.[8] Fine emulsions of a particle size less than 0.4 μm are eliminated more slowly. Emulsions of FC-47 were eliminated slowly from exchange transfused rats so that retransfusion of shed blood was not necessary. Fluosol DA emulsions are eliminated more rapidly. The half-life was 4.2 hours for human subjects receiving 200 ml of Fluosol DA and 5.9 hours for subjects receiving 500-ml infusions.[12] Using fine emulsions of perfluorocytlbromide, in a dosage of 10 ml/kg of a 48% emulsion in rabbits, we observed a prolonged half-life of 32 hours (Fig. 2.2). Just as we do not yet have standards for elimination rates from the body, the ideal intravascular elimination rate is also not known. Different rates of elimination may be acceptable for different applications. In the controlled environment of open heart surgery, a half-life of 4 to 6 hours for synthetic blood may be satisfactory while longer intravascular dwell times may be needed when treating mass casualties.

SYNTHETIC BLOOD IN EXTRACORPOREAL CIRCULATION

Is There a Need?

Why should we be interested in erythrocyte substitutes for cardiopulmonary bypass? After all, large numbers of coronary bypass procedures are being performed with very low morbidity and mortality. In order to justify using such a radically new drug, one would have to demonstrate that the use of fluorochemicals somehow improves the care of patients subjected to cardiopulmonary bypass. Hemodilution techniques, well-engineered disposable oxygenators, and cell-savers have resulted in a significant decrease in the numbers of patients receiving blood transfusions for open heart surgery. Nevertheless, the large numbers of open heart sur-

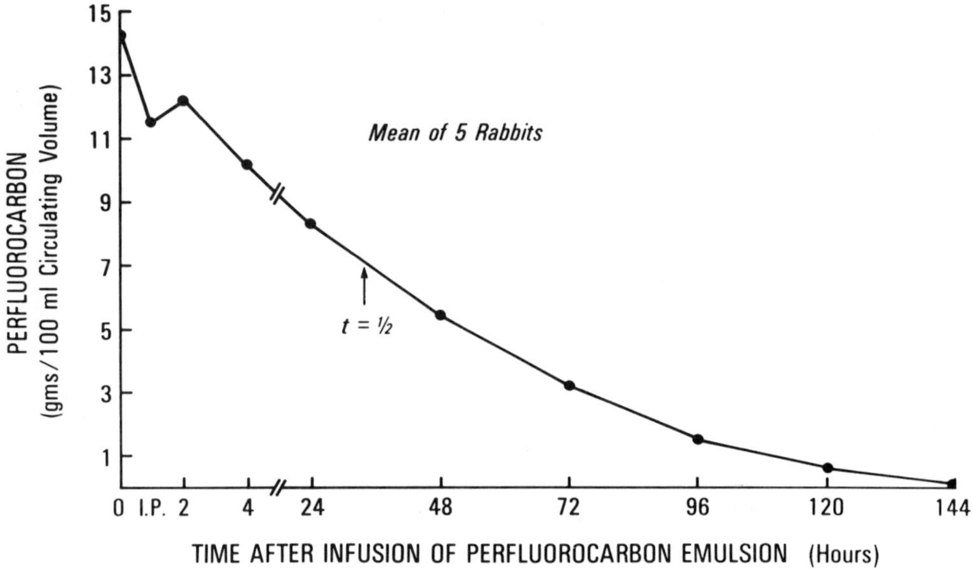

Figure 2.2. This graph depicts the concentration of perfluoroctylbromide in the blood of rabbits at different time periods after the i.v. administration of 9.26 g/kg of a fine emulsion (10 ml/kg of a 48% emulsion). The concentration of perfluoroctylbromide was determined by gas chromatography. Note that the intravascular half-life was about 32 hours.

gical procedures continues to place strains on our blood procurement programs. Trauma to formed elements has been decreased but not eliminated. The Alabama group[13] described complement activation due to surface energy effects during CPB with the most up to date techniques and apparatus and concluded that these inflammatory mediators may contribute to the "post-pump syndromes." We continue to face the problem of disease transmission by transfusions of blood components, even with the use of volunteer donors. Blood is expensive, but perfluorochemicals are also expensive, and this cost is increasing at about the same rate as other petroleum products. All things considered, synthetic blood is an attractive concept for CPB, but one must reserve judgment until there is definition of the risks involved, information that is still not available.

There have been a number of preliminary investigations in several applications of synthetic blood as related to cardiopulmonary bypass. These areas of application are as follows:

1. Liquid membrane oxygenators
2. Oxygenator prime and blood replacement
3. Myocardial preservation
4. Hypothermia
5. Isolated organ perfusion

Liquid Membrane Oxygenators

Howlett et al.[14] and later Wallace et al.[15] have used fluorocarbons as liquid membrane oxygenators. This novel and intriguing application continues to undergo modifications in design. The fluorochemical interface with blood is atraumatic, and gas exchange is efficient. Cost of the fluorochemicals as well as unsolved design problems appear to be major deterrents to the application of this concept.

Oxygenator Prime and Blood Replacement

Ochi et al.[16] used Fluosol DA to prime the oxygenator for 3 hours of CPB in dogs. Although metabolic acidosis developed, the microcirculation of the mesentery was maintained in a satisfactory state. The liver showed accumulation of fluorochemical vacuoles in the reticuloendothelial cells, but no other histological abnormalities were reported. Adachi et al.[17] used Fluosol DA-25 to replace blood temporarily during CPB in dogs. The autogenous blood was stored in a reservoir to be used to replace the Fluosol at conclusion of the CPB. The animals' hemoglobin concentration was reduced to 10% of the prebypass level, but oxygen consumption was kept at expected levels. Engleman et al.[18] tested the capacity of Fluosol DA-20 to maintain myocardial function and structural and biochemical integrity during CPB in pigs. Increased cardiac contractibility was attributed to high levels of ionized calcium. Myocardial metabolism and functional measurements were maintained during 1 hour of Fluosol DA-20 perfusion, indicating there was sufficient oxygen carrying capacity in Fluosol DA-20. The ultrastructure of the myocardial cells remained intact.

The temporary use of synthetic blood for its oxygen-carrying capacity during CPB circumvents the potential problems of reticuloendothelial blockade due to a massive dose of fluorocarbon emulsions. The phagocytosis of emulsion probably would not present a problem for 2 to 3 hours of bypass. The autogenous blood could be returned from the storage reservoir, and the synthetic blood could be largely removed at the termination of CPB. It will be important to obtain survival data on animals subjected to the use of synthetic blood during CPB before one can conclude anything regarding its utility. This data is still not available.

Myocardial Preservation

At this time, the most promising application for synthetic blood is as a cardioplegic medium. Kanter et al.[19] compared Fluosol 43, crystalloid, and blood as cardioplegic agents with 25 mEq/liter of K^+ added to each agent. A period of 100 minutes of cardiac arrest at 20°C was followed by a 45-minute recovery period at 37°C in perfused rabbit hearts. Cardioplegic solution was given every 20 minutes during the ischemic period. The hearts arrested with Fluosol 43 showed significantly greater myocardial oxygen tensions during the arrest period. The myocardial oxygen consumption with Fluosol was approximately ten times greater than that with crystalloid and five times greater than the O_2 consumption with blood cardioplegia. Cardiac performance was also significantly better during the reperfusion period, and there was less myocardial edema in the hearts arrested with Fluosol. These results were interpreted as indicative of enhanced O_2 delivery and utilization during hypothermic ischemia with perfluorocarbon. With the blood cardioplegia solution, only 10% of the available oxygen was actually delivered to the myocardium, probably due to the leftward shift of the oxyhemoglobin dissociation curve associated with hypothermia.

Since most cardiac surgery is performed in patients with ischemic heart disease, it is important to mention the studies of Rude et al.,[20] who compared synthetic blood and saline in dogs with coronary artery occlusion while breathing 20% O_2 or 100% O_2. The fluorocarbon treated dogs showed reduced ischemic injury with and without supplemental O_2. Fluorocarbon and O_2 in combination led to an increased myocardial oxygen tension in the ischemic zones. This is the first experimental maneuver that has produced this effect! Glogar et al.[21] found a significant decrease in myocardial infarction size in animals treated with synthetic blood.

These experimental findings as well as theoretical considerations lead me to believe that a fluorocarbon cardioplegic medium could be used with clear advantage. Because the cardioplegic solution can be retrieved from the right atrium, there would be very little risk of fluorocarbon toxicity, if such a thing is in fact possible.

Hypothermia

Profound systemic hypothermia is a valuable tool for specific types of cardiovascular surgery. The reason this modality is not used more commonly is because of the production of significant pathophysiologic states such as coagulopathies, the no-reflow phenomenon, and the failure of hemoglobin to release oxygen stores during hypothermia, except at very low partial pressures of oxygen. Perfluorocarbon emulsions may provide a solution to some of these problems. As noted above, the oxygen dissociation curve for fluorochemicals is linear rather than sigmoidal as with hemoglobin. Therefore, there is a more uniform release of O_2 when synthetic blood is substituted for natural blood. The O_2 solubility of fluorocarbons at low temperatures increases significantly with about 50% more O_2 dissolved at 0°C compared with 40°C.[22]

The thermal heat capacity of fluorochemicals is as unique as that of the oxygen solubility. The high thermal heat capacity has been exploited in industrial applications, but has been tested only once in biomedical research. This singular experiment was probably the first biological application of perfluorocarbons. In 1964, while developing techniques for gastric cooling, we evaluated new liquids for more rapid and efficient cooling than that obtained with saline or with combinations of water and alcohol. We were familiar with the properties of fluorochemicals as a result of earlier research work on heart valves and drug release mechanisms. FC-75 was obtained from the 3M Company and used to freeze the stomachs of four dogs very rapidly and efficiently. Each dog was dead when we arrived in the laboratory the next morning, and high concentrations of FC-75 were measured in lung tissue due to intravascular migration of the fluorochemical through the injured gastric mucosa. Fortunately, this experiment was terminated rapidly without publication but not without some choice and characteristic comments by Dr. Wangensteen. We should not forget the potential value of this property of thermal heat capacity, however. This property should enable more rapid and uniform exchange of calories between tissues and the perfusate. The result should be a more reliable and safer method for maintaining hypothermia. Fluorochemicals are also noteworthy for their stable physical properties over a wide range of temperatures. Viscosity of pure fluorocarbon changes very little during hypothermia. Since water represents the bulk of the emulsions of synthetic blood, the viscosity temperature relationships of synthetic blood closely resemble those of natural blood.[22]

Isolated Organ Perfusion

Preservation of individual organs for transplantation purposes is also a promising area of application. The isolated organs successfully perfused with synthetic bloods include heart, brain, liver, and kidney. Geyer[23] has found the isolated perfused heart preparation to be a sensitive tool for testing toxicity of fluorochemical emulsions. Mouse hearts perfused with "good" emulsions performed better than hearts perfused with shed blood or "bad" emulsions. Honda et al.[24] used Fluosol DA to preserve cadaver kidneys for transplantation into humans. No toxic effects were found in the kidneys or the recipients. There are a number of investigations under way with synthetic blood in organ perfusion and preservation at the present time. Theoretical considerations alone suggest these will be fruitful endeavors.

CHEMICAL AND BIOLOGICAL REACTIVITY AND TOXICITY

Literally hundreds of fluorochemicals have been screened in the research and development work for a synthetic blood. The chemicals mentioned in this paper enjoy a remarkable chemical stability at physiological temperatures. These fluorochemicals are not altered in the body as indicated by the absence of excessive fluoride ion in the urine and the chemical similarity of the fluorocarbon retained in the tissues with those of the standard. In this respect, these compounds resemble Teflon, a fluorocarbon polymer.

Recent evidence indicates that the perfluorocarbons are *not* biologically inert. Miller et al.[25] have described the histological changes observed in the liver and other organs after dosing with synthetic bloods. These changes included histiocyte clusters and extramedullary hemopoiesis in the liver. Hepatocytes showed no ultrastructural changes, except for the volume density increase due to phagocytosed emulsion particles. Splenic white pulp diminished while red pulp and marginal zones were enlarged and transforming lymphocytes and mitoses increased. This histochemical response to fluorochemicals was considered to be more or less innocuous. Miller et al.[26] also observed augmentation of the tumoricidal potential of peritoneal macrophages from rats receiving perfluorocarbon emulsions intravenously or intraperitoneally.

We have observed augmentation of the antimicrobial function of peritoneal exudate in rats receiving intraperitoneal fluorochemicals. Figure 2.3 illustrates the "protective" effects of perfluorohexylbromide (PFHB) provided in a standard *Escherichia coli* peritonitis model. In this experiment, rats received neat PFHB or emulsions of PFHB intraperitoneally in the doses shown on the

E COLI PERITONITIS PERFLUOROHEXYLBROMIDE (PFHB) $C_6 F_{13} Br$

	TREATED							
	NEAT				EMULSION			
ml/kg	1	5	10	20	1	5	10	20
Deaths	10	1	5	0	1	3	1	3
Total	17	18	27	15	24	18	18	9
% Mortality	59	6	19	0	4	17	6	33

	CONTROL							
	NEAT				EMULSION			
ml/kg	1	5	10	20	1	5	10	20
Deaths	15	15	22	9	15	15	13	9
Total	17	17	27	9	17	17	18	9
% Mortality	88	88	81	100	88	88	72	100

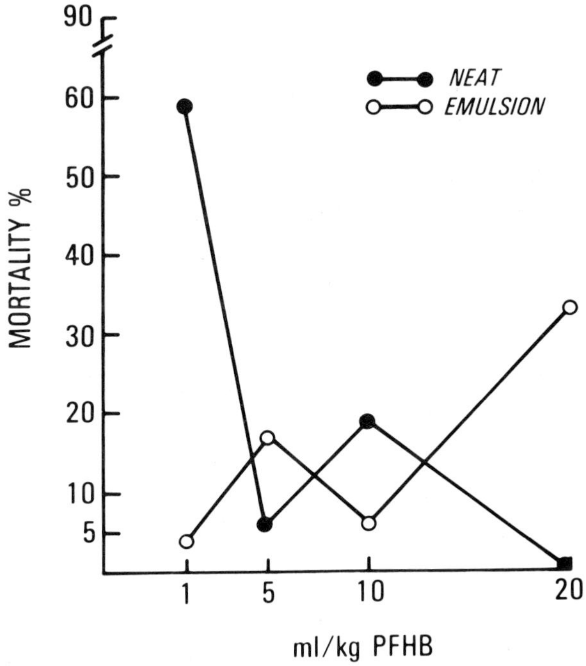

Figure 2.3. Tabular and graphic representation of the mortality rates of rats subjected to a standardized challenge of intraperitoneal *E. coli.* The treated animals received an intraperitoneal injection of perfluorohexylbromide *(PFHB)* as either the neat liquid or large particle size emulsion 24 hours prior to the intraperitoneal injection of *E. coli.* Mortality was counted up to 48 hours after the dose of bacteria. Note that the mortality rate decreased with increasing doses of neat PFHB. The mortality rates were lowest with a 1 ml/kg dose of PFHB emulsion and increased with higher doses of emulsion. The differences in mortality between treated and control animals were statistically significant ($p < 0.05$) at all dose levels except 1 ml/kg of neat PFHB. The term total refers to the number of rats in each dosage group. The treatment and control groups were performed at the same time to allow for fluctuations in the lethality of the bacterial culture.

abscissa, and control rats received saline. Twenty-four hours later, the rats were challenged with a dose of *E. coli* that produced a high mortality in matched control rats, as shown in the tables above the graph. Pretreatment of rats with PFHB transtracheally has also improved survival with induced pseudomonas pneumonia. We observed addi-

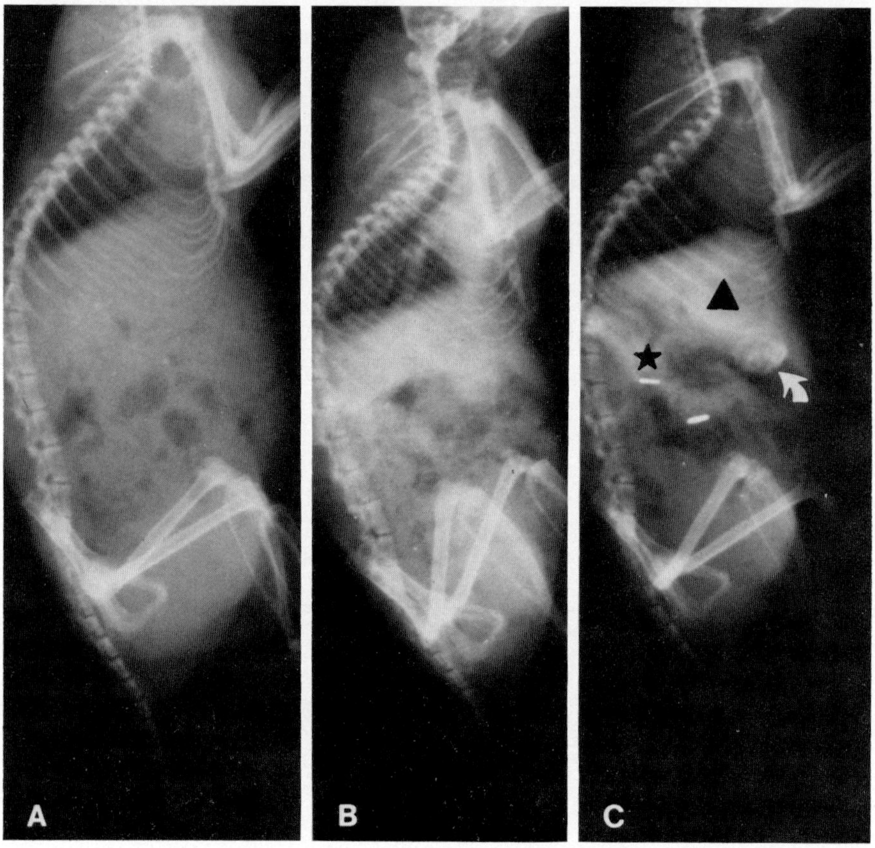

Figure 2.4. X-rays of a hamster with induced adenocarcinoma of the pancreas with a single metastatic tumor nodule in the right lobe of the liver. *A* is the control x-ray. *B* is the x-ray taken 5 hours after the intravenous injection of synthetic blood emulsion of PFOB in a dose of 14 g/kg. Note that the heart and great vessels are radiodense and there is beginning radiopacification of the liver and spleen which illustrates the intravascular persistence of the fluorochemicals as well as the initial stages of phagocytosis of emulsion particles by the reticuloendothelial (RE) system. *C* is an x-ray taken 48 hours later and after 2 mm surgical metallic clips were placed on the proximal and distal poles of the pancreas. The *arrow* points to the metastatic nodule, the *triangle* is superimposed on the liver, and the *star* is superimposed on the spleen. The increased radiodensity of the tumor is nonhomogenous and is distinct from that of the liver and spleen. The multiple primary tumors of the pancreas were less than 1 mm in diameter and below the limits of resolution of the technique. These x-rays illustrate pictorially the uptake of fluorochemicals by the normal reticuloendothelial tissues of the spleen and liver and by macrophages of abnormal tissues such as malignant tumors. This experiment also suggests potential future uses for synthetic bloods containing brominated perfluorocarbons; namely, diagnostic angiography and imaging of small foci of malignant tumors. When the more sensitive modality of computerized tomography is used, the dose of radiopaque fluorocarbon required is a fraction of that used with conventional radiography.

tional evidence of biological activity of fluorochemical emulsions in a series of tumor-imaging experiments. When the synthetic blood is prepared with perfluorocytlbromide rather than other fluorochemicals, the reticuloendothelial structures, such as the liver and spleen, become radiopaque.[27] The brominated fluorochemicals are avidly endocytosed by the monocytic phagocytes. When brominated perfluorocarbon emulsions are given to animals with malignant tumors, the tumors become radiopaque[28] (Fig. 2.4). The fluorochemicals are, therefore, excellent for tumor imaging using conventional radiography and even more so with computed tomography.[29] What is particularly interesting is the different imaging patterns for different structures. The spleen becomes radiopaque in a matter of minutes, and the liver is radiodense within an hour after intravenous injection of PFOB emulsions. After the radiodensity of the spleen and liver peaks and then decreases over the first 2 to 4 days, the malignant tumors show increased radiodensity which continues to increase for 1 to 2 weeks. The radiodensity of the tumors persists for up to 6 weeks. Tumor imaging is due to the uptake of PFOB by tumor macrophages. The gradual increase in tumor radiodensity is thought to be due to the localization of PFOB-labeled macrophages which have been "loaded" in another location, such as the marrow or spleen, and then these fluorocarbon labeled monocytes are recruited to the tumors. Immunodepression was implicated in the mortality of tumor-bearing rabbits receiving large doses of the perfluorochemicals.[28]

Further evidence for the biological effects on the reticuloendothelial system were provided by the experiments of Lutz.[30] After large doses of Fluosol, the peak concentrations of fluorochemicals were seen in the spleen at 12 hours and in the liver at 2 days. Maximum increase in weight of the spleen occurred at 4 days and of the liver on the 8th day. The delayed increases in weight were attributed to both hypertrophy and hyperplasia. The function of the reticuloendothelial system, as measured by the clearance of colloidal carbon, decreased after a large dose of 4.4 g/kg of perfluorocarbon. Lutz et al.[31] also noted a susceptibility to endotoxin shock following treatment with Fluosol.

Although perfluorocarbons have been described as biologically inert substances, recent evidence indicates they are biologically reactive with a significant effect on monocytic phagocytes. In low or moderate doses, the perfluorocarbons appear to produce immunostimulation. Large doses appear to cause reticuloendothelial blockade with resultant immunodepression. The duration and magnitude of these "constructive" and "destructive" influences have not been defined. The constructive influence or immunostimulation may be used therapeutically. Reticuloendothelial blockade or immunodepression is probably the principle risk to be considered in the administration of synthetic bloods. It is imperative that future investigations be directed toward a better description of the risks in terms of alterations of host resistance to infection and neoplasia.

SUMMARY

Perfluorocarbon emulsions or synthetic bloods have potential for use in cardiopulmonary bypass in the following ways:

1. Cardioplegic Medium. Synthetic blood appears to be superior to blood cardioplegia as a cardioplegic agent. Small quantities would be needed for this purpose and most could be recovered and discarded.

2. Perfusion of Organs for Transplantation. The function of isolated organs is well preserved by perfusion with synthetic blood. The recipients of the transplanted organs would receive very little perfluorochemical in the final washout.

3. Blood Replacement during CPB. Synthetic blood should be effective for total body perfusion during open heart surgery to avoid the trauma to formed elements and proteins. The patients' blood can be reinfused at the conclusion of the surgical procedure, and a major portion of the perfluorocarbon can be recovered.

4. Erythrocyte Substitute following Surgical Procedure. Limited quantities of synthetic blood might be used as erythrocyte replacement in the postoperative period when natural blood was not available or could not be used for some reason.

Additional studies are needed to define the maximal dose of different fluorochemicals under different conditions such as surgical stress, sepsis, and the presence of malignant neoplasms.

ACKNOWLEDGMENTS

The research work wth halogenated perfluorocarbon compounds was conducted with the support of NIH Grant GM 25723-04. The author wishes to express his appreciation to Frances Multer for her assistance in the conduct of experiments and to Marilyn Rose and Barbara Clayton for preparation of the manuscript.

References

1. Clark LC Jr, Gollan F: Survival of mammals breathing organic liquids equilibrated with oxygen at atmospheric pressure. Science 152:1755, 1966.
2. Gollan F, Clark LC Jr: Organ perfusion with fluorocarbon fluid. Physiologist 9:191, 1966.
3. Sloviter HA, Kamimoto T: Erythrocyte substitute for perfusion of brain. Nature 216:458, 1967.
4. Geyer RP, Monroe RG, Taylor K: Survival of rats totally perfused with a fluorocarbon-detergent preparation. In *Organ Perfusion and Preservation*, edited by JC Norman. New York, Appleton-Century-Crofts, 1968, p. 85.
5. Geyer, RP: Fluorocarbon-polyol artificial blood substitutes. N Engl J Med 289:1077, 1973.
6. Clark LC Jr, Kaplan S, Becattini F: The physiology of synthetic blood. J Thorac Cardiovasc Surg 60:757, 1970.
7. Yokoyama K, Yamanouchi K, Watanabe M, Matsumoto T, Murashima R, Diamoto T, Hamano T, Okamoto H, Suyama T, Watanabe R, Naito R: Preparation of perfluorodecalin emulsion, an approach to the red cells substitute. Fed Proc 34: 1478, 1975.
8. Yokoyama K, Yamanouchi K, Ohyanagi H, Mitsuno T: Fate of perfluorochemicals in animals after intravenous injection or hemodilution with their emulsions. Chem Pharm Bull 26:956, 1978.
9. Ghosh A, Janic V, Sloviter HA: Enzymic method for measuring dissolved oxygen in nonaqueous materials. Anal Biochem 38:270, 1970.
10. Tremper KK, Lapin R, Levine E, Friedman A, Shoemaker WC: Hemodynamic and oxygen transport effects of a perfluorochemical blood substitute, Fluosol-DA (20%). Crit Care Med 8:738, 1980.
11. Clark LC Jr, Moore RE, Diver S, Miller ML: A new look at the vapor pressure problem in red cell substitutes. Proceedings of the 4th International Symposium on Perfluorochemical Blood Substitutes. Kyoto, Japan, p. 55, 1978.
12. Ohyanagi H, Toshima K, Sekita M, Okamoto M, Itoh T, Mitsuno T, Naito R, Suyama T, Yokoyama K: Clinical studies of perfluorochemical whole blood substitutes: Safety of Fluosol-DA (20%) in normal human volunteers. Clin Therap 2:306, 1979.
13. Chenoweth DE, Cooper SW, Hugli TE, Stewart RW, Blackstone EH, Kirklin JW: Complement activation during cardiopulmonary bypass. N Engl J Med 304: 497, 1981.
14. Howlett S, Dundas D, Sabiston DC Jr: Fluid fluorocarbon as oxygenator in experimental extracorporeal circulation. Arch Surg 91:643, 1965.
15. Wallace HW, Asher WJ, Zubrow MT, Stein TP, Brooks H: Liquid membrane oxygenator. J Thorac Cardiovasc Surg, 66:887, 1973.
16. Ochi S, Sakabe H, Sasaki Y, Nakaji S, Nakamura A, Oga K, Hashimoto I: Cardiopulmonary bypass with perfluorochemicals by a pulsitile pump. Proceedings of the 4th International Symposium on Perfluorochemical Blood Substitutes. Kyoto, Japan, p. 331, 1978.
17. Adachi S, Mori T, Kitamura S, Miyamoto K, Murata H, Okuda A, Kawashima Y: Cardiopulmonary bypass primed with 35 W/V% PFC emulsion after removal of 75% autologous blood. Proceedings of the 4th International Symposium on Perfluorochemical Blood Substitutes, Kyoto, Japan, p. 318, 1978.
18. Engleman RM, Rousow JH, Dobbs WA: Fluosol DA, an artificial blood for total cardiopulmonary bypass. Ann Thorac Surg, in press, 1981.
19. Kanter KR, Jaffin JH, Ehrlichman RJ, Flaherty JT, Gott VL, Gardner TJ: Superiority of perfluorocarbon over blood and crystalloid cardioplegia. Circulation 62(III):323, 1980.
20. Rude RE, Glogar DH, Khuri SF, Karaffa S, Kloner RA, Clark LC Jr, Muller JE, Braunwald E: Effects of fluorocarbons and supplemental oxygen on acute myocardial ischemia assessed by intramyocardial gas tension measurement. Am J Cardiol, 47:436, 1981.
21. Glogar DH, Rude RE, Clark LC Jr: Reduction in myocardial infarct size with fluorocarbons. Science, in press, 1981.
22. Naito R, Yokoyama K: Perfluorochemical blood substitutes (Fluosol 43) (Fluosol DA, 20% and 35%). The Green Cross Corp., Osaka, Japan. Technical Information Series No. 5, 1978.
23. Geyer RP: Personal communication, 1980.
24. Honda K, Motoki R, Hoshino S, Inque H, Hamada O, Iwaya F, Ando M: Use of perfluorochemical artificial blood (Fluosol-DA) for perfusion of cadaveric kidneys for transplantation. Curr Ther Res 28: 306, 1979.
25. Miller ML, Wessler EP, Jones SC, Clark LC Jr: Some morphologic effects in "inert" particulate loading on hemopoietic elements in mice. J Reticuloendothel Soc 20:385, 1976.
26. Miller ML, Stinnett JD, Clark LC Jr: Ultrastructure of tumoricidal peritoneal exudate cells stimulated *in vivo* by perfluorochemical emulsions. J Reticuloendothel Soc 27:105, 1980.
27. Long DM Jr, Lasser EC, Sharts CM, Multer FK, Nielsen M: Experiments with radiopaque perfluorocarbon emulsions for selective opacification of organs and total body angiography. Invest Radiol 15:242, 1980.
28. Long DM, Multer FK, Greenburg AG, Peskin GW,

Lasser EC, Wickham WG, Sharts CM: Tumor imaging with X-rays using macrophage uptake of radiopaque fluorocarbon emulsions. Surgery 84:104, 1978.

29. Young SW, Enzmann DR, Long DM, Muller HH: Perfluoroctylbromide contrast enhancement of malignant neoplasms: Preliminary observations. Radiology, in press, 1981.
30. Lutz J, Metzenauer P: Effects of potential blood substitutes (perfluorochemicals) on rat liver and spleen. Pfluegers Arch 387:175, 1980.
31. Lutz J, Barthel U, Metzenauer P: Increased susceptibility to endotoxin shock following treatment with perfluorochemicals: Its time course and modification by drugs. Pfluegers Arch 384:R6, 1980.
32. Wesseler EP, Iltis R, Clark LC Jr: The solubility of oxygen in highly fluorinated liquids. J Fluorine Chem 9:137, 1977.

CHAPTER 3

ENDOCRINE RESPONSES TO CARDIOPULMONARY BYPASS

Julie A. Swain, M.D.

Cardiopulmonary bypass introduces significant alterations in physiological homeostasis not found in other major surgical procedures. With the use of cardiopulmonary bypass, the heart and lungs are not perfused and are removed from participation in hormonal secretion and degradation. Also, the blood is in contact with the foreign surfaces of the oxygenator and its tubing and is subjected to the trauma of this interaction as well as adsorbing plasma proteins. Systemic heparinization must be used, which results in altered tissue release of hormones, cellular affinities, and globulin binding properties. Moderate to profound hypothermia is generally used and affects the rate of enzymatic processes for synthesis and degradation as well as most other metabolic processes. With the trend toward nonblood priming solutions, the hemodilution produced during cardiopulmonary bypass dilutes the serum concentrations of electrolytes, hormones, and serum proteins, which shifts the free *vs.* protein-bound ratios of many hormones, thus alterating their effects. One of the most potent forces which disrupts hormonal function is nonpulsatile flow. Organ perfusion, as well as the distribution of blood flow in the organ, is changed when nonpulsatile cardiopulmonary bypass is used. Many of these changes can be lessened or reversed by utilization of pulsatile perfusion systems during cardiopulmonary bypass. In evaluating the current literature relating to endocrine responses to cardiopulmonary bypass, difficulties arise when comparing studies because of markedly different conditions of bypass including temperature, priming solution, drugs, and whether cardioplegia was used.

CATECHOLAMINES

The catecholamine response to cardiopulmonary bypass is important in controlling the peripheral circulation. Catecholamines are secreted from postganglionic adrenergic nerve endings and from the adrenal medulla. Besides being dependent on cardiopulmonary bypass stress catecholamine secretion is very dependent on the choice of anesthetic the patient's volume status, and the body temperature. Catecholamines are responsible for heat production during abnormally low body temperatures. With moderate hypothermic bypass, the plasma epinephrine is increased over ten times prebypass levels, while norepinephrine rose to a lesser extent (four times prebypass levels)[1, 2] (Fig. 3.1). Therefore, it appears that epinephrine is more important than norepinephrine in the response to hypothermic stress because the change is proportionally greater in epinephrine levels. The hypotension that generally occurs at the initiation of cardiopulmonary bypass may be a potent stimulus for reflex catecholamine release. It is possible that the acute hemodilution occurring during this time is responsible for this transient hypotension by decreasing the concentration of circulating plasma catecholamines and, there-

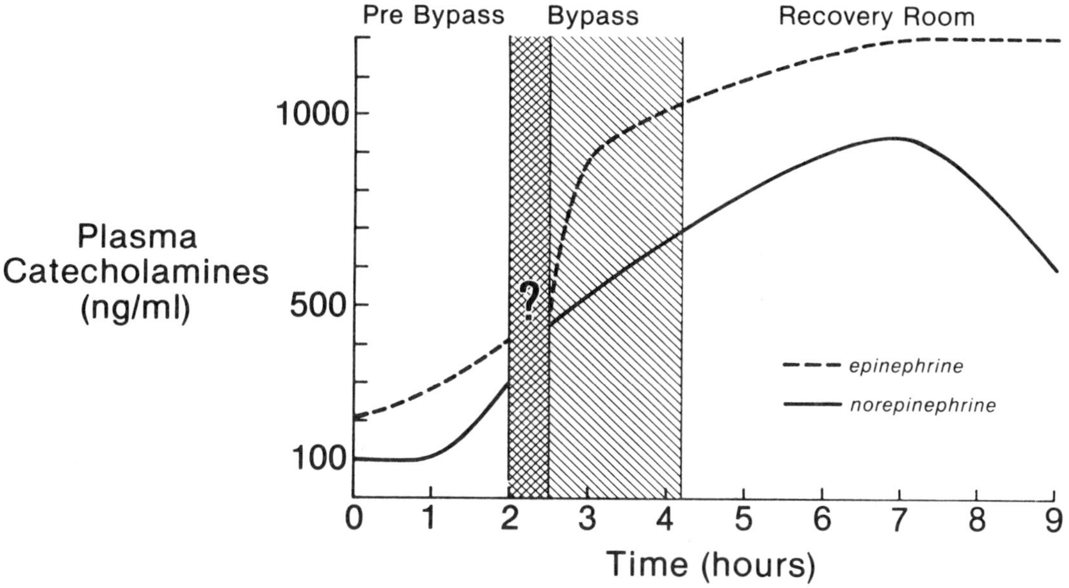

Figure 3.1. Plasma catecholamine levels during bypass. The cross-hatched area represents the time during initiation of bypass when dilution of catecholamines may cause hypotension. (Adopted from R. Landymore et al.[1])

fore, decreasing peripheral vascular resistance.[3] These elevations of catecholamines may be responsible for the peripheral vasoconstriction and shifts in intraorgan blood flow occurring with cardiopulmonary bypass. Since catecholamine levels remain elevated for several hours after bypass,[1] catecholamines may also be responsible for hemodynamic alterations in the early postoperative period where hypertension is commonly seen and may result in endocardial ischemia, decreased cardiac output, and depressed renal function. The substitution of pulsatile perfusion has no effect on the catecholamine elevations found during cardiopulmonary bypass.[1]

VASOPRESSIN

Vasopressin, or antidiuretic hormone (ADH), is a potent determinant of sodium and water homeostasis and peripheral vascular resistance in the surgical patient. Vasopressin leads to decreased cardiac output, decreased contractility, and coronary and renal vasoconstriction,[4] which may lead to myocardial ischemia or renal failure. The massive increase in vasopressin produced by cardiopulmonary bypass far exceeds that seen during major general surgical procedures.[5, 6] Paradoxical effects on renal function occur when vasopressin levels are this high. A sodium and water diuresis is produced that may be secondary to altered intrarenal blood flow distribution. Thus, decreased urine osmolality is coupled with increased vasopressin, a form of inappropriate ADH syndrome.

General anesthesia and surgical stress are known to produce moderate increases in vasopressin.[7] With cardiopulmonary bypass, massive increases up to 20 times basal values in vasopressin are produced, and these elevations persist postoperatively[5, 6] (Fig. 3.2). Vasopressin levels differ in valve replacement and coronary artery bypass patients, in that coronary bypass patients have persistently higher levels of vasopressin than valve patients.

The reasons for the increased vasopressin are complex because vasopressin is initiated by many stimuli. Volume receptors and left atrial stretch receptors influence vasopressin secretion.[8] The large vasopressin increase with bypass may be secondary to a transient blood volume decrease at the initiation of bypass. Also, with left ventricular venting,

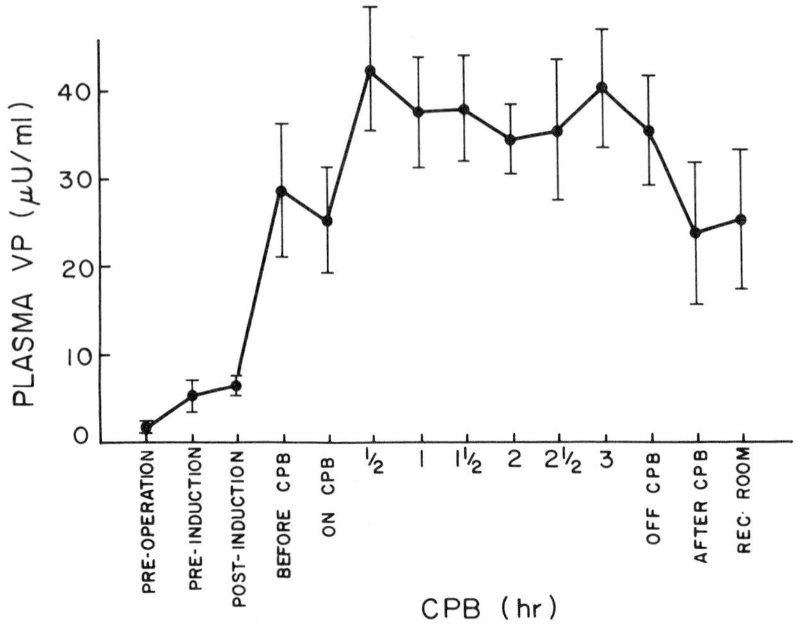

Figure 3.2. Plasma vasopressin (*VP*) concentrations in coronary bypass patients during cardiopulmonary bypass (*CPB*). (Adopted with permission from W. Wu et al.[5])

left atrial pressure is markedly decreased in the decompressed heart and may simulate volume depletion, which is known to be a potent initiator of vasopressin release.[8] Also, the transient hypotension that normally occurs at the initiation of bypass, possibly secondary to catecholamine dilution,[3] may lead to increased vasopressin secretion. Studies using pulsatile bypass demonstrate a significant decrease in vasopressin release when compared to nonpulsatile flow, although vasopressin is still elevated over normal values.[1, 6] With pulsatile bypass, less peripheral vasoconstriction and increased flow rates are seen, as well as increased urinary output.[6] Osmoreceptors also regulate vasopressin secretion. In studies of vasopressin release, there was either no change or a decrease in serum osmolarity, which should not increase vasopressin levels.[5] Pain increased vasopressin,[5] and the practice of maintaining light anesthesia in cardiac patients may be partly responsible for the increased vasopressin levels.

One of the most important influences on vasopressin levels is the increased catecholamine secretion occurring during bypass. Vasopressin and catecholamines potentiate each other's vasoconstricting effects and lead to intense peripheral vasoconstriction.[9]

Clinically, few measures are available to decrease this large vasopressin response. Pulsatile bypass, adequate anesthetic to prevent painful stimuli, anesthetic agents that suppress vasopressin secretion (diazepam, fentanyl, and morphine), and prevention of large variations in vascular volume and blood pressure may be beneficial.

CARBOHYDRATE METABOLISM

Carbohydrate metabolism is markedly deranged during and after cardiopulmonary bypass. The magnitude of these changes depends on the degree of hypothermia and the method of bypass. Following the onset of bypass, serum glucose rises to over 400 mg% with an insulin response of 200 MU/ml. In the normal patient, an expected insulin level of 500 MU/ml follows with this degree hyperglycemia[10–13] (Fig. 3.3). Therefore, both hyperglycemia and impaired insulin response are produced by cardiopulmonary bypass.[11] These peak values of serum glucose and insulin occur during cardiopulmonary bypass and hypothermia, but with the conclusion of bypass and rewarming, these values rapidly return to normal within 12 hours.

Normal glucose utilization is dependent on appropriate insulin synthesis and release and on normal glucose uptake by the skeletal muscle. Pancreatic islet cell function depends on pancreatic blood flow and distribution,[14] body temperature,[15] and the presence or absence of insulin antagonists, such as growth hormone, which is increased during take over bypass.[16, 17] Body temperature is probably the most important determinant of pancreatic response since there is no evidence that total pancreatic blood flow is abnormal during bypass. Other factors responsible for decreased insulin levels are binding by the oxygenator and tubing and alterations at the blood/gas interface.[18] Also, it has been shown that epinephrine suppress insulin release by the pancreas in response to glucose.[19] During cardiopulmonary bypass, epinephrine levels are abnormally high.[1] Epinephrine also increases glycogenolysis and contributes to hyperglycemia. When exogenous insulin is supplied, the hyperglycemia is unaffected,[20] indicating that an additional mechanism must be responsible for these changes.

Glucose uptake by cells is dependent on serum insulin concentrations, membrane transport of glucose, and glucose phosphorylation. Adequate insulin is required for normal membrane transport of glucose because it binds the cell wall and allows glucose transfer to occur at a rapid rate.[21] This process is energy dependent, requiring enzymatic processes and, like all enzyme systems, is affected by hypothermia. Hyponatremia secondary to hemodilution may be partly responsible for the decreased sensitivity to insulin since sodium is required for insulin-initiated intracellular transport of glucose.[22] Although the insulin response is abnormal, the persistently elevated glucose, concentrations coupled with a high circulating insulin concentration, indicate that the peripheral utilization of glucose is abnormal. Since most of glucose utilization occurs in skeletal muscle, the intense peripheral vasoconstriction

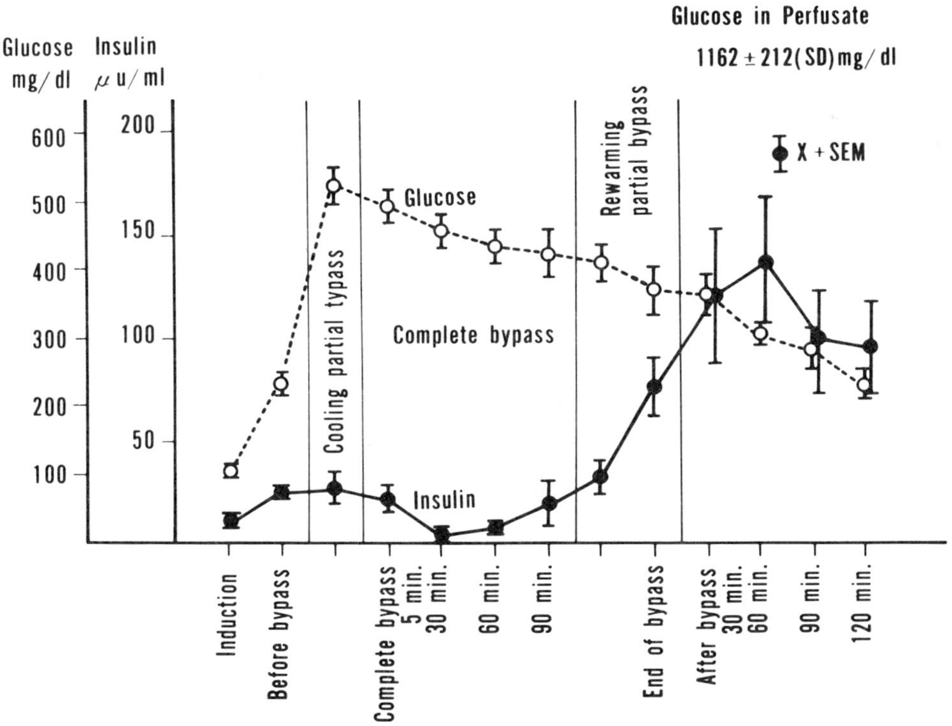

Figure 3.3. Plasma glucosea and insulin response to cardiopulmonary bypass. (Adopted with permission from T. Abe[10].)

produced by bypass may reduce glucose availability to the cell.[11] Thus, the combined effect of impaired transport mechanisms and decreased peripheral perfusion is responsible for the marked hyperglycemia.

Another important consequence of these changes in glucose utilization is large swings in potassium concentrations. During hypothermia, hyperkalemia may result partly because normal potassium transport into cells is dependent on both insulin and glucose transport.[23] New evidence suggests that potassium ion must be present for normal pancreatic insulin secretion.[24] Conversely, in the early postoperative period when glucose transport is accelerated because of the profound hyperglycemia, hypokalemia may occur. Hypokalemia is aggravated by occurrence of osmotic diuresis secondary to hyperglycemia with obligatory urinary potassium loss.

In summary, cardiopulmonary bypass causes an abnormal pancreatic insulin response and impaired glucose transport and utilization, which may have widespread effects on metabolic homeostasis. The clinical implications of these changes are important, especially in the diabetic patient. Two fatal cases of hyperosmotic hyperglycemic nonketotic coma after cardiopulmonary bypass have been reported.[20]

LIPID METABOLISM

Cardiopulmonary bypass causes extensive metabolic changes and converts the metabolic state to one of catabolism.[25] Glucose transfer is deranged during bypass, creating a need for alternate sources of substrate for energy production. Lipid metabolism is dominant[26] with free fatty acids serving this purpose until glucose utilization and carbohydrate metabolism return to normal.[17] During bypass elevated concentrations of norepinephrine and epinephrine cause lipolysis in adipose tissue and release free fatty acids. Free fatty acids are elevated two to four times above basal levels with bypass and do not return to normal until after the first postoperative day.[2, 10, 27, 28] Serum triglycerides are reduced, having been mobilized as free fatty acids for energy production.[27] The myocardium obtains much of its energy from fatty acids when glucose is not available.[29] Heparinization prior to cardiopulmonary bypass increases the activity of lipoprotein lipase and contributes to the production of free fatty acids.[30] In addition, the elevated levels of growth hormone[17] and catecholamines found during bypass increase free fatty acids. Proteolysis from protein catabolism during bypass liberates alpha amino acids that may be used as an alternate energy substrate.[10]

Several studies have shown that free fatty acids are arrhythmagenic in nature and may possibly lead to the arrhythmias commonly found after cardiopulmonary bypass.[31] Interest in lipid metabolism was stimulated by the theory that microembolization played a dominant role in production of neurological and pulmonary complications following bypass. Lipid microemboli could result from mechanical factors including transfused blood, fat aspirated in the pump suction, and sternal trauma. A correlation has been shown between capillary fat embolization and lipid breakdown products.[32] One study has shown a correlation between "long duration" extracorporeal circulation and histological evidence of lung fatty emboli.[33] However, other research has not shown a correlation between serum lipid levels and evidence of microemboli, although the incidence of microemboli was again correlated with the duration of cardiopulmonary bypass.[28]

ADRENAL

Secretion of cortisol is one of the features in the metabolic stress response. During nonpulsatile cardiopulmonary bypass cortisol secretion differs from that seen during general surgical procedures, where cortisol rises quickly to a maximum and slowly returns to baseline at 24 hours. Synthetic ACTH stimulation at the peak of cortisol secretion fails to provide any further rise in secretion of cortisol in these general surgical patients, indicating that the adrenal response is maximal.[34]

Taylor et al.[35, 36] has shown that during cardiopulmonary bypass, total plasma cortisol values fall from the level attained prebypass secondary to the initial surgical trauma (Fig. 3.4). Plasma-free cortisol concentration rises during bypass, probably secondary to

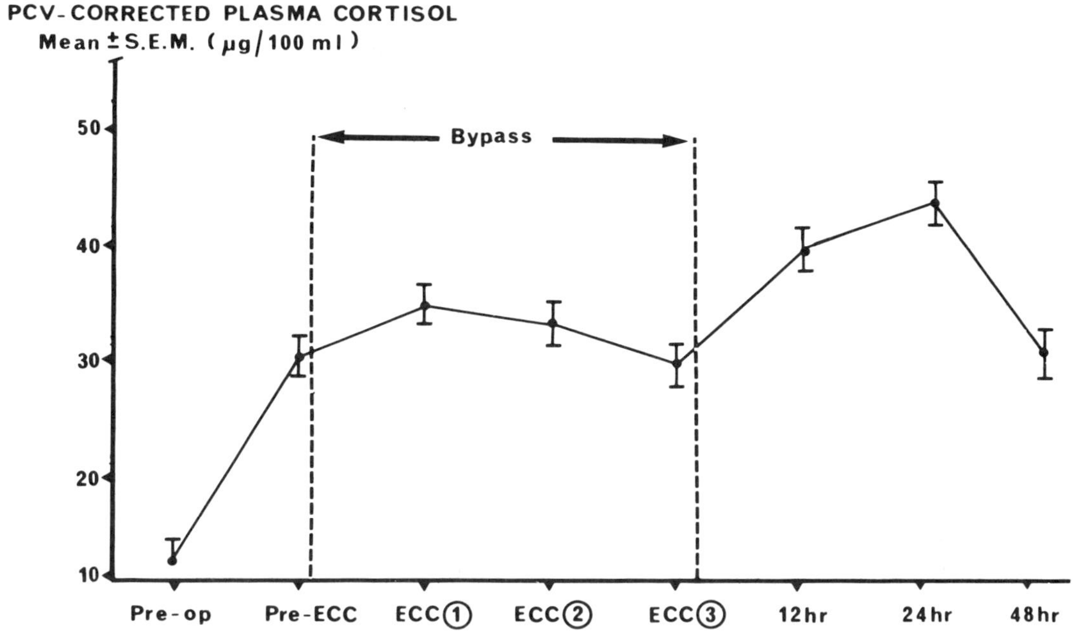

Figure 3.4. Packed cell volume (PCV)—corrected mean total plasma cortisol during cardiopulmonary bypass. (Adopted with permission from K. Taylor et al.[35])

hemodilution and liberation of free steroid from binding sites, but this rise only partly compensates for the drop in total cortisol.[37] Postoperatively, bypass patients exhibit a marked elevation of total and hemodilution-corrected total cortisol persisting past 48 hours, and plasma-free cortisol remains elevated at 24 hours.

In order to determine the cause of this depression of cortisol release, synthetic ACTH was given to patients during bypass. Surgical patients not undergoing bypass showed no rise in cortisol with administration of ACTH, thus indicating a maximal secretory response.[34] In contrast, the bypass patients had a positive response to ACTH,[35] indicating either a primary failure of pituitary secretion of ACTH or suppression of circulating ACTH. Taylor et al.[38] has reported a progressive fall in serum ACTH levels during bypass with a secondary ACTH response occuring 1 hour after the end of bypass.

When pulsatile bypass is used, these alterations are prevented.[36] Total plasma cortisol rose during pulsatile bypass in contrast to the nonpulsatile bypass patients where it fell dramatically as described above.

Adrenocortical hypofunction is significant in that a potential steroid inadequacy may exist during and after bypass when stress and metabolic derangements may be at their maximum. Dietzman et al.[39] has shown improvement in tissue perfusion and a decrease in peripheral vascular resistance when a large dose of steroids was given just prior to bypass. Steroids are known to reduce α-mediated vasoconstriction[40] and improve cell membrane integrity.[41]

THYROID

Cardiopulmonary bypass affects the hypothalmo-pituitary-thyroid axis. Major general surgical procedures produce small increases in protein-bound iodine and thyroxin, probably secondary to release from the liver.[42] Bypass produces a seven-fold increase in free thyroxine (T_4) while total T_4 remains unchanged.[43] However, free triiodothyronine (T_3) and total T_3 drop precipitously with bypass and remain depressed.[43] Part of the large increase in free T_4 is due to heparinization, which has been shown to increase free T_4 levels by a factor of four.[43–46] Heparin may act by displacing free T_4 from the liver, by reducing cellular binding of T_4, or by affecting thyroxin-binding globulin.[47] However, the increase in free T_4 is higher than that produced by heparinization and may be due to liver displacement of T_4 secondary to hemodynamic and metabolic changes in the liver. Additional free T_4 may be released at cellular level due to the effects of hemodilution and nonpulsatile flow on the cell.[43]

The precipitous drop in total T_3 may be more important than changes in T_4 because T_3 is thought to be the main metabolically active thyroid hormone.[48] This fall may be due to inadequate tissue release from the liver or other cells or an increase in peripheral utilization of T_3, the "stress response."[49] Since T_3 is synthesized by conversion of T_4 to T_3, impairment of this peripheral conversion could be responsible for the supranormal T_4 values and the lack of T_3.

The central regulating mechanism for thyroid hormone is the TRH (thyrotropin-releasing hormone)-TSH (thyroid-stimulating hormone) axis. TSH levels are unchanged during normothermic bypass;[43] however, when the temperature drops below 28°C, TSH increased.[50] The alterations in T_3 and T_4 described above are independent of TSH secretion since normal increases in T_3 and T_4 take 2 to 4 hours after TSH administration to occur.[51] Taylor has shown that during cardiopulmonary bypass, exogenous administration of TRH produces a very subnormal TSH response.[52] Because of the inadequate T_3 levels during bypass, there should be an increased sensitivity to TRH. This pituitary hypofunction may be secondary to inhibition by the markedly elevated total T_4 or effects of nonpulsatile flow on the anterior pituitary.

Pulsatile flow during bypass reverses the abnormal pituitary response to TRH, and normal levels of TSH are seen after exogenous TRH is administered during pulsatile bypass.[53] The reason for this anterior pituitary hypofunction is not known, but it may be related to improved capillary blood flow in the cerebral microcirculation during pulsatile flow.[54]

The clinical implications of these endocrine changes are important. Thyroid hormones have many effects on the myocardium and may act through adrenergic receptors in the myocardium. Two adenyl cyclase systems have been isolated in the myocardium, one of which is stimulated by catecholamines, the other by thyroid hormone and glucagon. These enzyme systems are responsible for the regulation of intracellular calcium and myocardial contractility.[55, 56] Currently, there is no evidence that acute drops in thyroid hormones alter myocardial adenyl cyclase. In some patients, poor myocardial contractility after bypass may be due to deficiencies in circulating T_3. The preoperative thyroid status of patients should be considered when poor contractility is encountered postoperatively.

CALCIUM

Calcium ions are important in regulating myocardial contractility as well as skeletomuscular activity. The content and distribution of the ionized calcium fraction of the total calcium is the physiologically active component. Availability of ionized calcium in the sarcoplasmic reticulum determines the calcium influx during depolarization and, therefore, because calcium is necessary for enzyme activation, membrane permeability, and excitation-contraction coupling, determines the inotropic state and the effectiveness of inotropic agents on the heart.[57] Calcium is also necessary for normal electrical conduction and rhythm of the heart.

The total and ionized calcium fraction changes during and after cardiopulmonary bypass are complex and are influenced by exogenous calcium in the pump prime solution or blood prime and by additional calcium given at the time of discontinuation of cardiopulmonary bypass. Large calcium shifts between the intra- and extracellular spaces occur. When crystalloid priming solutions are used during bypass, total caclcium is decreased, but ionized calcium is increased.[58] This reflects the effect of hemodilution on the concentration of both total caclcium and the dilutional effects on plasma proteins. After bypass there is a marked increase in both total and ionized calcium that peaks at 30 minutes and persists for 5 hours.[58] However, a bolus of calcium was given at the time of discontinuation of cardiopulmonary bypass in the above described studies that may be responsible for the elevations of total and ionized calcium.

There are important clinical implications from these studies. Ionized calcium changes produced no adverse effects during the study.[58] The empirical use of calcium supplements at the end of cardiopulmonary bypass for their ionotropic effects appears to have no harmful effects; however, during cardiopulmonary bypass, supplemental calcium may lead to accelerated adenosine triphosphate (ATP) breakdown since this is a calcium-dependent process. Hypocalcemia during cardiopulmonary bypass coupled with anoxic arrest and noncalcium-containing cardioplegia lead to slower ATP breakdown and may be beneficial.[59] The reperfusion period after the aortic clamp is removed and while cardiopulmonary bypass is mechanically assisting the heart is important for the resynthesis of the high energy phosphates. It is important to minimize myocardial oxygen consumption during this time. Exogenous calcium during this time will increase the ionotropic state of the myocardium and lead to further depletion of ATP. Exogenous calcium should be used only when bypass is about to be terminated, and a high ionotropic state is needed for resumption of full myocardial activity.

MAGNESIUM

Serum magnesium is altered during and after cardiopulmonary bypass. Magnesium is the second most abundant intracellular cation and is a key cofactor in enzyme systems, especially those essential for oxidative phosphorylation. Because there is a dynamic equilibrium between serum and intracellular magnesium, serum magnesium may be normal at the expense of intracellular ions. Preoperative cardiac surgery patients have been found to have intracellular depletion of magnesium, which may be due to insufficient dietary intake or increased excretion secondary to diuretics.[60] Serum magnesium is decreased in the intra- and postbypass periods, and urine excretion of magnesium is decreased.[60, 61] This may be due to loss to cardiopulmonary bypass priming solutions, intracellular transfer, hemodilution, or binding to chelating agents found in bank blood.

Clinically, magnesium depletion may be manifest in the postbypass period as hyperreflexia, muscular twitching, a prolongation of digitalis toxicity, and cardiac arrhythmias. Three postoperative cardiac surgery patients with ventricular fibrillation refractory to normal measures have been successfully defibrillated after magnesium administration. Magnesium depletion may occur after blood transfusions, with citrate anticoagulated blood causing chelation of serum magnesium. Calcium and magnesium are synergistic; magnesium depletion can cause hypocalcemia refractory to exogenous calcium replacement until magnesium is administered.

CONCLUSIONS

Cardiopulmonary bypass produces widespread alterations in all endocrine functions, some of which may be lessened by the use of pulsatile cardiopulmonary bypass. The magnitude and direction of these changes may be affected by the duration and conditions present at bypass (such as the degree of hypothermia, cardiac venting, and priming solution). For the most part, the reasons for these metabolic changes are poorly understood and must await further research in these areas. However, these changes may be very important in selected patients, and awareness of potential complications related to endocrine alterations may represent the difference between success and failure in a particular patient. The importance of these changes increases when long-term bypass and artificial heart replacements are considered.

References

1. Landymore RW Murphy DA, Kinley CE, Parrott JC, Moffitt EA, Longley WJ, Qirbi AA: Does pulsatile flow influence the incidence of postoperative hypertension? Ann Thorac Surg 28:261, 79.
2. Hirvonen J, Huttunen P, Nuutinen L, Pekkarinen A: Catecholamines and free fatty acids in plasma of patients undergoing cardiac operations with hypothermia and bypass. J Clin Pathol 31:949, 1978.
3. Balasaraswathi K, Glisson SN, El-Etr AA, Azad C: Effect of priming volume on serum catecholamines during cardiopulmonary bypass. Can Anaesth Soc J 27:135, 1980.
4. Heyndrickx GR, Boettcher DH, Vatner SF: Effects of angiotensin vasopressin, and methoxamine on cardiac function and blood flow distribution in conscious dogs. Am J Physiol 231:1579, 1976.

5. Wu W, Zubuzek VK, Bellevue C: Vasopressin release during cardiac operation. J Thorac Cardiovasc Surg 79:83, 1980.
6. Philbin DM, Levine FH, Emerson CW, Coggins CH, Buckley MJ, Austin WG: Plasma vasopressin levels and urinary flow during cardiopulmonary bypass in patients with valvular heart disease. J Thorac Cardiovasc Surg 78:779, 1979.
7. Moses AM, Miller M, Streeten DHP: Effect of pulsatile flow. Pathophysiologic and pharmacologic alterations in the release and action of ADH. Metabolism 25:697, 1976.
8. Share L: Vasopressin, its bioassay and the physiological control of its release. Am J Med 42:701, 1967.
9. Bartelstone HJ, Nasmyth PA: Vasopressin potentiation of catecholamine actions in dog, rat, cat, and rat aortic strip. Am J Physiol 208:754, 1965.
10. Abe T: Influence of cardiac surgery using cardiopulmonary bypass on metabolic regulation. Jap Circ J 38:13, 1974.
11. Landymore RW, Murphy DA, Longley WJ: Effect of cardiopulmonary bypass and hypothermia on pancreatic endocrine function and peripheral utilization of glucose. Can J Surg 22:248, 1979.
12. Allison SP: Changes in insulin secretion during open heart surgery. Br J Anaesth 43:138, 1971.
13. Hewitt RL, Woo RD, Ryan JR, Drapanas T: Plasma insulin and glucose relationships during cardiopulmonary bypass. Surgery 71:905, 1972.
14. Mandelbaum I, Morgan CR: Pancreatic blood flow and its relationship to insulin secretion during extracorporeal circulation. Ann Surg 170:753, 1969.
15. Baum D, Dillard DH, Porte D Jr: Inhibition of insulin release in infants undergoing deep hypothermic cardiovascular surgery. N Engl J Med 279:1309, 1968.
16. Salter CP, Fluck DC, Stimmler L: Effect of open-heart surgery on growth-hormone levels in man. Lancet 2:853, 1972.
17. Macdonald RG, Buckler JMH, Deverall PB, Watson DA, Ballint M: Growth hormone and blood-glucose concentrations during cardiopulmonary bypass. Br J Anaesth 47:713, 1975.
18. Lee WH Jr, Krumhaar D, Fonkalsrud EW, Schjeide OA, Maloney JV Jr: Denaturation of plasma proteins as a cause of morbidity and death after intracardiac operations. Surgery 50:29, 1961.
19. Porte D Jr, Graber AL, Kuzuya T, Williams RH: The effect of epinephrine on immunoreactive insulin levels in man. J Clin Invest 45:228, 1966.
20. Mills NL, Beaudet RL, Isom OW, Spencer FC: Hyperglycemia during cardiopulmonary bypass. Ann Surg 177:203, 1973.
21. Clausen T: The effect of insulin on glucose transport in muscle cells. Curr Topics Membr Transport, p. 209, 1975.
22. Fulton RL, Ridolpho P: Physiologic effects of acute sodium depletion. Ann Surg 173:344, 1971.
23. Mandelbaum I, Morgan CR: Effect of extracorporeal circulation upon insulin. J Thorac Cardiovasc Surg 55:526, 1968.
24. Levine R: Mechanisms of insulin secretion. N Engl J Med 283:522, 1970.
25. Manners JM: Nutrition after cardiac surgery. Anaesthesia 29:675, 1974.
26. Moffitt EA, Rosevear JW, Molnar GD, McGoon DD: Myocardial metabolism in open-heart surgery. Correlation with insulin response. J Thorac Cardiovasc Surg 59:691, 1970.
27. Nuutinen L, Mononen P, Kairaluoma M, Tuononen S: The effect of cardiopulmonary bypass time on plasma lipids. Ann Chir Gynaecol 66:90, 1977.
28. Arrants JE, Gadsden RH, Huggins MB, Lee WH Jr: Effects of extracorporeal circulation upon blood lipids. Ann Thorac Surg 15:230, 1973.
29. Williamson J, Krebs H: Acetoacetate as fuel of respiration in the perfused rat heart. Biochem J 80:540, 1961.
30. Goodman L, Gilman A: *The Pharmacological Basis of Therapeutics.* New York, Macmillan, 1975.
31. Kurien VA, Olive MF: A metabolic cause for arrhythmias during acute myocardial hypoxia. Lancet 1:813, 1970.
32. Owens G, Adams JE, McElhannon FM, Youngblood RW: Experimental alternations of certain colloidal properties of blood during cardiopulmonary bypass. J Appl Physiol 14:947, 1959.
33. De Gasperis C: Human lung fat microembolism associated with cardiopulmonary bypass: Electron microscopic evidence. Scand J Thorac Cardiovasc Surg 2:84, 1968.
34. Hume DM, Bell CC, Bartter F: Direct measurement of adrenal secretion during operative trauma and convalescence. Surgery 52:174, 1962.
35. Taylor KM, Jones JV, Walker MS, Rao S, Bain WH: The cortisol response during heart-lung bypass. Circulation 54:20, 1976.
36. Taylor KM, Wright GS, Reid JM, Bain WH, Caves PK, Walker MS, Grant JK: Comparative studies of pulsatile and nonpulsatile flow during cardiopulmonary bypass. II. The effects on adrenal secretion on cortisol. J Thorac Cardiovasc Surg 75:574, 1978.
37. Uozumi T, Manabe H, Kawashima Y, Hamanaka Y, Monden Y, Matsumoto K: Plasma cortisol, corticosterone, and non-protein-bound cortisol in extracorporeal circulation. Acta Endocrinol 69:517, 1972.
38. Taylor KM, Walker MS, Rao LGS, Jones JV, Gray CE: Plasma levels of cortisol, free cortisol, and corticotropin during cardio-pulmonary by-pass. J Endocrinol 67:29p, 1975.
39. Dietzman RH, Lunseth JB, Goott B, Berger EC: The use of methylprednisolone during cardiopulmonary bypass. A review of 427 cases. J Thorac Cardiovasc Surg 69:870, 1975.
40. Motsay GJ, Alho A, Jaeger T, Shultz LS, Dietzman RH, Lillehei RC: Effects of methylprednisolone, phenoxybenzamine, and epinephrine tolerance in canine endotoxin shock: Study of isogravimetric capillary pressures in forelimb and intestine. Surgery 70:271, 1971.
41. Weissmann G, Thomas L: Effects of corticosteroids upon connective tissue and lysosomes. Recent Prog Horm Res 20:215, 1964.
42. Oyama T, Shibata S, Matsuki A, Kudo T: Serum endogenous throxine levels in man during anaesthesia and surgery. Br J Anaesth 41:103, 1969.
43. Bremner WF, Taylor KM, Baird S, Thomson JE, Thomson JA, Ratcliffe JG, Lawrie TDV Bain WH: Hypothalamo-pituitary-thyroid axis function during

cardiopulmonary bypass. J Thorac Cardiovasc Surg 75:392, 1978.
44. Saeed-Uz-Zafar M, Miller JM, Breneman GM, Mansour J: Observations on the effect of heparin on free and total thyroxine. J Clin Endocrinol Metab 32:633, 1971.
45. Hershman JM, Jones CM, Bailey AL: Reciprocal changes in serum thyrotropin and free thyroxine produced by heparin. J Clin Endocrinol Metab 34: 574, 1972.
46. Oppenheimer JH: Thyroid hormones in liver. Mayo Clin Proc 47:854, 1972.
47. Schwartz HL, Schadlow AR, Faierman D, Surks MI, Oppenheimer JH: Heparin administration appears to decrease cellular binding of thyroxine. J Clin Endocrinol Metab 36:598, 1973.
48. Hollander CS, Shenkman L: The physiological role of triiodothyronine. Am J Med Sci 264:4, 1972.
49. Sullivan PRC, Bollinger JA, Reichlin S: Selective deficiency of tissue triiodothyronine. A proposed mechanism of elevated free thyroxine in the euthyroid sick. J Clin Invest 52:83a, 1973.
50. Wilber JF, Baum D: Elevation of plasma TSH during surgical hypothermia. J Clin Endocrinol Metab 31: 372, 1970.
51. Lawton NF, Ellis SM, Sufi S: The triiodothyronine and thyroxine response to thyrotrophin-releasing hormone in the assessment of the pituitary-thyroid axis. Clin Endocrinol 2:57, 1973.
52. Taylor KM: Pituitary-adrenal axis during cardiopulmonary bypass. Br Heart J 38:321, 1976.
53. Taylor KM, Wright GS, Bain WH, Caves PK, Beastall GS: Comparative studies of pulsatile and non-pulsatile flow during cardiopulmonary bypass. III. Response of anterior pituitary gland to thyrotropin-releasing hormone. J Thorac Cardiovasc Surg 75:579, 1978.
54. Matsumoto T, Wolferth CC Jr, Perlman MH: Effects of pulsatile and non-pulsatile perfusion upon cerebral and conjuctival microcirculation in dogs. Am Surg 37:61, 1971.
55. Levey GS: Catecholamine sensitivity, thyroid hormone and the heart. A reevaluation. Am J Med 50: 413, 1971.
56. Epstein SE, Skelton CL, Levey GS, Entman M: Adenyl cyclase and myocardial contractility. Ann Intern Med 72:561, 1970.
57. Langer GA: Ion fluxes in cardiac excitation and contraction and their relation to myocardial contractility. Physiol Rev 48:708, 1968.
58. Westhorpe RN, Varghese Z, Petrie A, Wills MR, Lumley J: Changes in ionized calcium and other plasma constituents associated with cardiopulmonary bypass. Br J Anaesth 50:951, 1978.
59. Fleckenstein A, Janke J, Doering HJ, Leder O: The "key-role" of calcium in the production of non-coronarogenic myocardial necrosis. Sixth Annual Meeting of the International Study Group for Research in Cardiac Metabolism, Freiburg, German Federal Republic, 1973.
60. Turnier E, Osborn J, Gerbode F, Popper R: Magnesium and open-heart surgery. J Thorac Cardiovasc Surg 64:694, 1972.
61. Scheinman M, Sullivan R, Hyatt K: Magnesium metabolism in patients undergoing cardiopulmonary bypass. Circulation 39–40 (suppl.):235, 1969.

CHAPTER 4

PERIOPERATIVE HYPERTENSION: PATHOGENESIS AND TREATMENT

DANIEL J. ULLYOT, M.D.

Perioperative hypertension has become a relatively recent concern to the cardiac surgeon coinciding with the large number of patients undergoing myocardial revascularization. Previously, *hypotension* associated with a low output syndrome following repair of congenital and vascular heart disease was the major concern in the perioperative period.

Although the inclusion of this topic in a symposium on "Pathophysiology and Techniques of Cardiopulmonary Bypass" implies, perhaps, a causal relation between extracorporeal circulation (ECC) and elevated blood pressure in the perioperative period, support for such an exclusive relationship is lacking. In fact, the evidence seems to suggest a predilection to hypertension among patients with coronary atherosclerosis under the circumstances of anesthesia and cardiac surgery with or without ECC. It has been shown, for example, that patients having internal mammary implantation (Vineberg) have an incidence of perioperative hypertension similar to that of those having coronary bypass using ECC.[1] Furthermore, patients having ECC for coronary artery surgery have a much higher incidence of perioperative hypertension than do, for example, patients having ECC for repair of valvular heart lesions.[2, 3]

Nonetheless, it is appropriate to discuss this topic here because the hypertensive response may occur during the conduct of ECC requiring appropriate intervention.

DEFINITION

Postoperative hypertension has been defined variously by different investigators. There is general agreement, however, that hypertension secondary to a variety of conditions seen in the postoperative period such as pain, apprehension, shivering, bucking the ventilator, inadequate ventilation (hypoxia, hypercarbia), intolerance of the endotracheal tube, and overtransfusion must be excluded.

Postoperative hypertension can be defined as a sustained (20 minutes or more) blood pressure elevation without obvious cause in a well-sedated patient in whom the diastolic pressure is increased 20 mm Hg or the systolic pressure is increased 30 mm Hg above preoperative values. For the majority of patients, blood pressures exceeding 160/90 mm Hg satisfy these criteria. During ECC, mean arterial pressure exceeding 90 mm Hg is considered in the hypertensive range.

PATHOGENESIS

One third to one half of patients undergoing myocardial revascularization manifest hypertension as defined above in the perioperative period.[2, 4] Hypertension occurs during the first 6 to 8 hours following surgery, and most commonly begins approximately 1 hour after the termination of ECC. Hypertension may be seen prior to, during, or immediately after ECC.

Hemodynamic studies have established that the hypertensive response is due to an increase in systemic vascular resistance (SVR).[4-6] It is beyond the scope of this discussion to review in detail the regulation of systemic vascular resistance. The simple hemodynamic relations are as follows:

$$SVR = \frac{\overline{AP} - \overline{RAP}}{CO}$$

where SVR = systemic vascular resistance
$\overline{AP}$ = mean systemic arterial pressure
$\overline{RAP}$ = mean right atrial pressure
CO = cardiac output

Systemic arterial pressure is determined by the relationship between cardiac output and systemic vascular resistance. Blood pressure and cardiac output are measured directly; systemic vascular resistance is a derived variable calculated according to the above formula.

Studies comparing normotensive and hypertensive patients in the postoperative period show a statistically significant difference in systemic vascular resistance but not in cardiac output between the two groups (Table 4.1).

The study of pathogenesis then becomes a study of the factors causing increased systemic vascular resistance in patients with coronary atherosclerosis during the conditions associated with anesthesia, ECC, cardiac manipulation, and surgical stimulation.

There are two ways of approaching the problem. One is to attempt to identify factors tending to raise systemic vascular resistance. These can be broadly classified into humoral and neurogenic. The other is to examine the

Table 4.1
Hemodynamic Comparison between a Group of Patients Who Developed Hypertension and a Group Who Remained Normotensive after Coronary Artery Bypass Operation[4]

	Hypertension group (N = 16)	Normotension group (N = 16)	p Values
Heart rate (beats/min)	90.5 ± 2.4	91 ± 3	NS
Systolic blood pressure (mm Hg)	176 ± 6.0	128 ± 4.6	$p < 0.005$
Diastolic blood pressure (mm Hg)	90 ± 3.7	72 ± 3.4	$p < 0.01$
Mean arterial pressure (mm Hg)	122 ± 4.3	90 ± 3.8	$p < 0.005$
Pulmonary artery systolic blood pressure (mm Hg)	25 ± 1.7	23 ± 1.6	NS
Pulmonary artery diastolic blood pressure (mm Hg)	10.3 ± 1.3	10.1 ± 0.9	NS
Mean pulmonary pressure (mm Hg)	17.1 ± 1.3	15.8 ± 1.2	NS
Left ventricular filling pressure (mm Hg)	9.3 ± 1.3	9.1 ± 0.9	NS
Right ventricular filling pressure (mm Hg)	9.7 ± 0.8	10.4 ± 1.2	NS
Cardiac output (L/min)	5.5 ± 0.36	4.98 ± 0.41	NS
Stroke volume (ml/beat)	60.2 ± 3.7	54.5 ± 5.8	NS
Systemic vascular resistance (resistance units)	21.1 ± 1.3	16.7 ± 1.2	$p < 0.01$
Left ventricular stroke work (gm-M)	97.8 ± 5.6	62.7 ± 3.4	$p < 0.005$
Right ventricular stroke work (gm-M)	6.7 ± 0.37	4.45 ± 0.46	$p < 0.01$
Pulmonary vascular resistance (resistance units)	1.5 ± 0.18	1.2 ± 0.14	NS
Systolic blood pressure × heart rate	16,145 ± 411	11,774 ± 456	$p < 0.005$

(Reproduced with permission from A. J. Roberts et al.[4])

homeostatic mechanisms which keep blood pressure within a narrow range. Normally, a tendency to hypertension is countered by reduction in cardiac output (bradycardia, decreased stroke volume) or reflex vasodilatation. Baroreceptors in the carotid sinus, atria, and at several points in the arterial tree send afferent fibers to the medulla in which are located "cardioaccelerator" and "vasoconstrictor" control centers which in turn counter hypertension by reducing sympathetic discharge to the heart and by inhibiting sympathetic vasoconstrictor outflow. Perioperative hypertension represents a temporary failure of these control systems.

Before looking closer at pathogenesis, it is useful to summarize what factors appear *not* to be important in causing perioperative hypertension. These include age, sex, NYHA clinical class, history of myocardial infarction, history of kidney disease, left ventricular function, cross clamp time, number of grafts placed, state of consciousness, anesthetic agents, and various hemodynamic indices such as central venous pressure (CVP), left atrial pressure (LAP), heart rate (HR), pulmonary artery (PA) pressure, and pulmonary vascular resistance.[1, 4] There is sharp disagreement as to whether history of hypertension is a predisposing factor.[2, 4]

HUMORAL FACTORS

Substances which circulate and tend to increase systemic vascular resistance include catecholamines (epinephrine and norepinephrine) and angiotensin, which is activated by plasma renin. Roberts and coworkers[4] found norepinephrine levels and plasma renin activity (PRA) elevated in patients with perioperative hypertension, compared to normotensive controls.[4] Moreover, the extent of hypertension correlated both with PRA and epinephrine levels.

Increased PRA may potentiate the vasoconstrictor effect of catecholamines; conversely, catecholamines have been shown to stimulate renin release.

More general studies of circulating vasoconstrictor substances in patients undergoing open heart surgery show conflicting results. Hoar and coworkers[7] found evidence of sympathetic activation in the form of increases in both epinephrine and norepinephrine in response to both surgical stimulation and ECC (Table 4.2). PRA did not rise in their study in which halothane anesthesia was used. Factors postulated to cause catecholamine release are cold, acute hemodilution, nonpulsatile flow, and isolation of the lung from the circulation during ECC.[7]

Landymore et al.[9] found increased catecholamines and increased PRA in patients anesthetized with halothane and managed with nonpulsatile ECC.[8] These authors found no increase in PRA in patients having pulsatile ECC who importantly had a decreased incidence of postoperative hypertension.

In patients anesthetized with morphine, Bailey et al.[9] reported increased PRA and unchanged catecholamine levels associated with ECC. Studies by Taylor and Morton[10]

Table 4.2
Plasma Catecholamine Concentration and Plasma Renin Activity in Patients Undergoing Myocardial Revascularization

	Period I: Awake (*N* = 14)	Period 11: Anesthesia (*N* = 15)	Period 111: Operation (*N* = 15)	Period IV: Conclusion of CPB* (*N* = 15)	Period V: Chest closed (*N* = 11)
Norepinephrine (pg/ml)	366 ± 38.0†	470 ± 113.0	825 ± 123.0‡	1767 ± 290‡	731 ± 112.0§
Epinephrine (pg/ml)	92 ± 27.0	17 ± 7.0§	81 ± 16.0‡	519 ± 81.0‡	88 ± 25.0§
Dopamine (pg/ml)	40 ± 17.0	97 ± 54.0	108 ± 23.0	151 ± 36.0	106 ± 37.0
Plasma renin activity (ng/ml/hr)	4.0 ± 1.1	53 ± 1.5	5.3 ± 1.2	4.2 ± 1.0	4.6 ± 1.3

(Reproduced with permission from P.F. Hoar et al.[7],)
* CPB, cardiopulmonary bypass.
† Values are mean ± SE. Statistical analysis was done by Student's *t* test for paired data comparing each study period to the one immediately preceding.
‡ $p < 0.05$.
§ $p < 0.01$.

similarly found increased angiotensin II levels in patients anesthetized with morphine undergoing ECC.[10]

The data, which are conflicting, suggest that both catecholamine release and activation of the renin-angiotension system may contribute to perioperative hypertension modified perhaps by the anesthetic agent used, by use of pulsatile ECC, and by pretreatment with propranolol.[11]

NEUROGENIC FACTORS

It is more difficult to study neurogenic activity in the pathogenesis of perioperative hypertension.

Considerable interest in a cardiogenic hypertensive reflex was stimulated by the observations that unilateral stellate ganglion blockade will prevent[12] and reverse[13] perioperative hypertension following coronary bypass surgery. James and co-workers[14] showed transient hypertension following injection of small amounts of serotonin in the proximal left coronary artery in dogs. Histological study of the left main coronary artery in these animals disclosed a structure resembling a chemoreceptor. Support for this mechanism in man is the observation by Roberts et al[4] that patients with greater than 50% stenosis of the left main coronary artery were more prone to the development of perioperative hypertension.

Since dopamine-β-hydroxylase (DBH) catalyzes the final step in the synthesis of the sympathetic transmitter norepinephrine, it was suggested that DBH might be a useful marker for sympathetic activity. Roberts et al.[4] found preoperative DBH levels significantly higher in patients developing postoperative hypertension than in control's and suggested an important role of the central nervous system in perioperative hypertension. This suggestion is rendered premature, however, by the work of Horwitz et al.,[15] who found serum DBH activity an unsatisfactory index of sympathetic function in man.

It is apparent from the foregoing that, whereas the pathophysiology of perioperative hypertension is not clear, both humoral and neurogenic mechanisms are important in the genesis of this response. It has been proposed that a heightened sympathetic response to stress is an important risk factor in the development of coronary atherosclerosis. Friedman and Rosenman[16] described behavioral characteristics associated with excessive aggressiveness, competitiveness, and time urgency which they termed "type A" behavior. It has subsequently been established in both prospective and retrospective studies that the type A behavior pattern is a significant predictor of coronary heart disease.[17, 18]

These studies suggest that an exaggerated sympathetic response to stress is present in a subgroup of patients developing coronary atherosclerosis and that this response may be contributory to the development of coronary heart disease. It is probable that this same heightened sympathetic response may account for the perioperative hypertension seen in association with the attempt to manage such patients surgically. Type A personality is a predictor of elevated norepinephrine concentrations during job stress testing[19]. Moreover, patients with atherosclerotic disease have been shown to respond to a cold pressor test with marked elevation in blood pressure.[20]

The anticipation of surgery, operative manipulation, and the physiological stimuli of ECC are potent stressors which might be expected to provoke heightened sympathetic responses in many patients with coronary atherosclerosis. Further elucidation of the pathogenesis of perioperative hypertension may depend on fundamental discoveries about the stress response and its aberrant forms in certain individuals.

CLINICAL SIGNIFICANCE

Hypertension in the early postoperative period increases bleeding and may cause myocardial injury, particularly in patients who, because of severe distal disease, have incomplete revascularization. Viljoen et al.[21] report increased hemorrhage in more than 50% of hypertensive patients. Estafanous et al.[1] describe disruption of a ventriculotomy closure in one patient and of a proximal vein graft suture line in another, both related to hypertension and both resulting in death.

Hoar et al.[5] showed depession in the ratio of diastolic pressure-time-index to the systolic-pressure-time-index, an expression believed to represent the subendocardial oxygen supply-demand relationship in postoperatively hypertensive patients (Fig. 4.1). These authors showed a statistically significant improvement in this ratio following treatment (Table 4.3).

Table 4.3
Cardiovascular Response to Epidural Anesthesia in Postoperatively Hypertensive Patients

Measurement	Postoperatively Hypertensive Patients* Before Drug Administration	After Drug Administration	Significance
Blood pressure			
systolic	156	105	$p < 0.001$
diastolic	89	62	$p < 0.001$
CI†	2.48	2.14	NS
SVR	22	17.5	$p < 0.005$
DPTI/SPTI	0.80	1.09	$p < 0.005$

(Reproduced with permission from P.F. Hoar et al.[5])
* N = 7.
† CI, cardiac index; SVR, systemic vascular resistance; DPTI/SPTI, diastolic pressure-time index/systolic pressure-time index.

TREATMENT

Because of increased bleeding, the threat of suture line disruption, and the possibility of ischemic myocardial injury, perioperative hypertension should be treated.

Several therapeutic approaches have been advocated. Bidwai et al.[12] describe unilateral stellate ganglion block using lidocaine. Hoar et al.[5] used thoracic epidural anesthesia both to treat hypertension and ameliorate incisional pain.

We favor intravenously administered sodium nitroprusside.[22] Roberts et al.[4] report an average duration of nitroprusside therapy of 12 hours (range 2–38 hours) suggesting that the hypertensive response may be prolonged in some patients. We have noted consistent control of hypertension using this agent and have not observed tachyphylaxis. We have found intermittent administration of intravenous propranolol a useful adjunct in patients with hyperdynamic left ventricular function. Caution must be exercised with nitroprusside therapy. Sudden and profound hypotension is not an uncommon occurrence. Arterial and central venous pressure monitoring in an ICU setting with one-on-one nursing is mandatory. Atrial pressures must be maintained by judicious volume replacement during this period in order to minimize the occurrence of sudden hypotension.

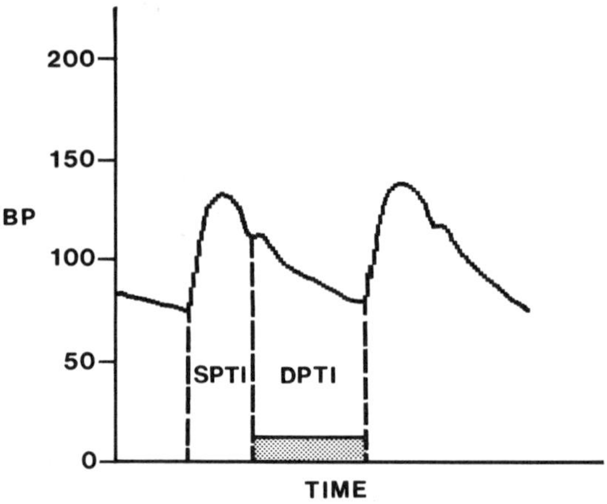

Figure 4.1. Systemic arterial pressure tracing describing the theoretical supply/demand relationship (*DPTI/SPTI*) of the subendocardial area of the left ventricle. *SPTI*, the estimate of myocardial oxygen needs (demand), is measured by the area under the systolic portion of the systemic arterial pressure tracing from the onset of systole to the dicrotic notch (closure of aortic valve). *DPTI*, the estimate of subendocardial flow (supply), is measured by the area between the closure of the aortic valve, to the onset of the next upstroke, minus the left atrial pressure (*LAP*). *BP*, blood pressure. (Reproduced with permission from P. F. Hoar et al.[5])

Another problem associated with nitroprusside therapy is arterial hypoxemia.[23] Normally segmental pulmonary atelectasis is matched by localized pulmonary arterial vasoconstriction to maintain favorable ventilation-perfusion relationships. Nitroprusside is a pulmonary vasodilator which may disrupt these relationships causing perfusion of poorly ventilated segments and resultant hypoxemia. One may compensate for this by increasing FIO_2 and by using positive and expiratory pressure.

Intravenous nitroglycerine or thorazine

may be used to control hypertension. The former is more difficult to prepare and the latter more difficult to control than nitroprusside.

CONCLUSION

Perioperative hypertension occurs in one third to one half of patients udergoing coronary artery bypass. This is a paroxysmal response with a peak incidence in the first 6 hours postoperatively and is due to an increase in peripheral vascular resistance. Increased circulating catecholamines, PRA, and neurogenic stimulation have been implicated in this response. The patient with coronary atherosclerosis is particularly prone to paroxysmal hypertension following cardiac surgical stimulation with or without ECC. Bleeding and ischemic myocardial injury are potential sequellae making treatment advisable. Intravenous propranolol and sodium nitroprusside provide effective treatment.

References

1. Estafanous FG, Tarazi RC, Viljoen JF, El Tawil MY: Systemic hypertension following myocardial revascularization. Am Heart J 85:732–738, 1973.
2. Estafanous FG, Tarazi RC: Systemic arterial hypertension associated with cardiac surgery. Am J Cardiol 46:685–694, 1980.
3. Estafanous FG, Tarazi RC, Buckley S, Taylor PC: Arterial hypertension in immediate postoperative period after valve replacement. Br Heart J 40:718–724, 1978.
4. Roberts JR, Niarchos AP, et al.: Systemic hypertension associated with coronary artery bypass surgery. Predisposing factors, hemodynamic characteristics, humoral profile, and treatment. J. Thorac Cardiovasc Surg 74:846–859, Dec 1977.
5. Hoar PF, Hickey RF, Ullyot DJ: Systemic hypertension following myocardial revascularization. A method of treatment using epidural anesthesia. J Thorac Cardiovasc Surg 71:859–864, 1976.
6. Wallach R, Karp RB, Renes JG, Oparil S, Smith LR, James JN: Pathogenesis of paroxysmal hypertension developing during and after coronary bypass surgery: A study of hemodynamic and humoral factors. Am J Cardiol 46:559–565, 1980.
7. Hoar PF, Stone JG, Faltas AN, Bendixen HH, Head RJ, Berkowitz BA: Hemodynamic and adrenergic responses to anesthesia and operation for myocardial revascularization. J Thorac Cardiovasc Surg 80: 242–248, Aug 1980.
8. Landymore RW, Murphy DA, Kinley CE, Parrott JC, Moffitt EA, Longley WJ, Quirbic AA: Does pulsatile flow influence the incidence of postoperative hypertension? Annals Thorac Surg 28: 261–268, 1979.
9. Bailey DR, Miller ED Jr, Kaplan JA, Rogers PW: The renin-angiotensin-aldosterone system during cardiac surgery with morphine-nitrous oxide anesthesia. Anesthesiology 42:538–544, 1975.
10. Taylor KM, Morton IJ, Brown JJ, Bain WH, Cones PK: Hypertension and the renin-angiotensin system following open-heart surgery. J Thorac Cardiovasc Surg 74:840–845, 1977.
11. Bühler FR, Laragh JH, Baer L, et al.: Propranolol inhibition of renin secretion. A specific approach to diagnosis and treatment of renin-dependent hypertensive diseases. NEJM 287:1209–1214, 1972.
12. Bidwai AV, Rogers CR: Preoperative stellate-ganglion blockade to prevent hypertension following coronary artery operations. Anesthesiology 51:345–347, 1979.
13. Fouad FM, Estafanous FG, Tarazi RC: Unilateral stellate block in the treatment of post-bypass hypertension: Implications of a new therapeutic approach. Hemodynamics of postmyocardial revascularization hypertension. Am J Cardiol 41:564–569, 1978.
14. James TN, Isobe JH: Analysis of components in a cardiogenic hypertensive chemoreflex. Circulation 52:179–192, 1975.
15. Horwitz D, Alexander RW, Lovenberg W, Keiser HR: Human serum dopamine-β-hydroxylase. Relationship to hypertension and sympathetic activity. Circulation Res. 32:594–599, 1973.
16. Friedman M, Rosenman RH: Assocation of specific overt behavior pattern with blood and cardiovascular findings. Blood cholesterol level, blood clotting time, incidence of arcus senilis, and clinical coronary artery disease. JAMA 169:1286–1296, 1959.
17. Rosenman RH, Brand RJ, Jenkins CD, et al.: Coronary heart disease in the Western Collaborative Group Study—Final follow-up experience of 8½ years. JAMA 233 (8):872–877, 1975.
18. Shekelle RB, Shoenberger JA and Stamler J: Correlates of the JAS type A behavior pattern score. J Chronic Dis 29:381–394, 1976.
19. Friedman M, St. George S, Byers So, and Rosenman RH: Excretion of catecholamines, 17-ketosteroids, 17-hydroxycorticoids and 5-hydroxyindole in men exhibiting a particular behavior pattern (A) associated with high incidence of clinical coronary artery disease. J Clin Invest 39:758–764, 1960.
20. Keys A, Taylor HL, Blackburn H, et al.: Mortality and coronary heart disease among men studied for 23 years. Arch Intern Med 128:201–214, 1971.
21. Viljoen JF, Estafanous FG, Tarazi RC: Acute hypertension immediately after coronary artery surgery. J Thorac Cardiovasc Surg 71:548–550, 1976.
22. Lappas DG, Lowenstein E, Waller J, Fahmy NR, and Daggett WM: Hemodynamic effects of nitroprusside infusion during coronary artery operation in man. Circulation 54 (Suppl. III):4–10, 1976.
23. Brodie TS, Gray R, Swan HJC, Matloff JM: Effect of nitroprusside on arterial oxygenation, intrapulmonic shunts and oxygen delivery. Am J Cardiol 37:123, 1976.

CHAPTER 5

RENAL EFFECTS OF CARDIOPULMONARY BYPASS

JOE R. UTLEY, M.D.

Renal dysfunction is a relatively common complication in patients undergoing cardiopulmonary bypass. Mild or transient renal failure occurs in 1.5 to 13% of patients postoperatively.[1–5] Severe forms of renal failure after cardiac surgery requiring dialysis have a mortality of 25 to 100%. Mortality increases with increasing severity of renal failure perioperatively (Fig. 5.1). Factors which may affect perioperative renal function include preoperative renal disease, nephrotoxic drugs, hemolysis, renal ischemia, and humoral effects of cardiopulmonary bypass and postoperative cardiac function. Successful perioperative management of renal function includes the recognition of preoperative and intraoperative risk factors, optimal management of operative interventions, including cardiopulmonary bypass, early detection of renal failure, use of appropriate osmotic, diuretic, and vasoactive drugs, and peritoneal dialysis or hemodialysis in severe renal failure.

PERIOPERATIVE RISK FACTORS

Patients with preoperative renal failure are at greater risk of renal failure postoperatively[1, 2, 6] (Fig. 5.2). If the renal dysfunction is due to prerenal factors associated with a correctible heart disease, renal function may improve dramatically postoperatively. Preoperative cardiac dysfunction, including New York Heart Association functional classification, ventricular end diastolic pressures, or cardiac output, is a significant risk factor for postoperative renal failure (Fig. 5.3). Patients with complex congenital cyanotic heart disease and patients with multiple valve disease due to rheumatic fever are at greatest risk of postoperative renal failure.[4, 7] The greater duration of cardiopulmonary bypass and the higher incidence of preoperative renal dysfunction is a significant factor in these two groups of patients (Fig. 5.4). Patients with rheumatic valve disease are often operated upon in a setting of chronic heart failure with prerenal azotemia. In addition they may have vascular and glomerular lesions due to rheumatic or embolic events. Patients with cyanotic congenital heart disease often have small kidneys with enlarged glomeruli which may be a cause of benign proteinuria. These changes have been attributed to polycythemia and hypoxia. Other renal abnormalities observed in cyanotic congenital heart disease include dilatation and elongation of capillary loops and afferent arterioles, hyalinization of arterioles, glomerular sclerosis, and thickening of glomerular basement membranes. Diminished clearance of para-aminohippuric acid has been observed in children with cyanotic congenital heart disease. The diminished blood flow is principally to the outer renal cotex and is probably related to the increased responsiveness of children's renal vessels to elevated catecholamines and renin. Increase in filtration fraction has been observed in all forms of congenital heart disease. Children with cyanotic heart disease have a diminished diuretic response to a sodium load. The diminished renal plasma flow does not return to normal with surgical cor-

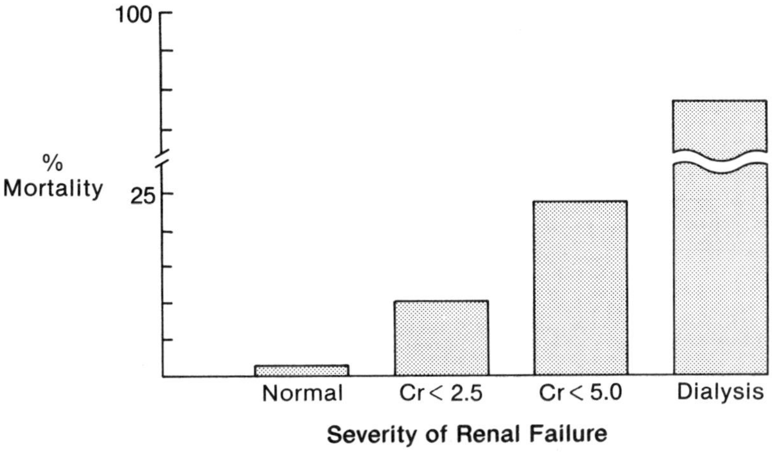

Figure 5.1. Mortality increases with increasing severity of perioperative renal failure. Perioperative renal failure was quantitated by the maximum serum creatinine concentration. Normal is less than 1.0 mg%, serum creatinine 1.0 to 2.5 mg%, serum creatinine 2.5 to 5.0 mg%, and the requirement for dialysis ($p < 0.05$). Cr = maximum serum concentration. (Reproduced with permission from R. M. Abel et al.[1,2])

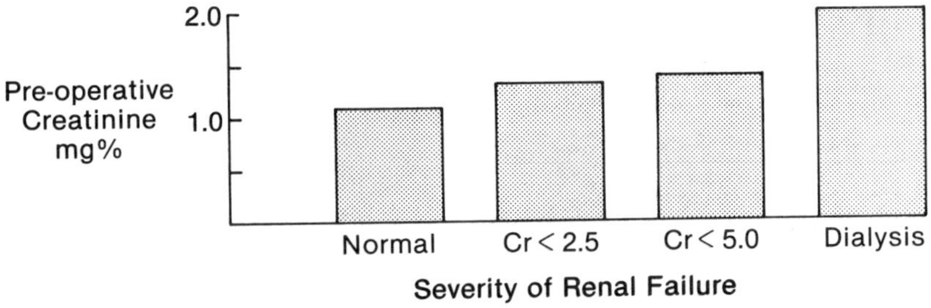

Figure 5.2. The mean preoperative serum creatinine concentration increased with increasing severity of postoperative renal failure ($p < 0.05$). (Reproduced with permission from R. M. Abel et al.[1,2])

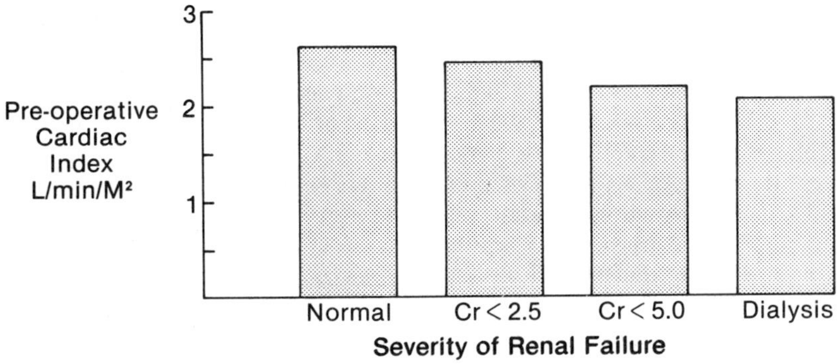

Figure 5.3. The mean preoperative cardiac index decreased with increasing severity of postoperative renal failure ($p < 0.05$). (Reproduced with permission from R. M. Abel et al.[1,2])

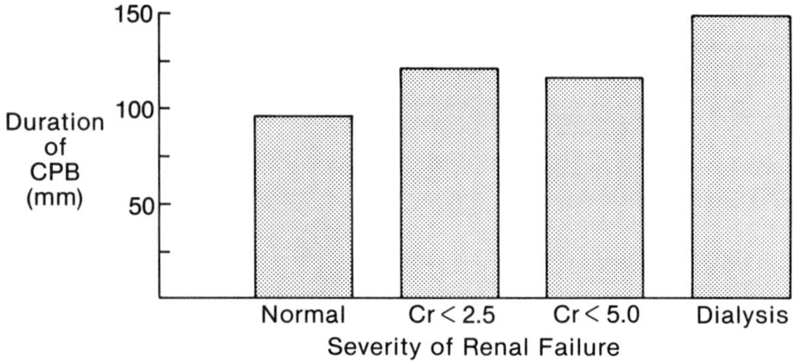

Figure 5.4. With increasing severity of postoperative renal failure, the mean duration of cardiopulmonary bypass (*CPB*) increased ($p < 0.05$).

rection.[8–10] The diminished glomerular filtration observed in patients with hematocrit greater than 50% returned to normal following surgical correction.[11] Congenital dysplasia of kidneys and coarctation was associated with an increased risk of renal failure in a group of infants studied by Chesney et al.[12] Our experience with cardiopulmonary bypass in the presence of uncorrected coarctation in older children shows the risk of renal failure is small.[13]

Patients with coronary artery disease and generalized atherosclerosis may have renal artery obstruction or arteriolar nephrosclerosis. Embolic lesions in renal arteries and glomeruli are common in patients with bacterial endocarditis. Immune globulins have been demonstrated in the glomerular lesions with bacterial endocarditis. Perioperative antibiotics may increase the risk of renal failure. These include cephalosporin, gentamycin, and methacillin.[14–16]

A major factor in the development of renal failure following cardiac surgical procedures is the cardiac performance postoperatively. Higher incidence of postoperative low cardiac output and longer periods of cardiopulmonary bypass contribute to the increased incidence of renal failure following correction of complex congenital heart disease and multiple valve rheumatic valve disease. The postoperative cardiac output is an important determinant of renal function (Fig. 5.5).

INTRAOPERATIVE FACTORS

The duration of cardiopulmonary bypass has been a significant determinant of postoperative renal function in most studies.[1, 2, 4, 6, 7, 17] The duration of aortic clamping and the total duration of operating also correlate with the risk of postoperative renal failure.[6] Perfusion pressure during cardiopulmonary bypass was less in patients who developed renal failure in one study.[6] In a retrospective study, Abel et al.[1, 2] did not show that perfusion pressure, flow rates, or presence of hemoglobulinemia had significant effects on postoperative renal function.

General Renal Effects

Ischemia has often been implicated as a major factor in renal dysfunction with cardiopulmonary bypass. Diminished renal blood flow, para-aminohippuric acid extraction, and decreased urine output become greater with longer periods of cardiopulmonary bypass.[7] Negative free water clearance and creatinine clearance are less in patients who have perfusion greater than 60 minutes, compared to patients with perfusion less than 60 minutes.[18] The depression of renal plasma flow, glomerular filtration rate, and sodium excretion was less at higher pressure and flow rates than at low flow rates.[19] The depressed renal plasma flow and glomerular filtration has been confirmed in children as well.[9]

Early Recognition of Renal Failure

Increased urine concentration of urea has been correlated with decreased renal perfusion during cardiopulmonary bypass and has been found to be a sensitive early indication of renal dysfunction.[20, 21] Free water clearance has been shown to be the most sensitive predictor of renal failure following cardiopulmonary bypass. Free water clearance is

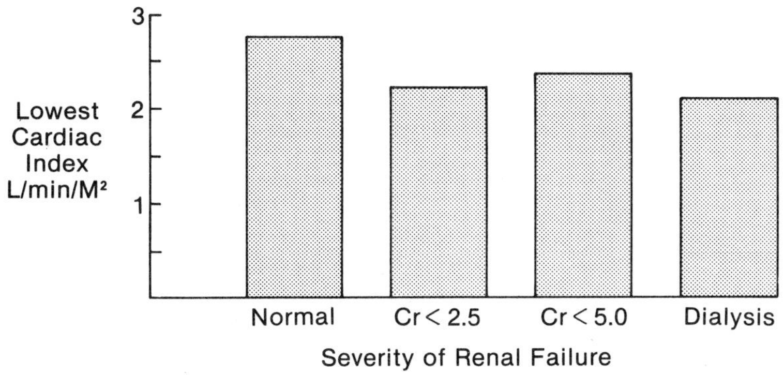

Figure 5.5. The lowest postoperative cardiac index decreased with increasing severity of postoperative renal failure ($p < 0.05$). (Reproduced with permission from R. M. Abel et al.[1, 2]). L/min/m^2 is liters per minute per square meter.

urine volume minus osmolar clearance:

$$C_{H_2O} = UV - C_{osm}$$

Patients who have C_{H_2O} greater than −20 ml/hr had no perioperative renal impairment. All patients with C_{H_2O} less than −8 ml/hr had acute renal insufficiency.[2, 23] Abnormal C_{H_2O} permitted the diagnosis of renal failure 1.5 days postoperatively. Diagnosis was done by means of urine urea (3 days), BUN (3.5 days), serum creatinine (4.5 days), oliguria (6.5 days).[24] Use of C_{H_2O} for early diagnosis after cardiopulmonary bypass allows better early management with fluid restriction, potassium restriction and diuretics.[23]

The effect of cardiopulmonary bypass on renal function may be caused by many factors accompanying the procedure, including vasoactive responses, nonpulsatile flow, endocrine effects, hypothermia, and hemodilution.

Vascular Effects

The fall in blood pressure at the onset of cardiopulmonary bypass may be related to a dilution of circulating catecholamines by the priming volume of the pump oxygenator. This is followed rapidly by an increase in adrenal catecholamine secretion and rise of circulatory catecholamines within 20 minutes.[25] The levels of circulatory catecholamine do not return to previous levels despite a return of blood pressure to normotensive levels.[26] The renin-angiotensin-aldosterone axis is stimulated at the onset of cardiopulmonary bypass, which contributes to the rise in renal vascular resistance.[27]

Pharmacologic Effects

Massive doses of steroids during cardiopulmonary bypass increase urine volume due to solute diuresis. The studies suggested that renal vasodilation was an important part of the effect.[28]

Furosemide has been shown to reverse the effect of cardiopulmonary bypass on renal blood flow. The effect of furosemide was more pronounced in the renal cortex than in juxtamedullary or medullary component of flow (Fig. 5.6).[29, 30] In a clinical study, furosemide was found to significantly increase creatinine clearance and lower serum creatinine in patients with greater than 60 minutes of cardiopulmonary bypass.

The addition of nitrous oxide to morphine and halothane, oxygen anesthesia has been found to lower blood pressure, decrease urine sodium/potassium ratio, and depress free water clearance. Postoperative creatinine and free water clearance were less in the nitrous oxide group.[31] The authors attributed the differences to depressed cardiac performance in the nitrous oxide group.

Microemboli

The pump oxygenator and cardiotomy suction apparatus may have important renal effects because of production of microemboli and hemolysis. Although microemboli have usually been implicated as a cause of post-

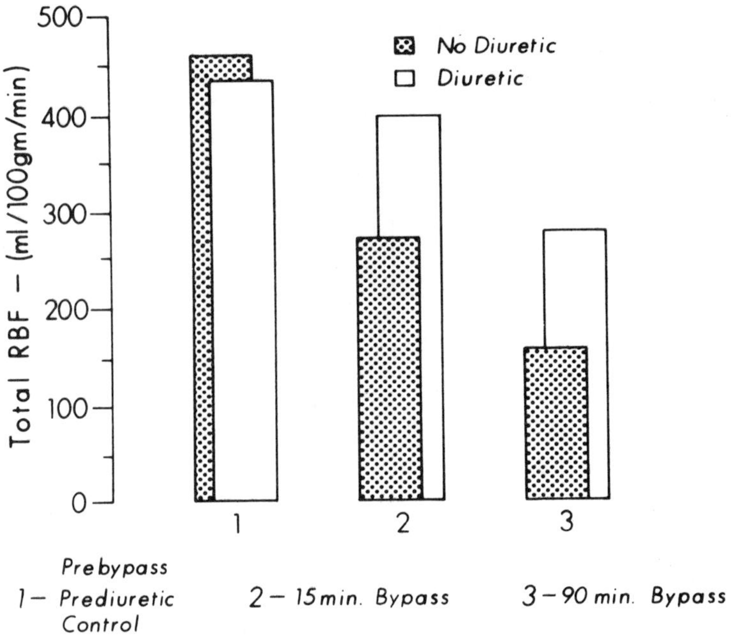

Figure 5.6. Furosemide-increased renal blood flow (*RBF*) during cardiopulmonary bypass.

operative cerebral dysfunction rather than renal failure, high levels of renal blood flow during hemodilution put the kidneys at risk of microembolic damage. Microemboli from oxygenators may be solid or gaseous. Increased number of microemboli are associated with high cardiotomy suction rates, use of nitrogen and physical disturbance of the oxygenator. Most microemboli are generated during the first 10 minutes of cardiopulmonary bypass. Particles contaminating disposable oxygenators are a common cause of microemboli.[32] Arterial filters decrease the numbers of microemboli. Microembolic rates progressively decrease in most patients during the period of perfusion.[33] The rate of microemboli production is greater with bubble oxygenators than disc oxygenators. More microemboli are produced at higher gas flow rates. The production of microemboli was least in bubble oxygenator when the gas flow was least, but oxygenator blood volume was greatest.[34] In a clinical study the mean concentration of microemboli was 2.3 per milliliter of circulating blood. The emboli were between 50 and 200 μg in diameter and were composed mainly of aggregates of platelets and white cells.[35]

Our studies of the effects of hemodilution, hypothermia, and cardiopulmonary bypass on renal function whos that the pump oxygenator diminishes blood flow and oxygen delivery to the outer renal cortex (Fig. 5.7). This is associated with increased water content of the renal medulla and diminished sodium, osmolar and free water clearances. The pump oxygenator also caused a fall in urine output and decreased urine concentration of sodium and increased urine concentration of potassium and creatinine.[36]

The diminished outer cortical flow caused by the pump oxygenator may be produced by axial migration of microemboli. Particles tend to migrate toward the center of flow in a vessel, and the axial migration is greater with larger particles. Thus particle poor blood is delivered to the inner cortex and particle rich blood is delivered to the outer cortex. Larger microspheres tend to be delivered to the outer cortex of the kidney (Fig. 5.8). This can explain the diminished outer cortical flow caused by the pump oxygenator.[37]

Hemolysis

Hemolysis has been recognized as an important effect of cardiopulmonary bypass.

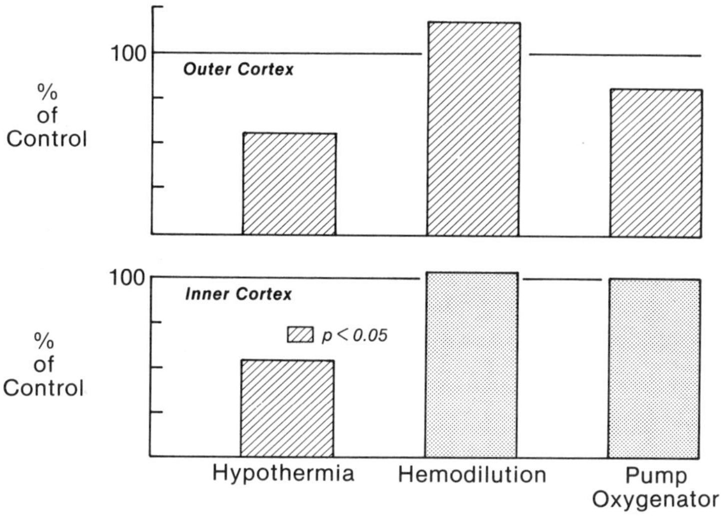

Figure 5.7. Studies of the separate effects of hypothermia, hemodilution, and pump oxygenator show that blood flow to the outer renal cortex is diminished by hypothermia and the pump oxygenator and is increased by hemodilution. Hypothermia decreased flow to inner cortex whereas hemodilution and the pump oxygenator had no significant effects.

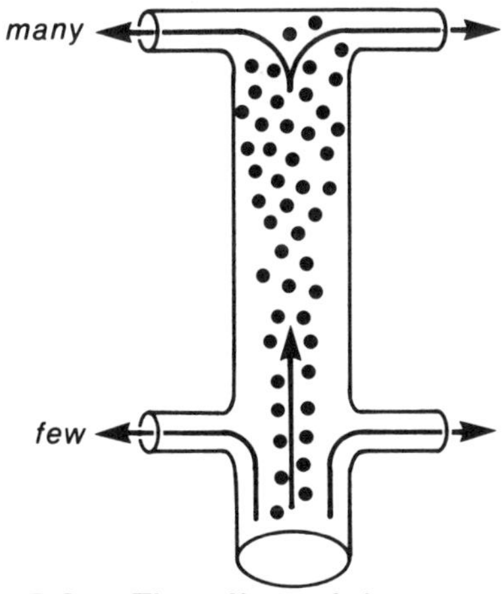

Figure 5.8. The effect of the pump oxygenator on distribution of renal blood flow is likely due to the selective delivery of microemboli to the outer renal cortex. Blood with fewer microemboli enters the proximal branches to the inner renal cortex.

Hemoglobin released from the destruction of red blood cells may be bound to proteins. Glomerular filtration of hemoglobin doesn't occur until the hemoglobin binding capacity in the plasma is saturated.

Hemoglobin is bound in plasma to haptoglobin, hemopexin, and as methemalbumin. Haptoglobin binds hemoglobin as a stable soluble complex. Haptoglobin is a symmetrical tetramer. Six forms have been recognized based on the electrophoretic characteristics of side chains. Hemoglobulinuria does not occur below serum concentrations of 100 to 150 mg/100 ml. The haptoglobin-hemoglobin complex is not filterable at the glomerulus. Hemoglobinuria occurs only after the haptoglobin binding is saturated. The haptoglobin-hemoglobin complex is taken up by the reticuloendothelial cells. The most active site of uptake is the liver, less is taken up in the bone marrow, and very little by the spleen. Haptoglobin levels are higher in men than women. Haptoglobin levels rise with fever or tissue injury.[38]

Hemopexin is a glycoprotein which binds heme. The hemopexin-heme complex is cleared slowly by hepatic parenchymal cells.

Methemalbumin is a complex of hematin and albumin which is found in the plasma when the haptoglobin and hemopexin carriers are saturated. The presence of methemalbumin is indicative of severe hemolysis.

The tetramer of hemoglobin may dissociate into dimers which are more readily filtered. Hemoglobin is absorbed by the proximal renal tubular cells and broken down into iron, globin, and porphyrin moieties. Hemoglobinuria occurs when the tubular capacity to reabsorb is exceeded.[38] The charge on the hemoglobin molecule is negative above its isoelectric pH. At pH below the isoelectric point of 6.99 the charge on the hemoglobin molecule is positive. A negatively charged protein (Tamm-Horsfall protein) in the distal renal tubule combines with hemoglobin to precipitate hemoglobulin-Tamm-Horsfall casts and induce renal failure. Keeping urine alkaline by bicarbonate infusion may diminish the rate of precipitation of hemoglobin in the tubules.[39]

In a study of mechanisms of hemoglobin clearance in heart surgery patients' free hemoglobin was cleared from the plasma faster than the hemoglobin-haptoglobin complex (Fig. 5.9). Appreciable free hemoglobin was present in serum before the onset of hemoglobinuria and after it ceased indicating the continued capacity of tubular reabsorption (Fig. 5.10). The majority of hemoglobin is cleared from the plasma by nonrenal mechanisms.[40, 41]

Early studies showed that cardiotomy suction was a greater source of hemolysis than the pump oxygenator. Factors found to be important are use of suction less than 60 mm Hg, negative pressure and design of suction tube to allow a longer entry area at low acceleration. The hemolysis for the pump oxygenator is mainly related to duration of perfusion.[42, 43] The rate of hemolysis in an oxygenator is greatly increased by gas flow compared to blood circulation without oxygenation.[29] Occlusive roller pumps produce greater hemolysis than nonocclusive pumps.[44] Turbulent flow in the pump oxygenator contributes to hemolysis.[44]

Hemodilution

Hemodilution decreases blood viscosity and oxygen-carrying capacity mainly because of lowered hematocrit. The effect of hemodilution on plasma colloidal oncotic pressure has important renal implications. The filtration of fluid at the renal glomerulus and its reabsorption from the renal glomerulus and its reabsorption from the renal tubules into the postglomerular capillaries depends on fil-

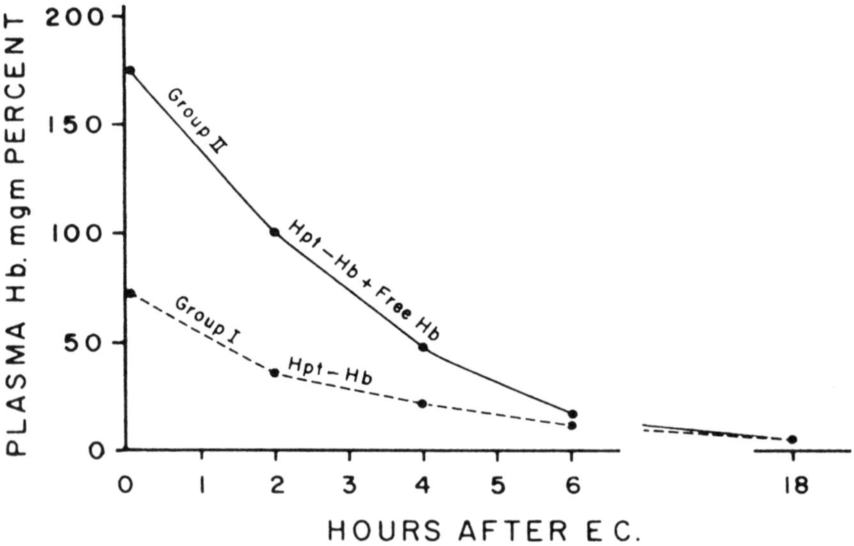

Figure 5.9. The rate of clearing of plasma hemoglobin is more rapid when free hemoglobin is present. In Group I all plasma hemoglobin is bound to haptoglobin. In Group II free hemoglobin, in addition to hemoglobin bound to haptoglobin, is present. *Hpt*, haptoglobin; *Hb*, hemoglobin; *EC*, extracorporeal circulation. (Reproduced with permission from M. N. Andersen et al.[40])

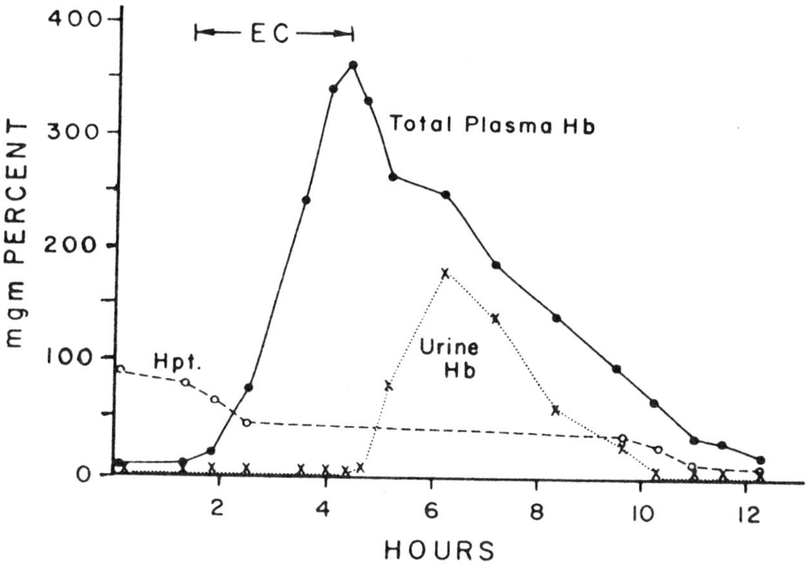

Figure 5.10. Haptoglobin (*Hpt.*) concentration falls progressively with rise in plasma hemoglobin (*Hb*) after the beginning of cardiopulmonary bypass. Urine excretion of hemoglobin begins only after the haptoglobin is saturated and the renal tubular reabsorption is exceeded. *Ec*, extracorporeal circulation. (Reproduced with permission from M. N. Andersen et al.[40])

tration gradients. Filtration is best understood with the Starling equation (Fig. 5.11). The filtration of plasma at the glomerulus is proportional to the difference between intravascular pressure in the glomerulus (P_c) and colloidal oncotic pressure in the glomerulus (π_c). The greater the difference between mean intravascular pressure and plasma colloidal oncotic pressure, the greater will be glomerular filtration (Fig. 5.12). The practical implication is that glomerular filtration will be sustained at lower perfusion pressure with hemodilution and lower plasma colloidal oncotic pressure (see Osmolar and Oncotic Agents).

Similarly, reabsorption of filtrate into the postglomerular capillary network is facilitated by lowered plasma colloidal oncotic pressure. Albumin increases tubular reabsorption and diminishes urine output because of this oncotic effect.

Hemodilution is probably the most important factor during cardiopulmonary bypass to protect against renal damage. Increased urine

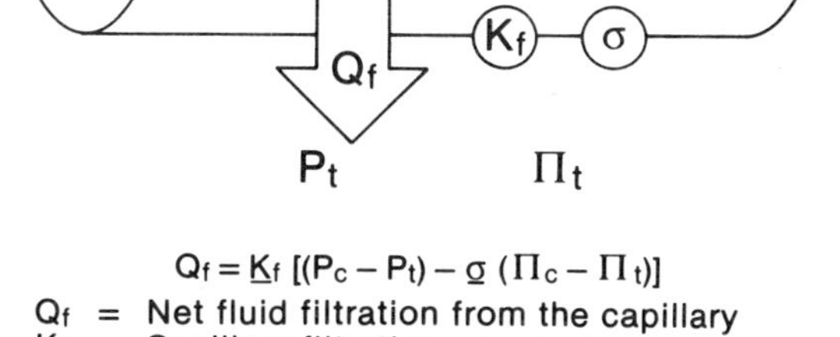

$$Q_f = \underline{K}_f\,[(P_c - P_t) - \underline{\sigma}\,(\Pi_c - \Pi_t)]$$

Q_f = Net fluid filtration from the capillary
$\underline{K}_f$ = Capillary filtration constant
$\underline{\sigma}$ = Capillary protein reflectance
P_c = Capillary hydrostatic pressure
P_t = Interstitial fluid hydrostatic pressure
Π_c = Serum colloidal osmotic pressure
Π_t = Interstitial fluid colloidal osmotic pressure

Figure 5.11. The Starling equation described the filtration of fluid across a semipermeable membrane.

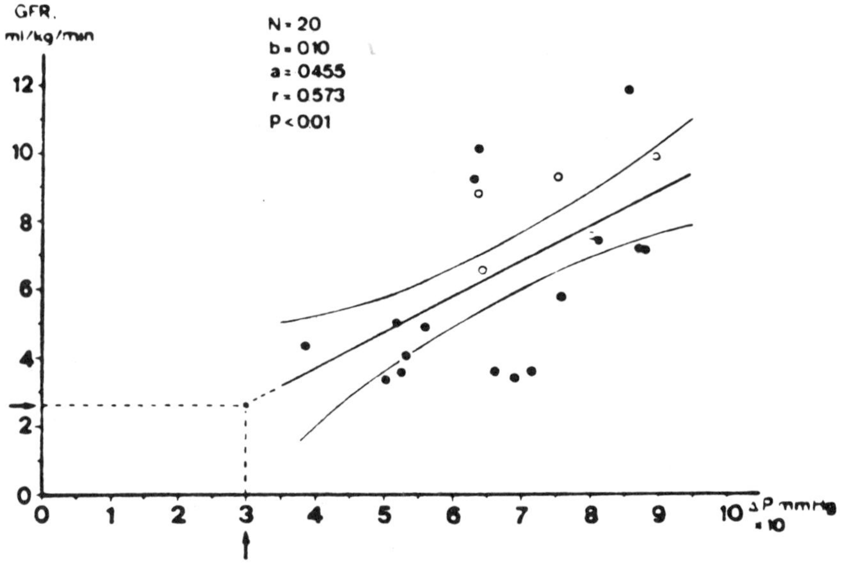

Figure 5.12. In this study glomerular filtration rate (*GFR*) was shown to be related to the difference between perfusion pressure and plasma colloidal oncotic pressure (Δ*P*). (Reproduced with permission from P. Schupbach et al.[57])

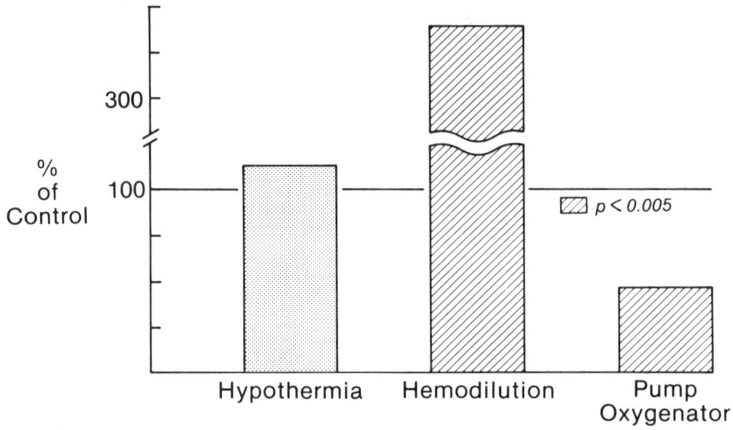

Figure 5.13. Studies in dogs of the separate effects of hypothermia, hemodilution, and pump oxygenator show that urine output is significantly increased by hemodilution and decreased by pump oxygenator.

output was recognized as an advantage of hemodilution early in its use (Fig. 5.13).[46] The diminished urine osmolarity with hemodilution has been demonstrated to protect renal tubular integrity.[47]

Hemodilution increases outer cortical blood flow, although outer cortical oxygen delivery is diminished because of greater decrease in oxygen-carrying capacity. The greater outer cortical flow is likely due to diminished blood viscosity rather than renal vasodilation because the distribution of small microspheres to the renal medulla is not increased by hemodilution.[36] Diminished medullary osmolarity was postulated as an important effect of hemodilution by Mielke. Increased medullary water content with hemodilution has recently been demonstrated

(Fig. 5.14).[36] Hemodilution increases renal plasma flow, but filtration fraction is decreased because glomerular filtration is not increased (Fig. 5.15 and 5.16). Renal clearance of sodium, potassium, osmolar, and free water clearance is increased by hemodilution (Fig. 5.17). Urine concentration of sodium is unchanged by hemodilution. Urine output is increased and urine concentration of sodium, potassium, and creatinine and osmolarity are diminished by hemodilution.[36] The clinical studies confirm the increased urine flow, increased osmolarity, creatinine, and sodium clearance with hemodilution.[47] Greater degrees of hemodilution are associated with higher urine output.[48] Hemodilution produces less hemolysis than whole blood priming.[49]

Hypothermia

Hypothermia has important renal effects which may contribute to renal dysfunction. Hypothermia depresses glomerular filtration rate and renal blood flow and osmolar clearance while it elevates filtration fraction and potassium excretion.[50] Hypothermia decreases inner and outer renal cortical blood flow in approximately equal proportions. Free water clearance is diminished by hypothermia. Microsphere studies show that hypothermia diminishes microspheres in the renal medulla, which suggests cortical vasoconstriction as the mechanisms.[36]

An important part of the mechanism of action of hypothermia is depression of tubular function.[51, 52] The vasoconstriction associated with hypothermia is opposed by the increased flow due to lowered viscosity with hemodilution. Thus, the combination of hemodilution and hypothermia produce satisfactory levels of renal perfusion.[36]

Osmolar and Oncotic Agents

Mannitol has been advocated as a component of priming solutions for several reasons. Hemolysis of red cells is diminished in the presence of mannitol.[53] Mannitol may affect renal function by causing renal vasodilation,

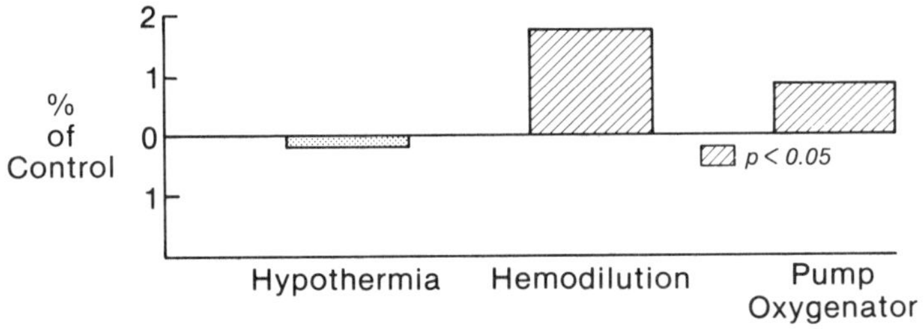

Figure 5.14. Significant increase in renal medullary water content occurred with hemodilution and pump oxygenator. Hypothermia caused no significant changes.

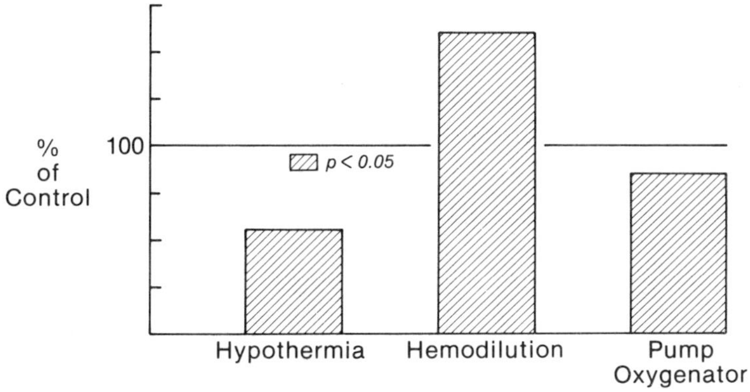

Figure 5.15. Both hypothermia and pump oxygenator caused a decrease in renal plasma flow. Hemodilution increased renal plasma flow.

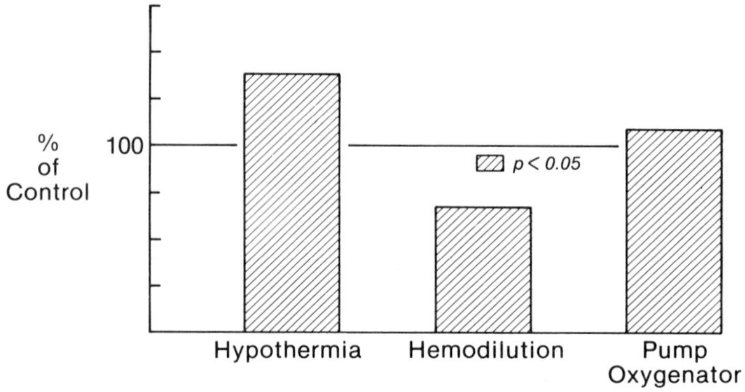

Figure 5.16. Filtration is increased with hypothermia and pump oxygenator. Hemodilution causes the opposite effect.

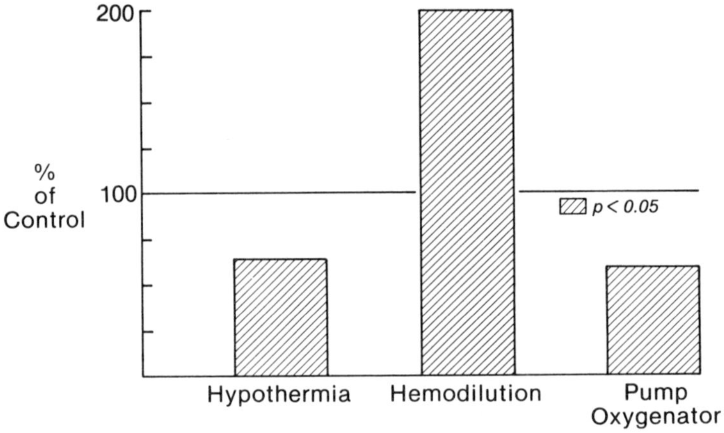

Figure 5.17. Both hypothermia and pump oxygenator cause significant decreases in free water clearance. Hemoglobin produced increases in free water clearances.

increased glomerular filtration, and increased urine flow by osmotic diuresis.[54] Our recent experimental studies show that, with hemodilution hypothermic cardiopulmonary bypass, mannitol decreased flow to the inner cortex of the kidney and diminished distribution of microspheres to the medulla suggests renal vasoconstriction (Fig. 5.18). Water content of outer cotex of kidney was diminished by mannitol. Our studies suggest that the effect of mannitol on glomerular and tubular function is not significant in the presence of hemodilution hypothermic cardiopulmonary bypass.[55]

Albumin has been used to diminish the interstitial edema that accompanies cardiopulmonary bypass. Early studies showed that albumin might augment urine output.[56] Studies of varying degree of perfusate oncotic pressure in rabbits have shown that lower levels of plasma oncotic pressure improve renal function during cardiopulmonary bypass. The investigators found a correlation between glomerular filtration and the differences between perfusion pressure and plasma colloidal oncotic pressure. The authors concluded that plasma oncotic pressure was a significant antagonist to renal ultrafiltration during hypotensive states.[57] Thus dilution of the plasma oncotic pressure may protect the kidney during hypotension. This is consistent with present concepts of glomerular function.[58] Our recent experimental studies show that albumin decreases urine output (Fig.

5.19). Albumin increases flow to the inner cortex of the kidney and increased the concentration of microspheres in the medulla, suggesting vasodilation rather than an effect on blood viscosity (Fig. 5.18). Albumin had no effect on water content of any region of the kidney. Albumin diminished urine sodium. Albumin also diminished sodium, osmolar, and free water clearance (Fig. 5.20).[55] Increased plasma oncotic pressure not only diminishes glomerular filtration but also increases reabsorption of fluid from the proximal renal tubule by an osmotic mechanism.[59,60] Thus, adding albumin to the priming solution reverses many of the desired effects of hemodilution (Fig. 5.21).

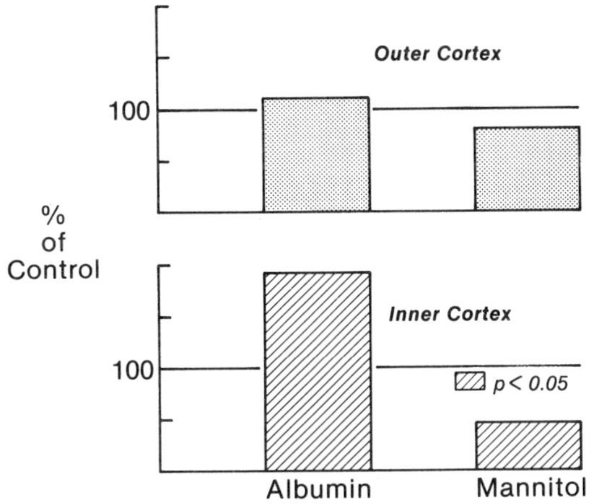

Figure 5.18. Renal blood flow to outer cortex was not affected by albumin or mannitol. Albumin increased flow to inner renal cortex. Mannitol decreased inner renal cortical flow.

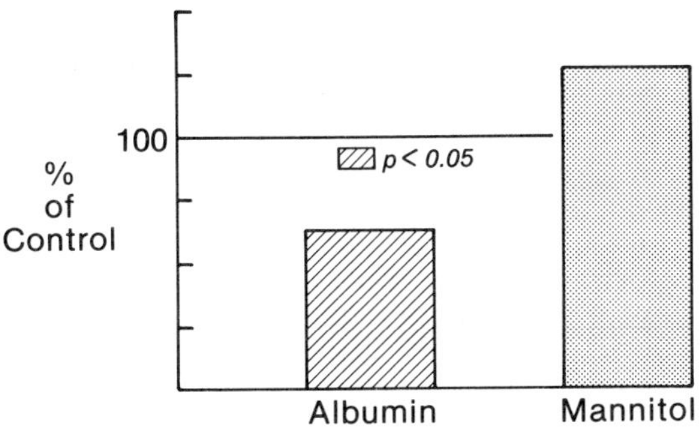

Figure 5.19. Albumin decreased urine output. Mannitol had no significant effect on urine output.

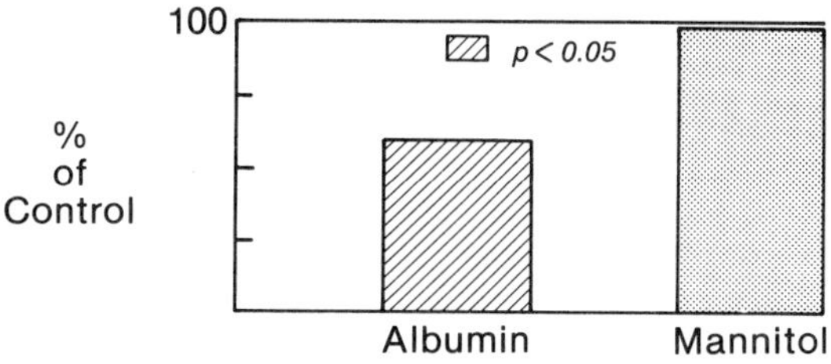

Figure 5.20. Free water clearance was diminished by albumin. Mannitol had no significant effect.

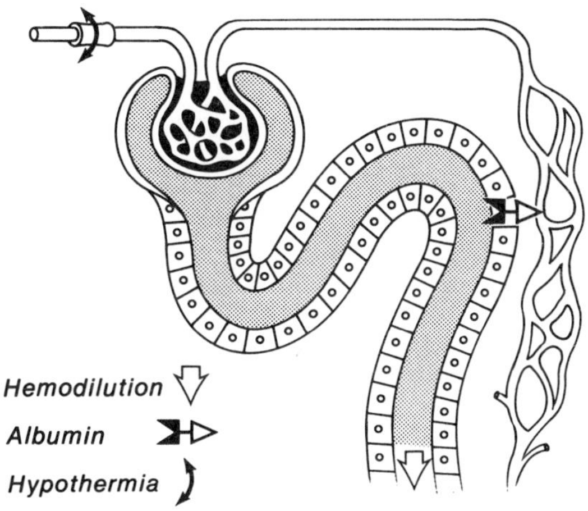

Figure 5.21. The general effects of hemodilution, hypothermia, and albumin are summarized. Hypothermia causes renal vasoconstriction. Hemodilution increased urine output and renal clearances because of increased renal plasma flow and lowered plasma colloidal oncotic pressure. Albumin diminishes urine output and clearances because of its oncotic effect in increasing tubular reabsorption.

Endocrine Effects

The effects of cardiopulmonary bypass involve most endocrine organs. The effect on renal function is most important in relationship to increased antidiuretic hormone (ADH) secretion. The rise in ADH secretion is greater during cardiopulmonary bypass than with operations not requiring cardiopulmonary bypass. The release of ADH is related to the low atrial pressures, hypotension, and nonpulsatile pressure that may accompany cardiopulmonary bypass.[63] The rise of ADH levels is greater in patients having coronary bypass graft than in those having valve operations. ADH is a potent renal vasoconstrictor, and the vasoconstriction is synergistic with the vasoconstriction of adrenergic drugs. ADH produces sodium diuresis at higher levels by a direct effect on tubular absorption. The stimulus for ADH during cardiopulmonary bypass is circulatory rather than osmotic.[61, 62] Some factors of nonpulsatile flow during cardiopulmonary bypass which cause ADH to rise also produce increases in epinephrine and renin-angiotensin release. Both angiotensin and epinephrine are important in the pathogenesis of hypertension, low cardiac output, and poor renal perfusion postoperatively.[64, 65]

The rise in plasma cortisol levels observed during or after cardiopulmonary bypass may contribute to the sodium retention and potassium diuresis occasionally observed after cardiopulmonary bypass.[66]

Prognosis of Renal Failure

Recently the prognosis of renal failure requiring hemodialysis which accompanies cardiac surgery appears to be improving. Early and frequent dialysis using peritoneal or hemodialysis techniques have lowered mortality to 27% in one series.[3] The factors which determine the outcome of renal failure may be different from those which produced renal dysfunction. Increasing age and the development of medical complications, particularly arrhythmias, cardiac failure, and bacteremia, are the most significant factors associated with mortality in these patients. If the renal failure is nonoliguric, the prognosis is improved. Factors which were not related to death included preoperative blood urea nitrogen, functional class, duration of cardiopulmonary bypass, blood pressure during bypass, blood used, and use of vasopressors.[67]

References

1. Abel RM, Buckley MJ, Austen WG, Barnett GO, Beck CH Jr, Fischer JE: Acute postoperative renal failure in cardiac surgical patients. J Surg Res 20:341, 1976.
2. Abel RM, Buckley MJ, Austen WG, Barnett GO, Beck CH Jr; Fischer JE: Etiology, incidence, and prognosis of renal failure following cardiac operations. Results of a prospective analysis of 500 consecutive patients. J Thorac Cardiovasc Surg 71:323, 1976.
3. Gailiunas P, Chawla R, Lazarus JM, Cohn L, Sanders J, Merrill JP: Acute renal failure following cardiac operations. J Thorac Cardiovasc Surg 79:241, 1980.
4. Krian A: Incidence, prevention, and treatment of acute renal failure following cardiopulmonary bypass. Int Anesth Clin 14:87, 1976.
5. Ogg CS, Cameron JS: Cardiovascular surgery and the kidney. Guy Hosp Rep 118:85, 1969.
6. Yeboah ED, Petrie A, Pead JL: Acute renal failure and open heart surgery. Br Med J 1:415, 1972.
7. Moghissi K, McMillan IKR: Acute renal failure and open heart surgery. Br Med J 32:228, 1972.
8. Aperia A, Bjarke B, Broberger O, Thorén C: Renal function in Fallot's tetralogy. Acta Paediatr Scand 63:398, 1974.
9. Bourgeois BFD, Donath A, Paunier L, Rouge J-C: Effects of cardiac surgery on renal function in children. J Thorac Cardiovasc Surg 77(2):283, 1979.
10. Gruskin AB: The kidney in congenital heart disease—an overview. Adv Pediatr 24:133, 1977.
11. Passwell J, Orda S, Modan M, Shem-Tov A, Aladjem M, Boichis H: Abnormal renal functions in cyanotic congenital heart disease. Arch Dis Child 51: 803, 1976.
12. Chesney RW, Kaplan BS, Freedom RM, Haller JA, Drummond KN: Acute renal failure: An important complication of cardiac surgery in infants. J Pediatr 87:381, 1975.
13. Utley JR, Noonan J, Kirkpatrick S: Cardiopulmonary bypass in the presence of uncorrected coarctation. J Thorac Cardiovasc Surg, in press, 1981.
14. Fillastre JP, Kleinknecht D: Acut renal failure associated with cephalosporin therapy. Am Heart J 89: 809, 1975.
15. Kiss J, Farago E, Gomory A, Homolay P, Kiss IS: Gentamycin in cardiac surgery. Acta Chir Acad Sci Hung 18:133, 1977.
16. Olsen S, Asklund M: Interstitial nephritis with acute renal failure following cardiac surgery and treatment with methicillin. Acta Med Scand 199:305, 1976.
17. Moghissi K, Machell ES, Munday KA: Changes in renal blood flow and PAH extraction during extracorporeal circulation of short and long duration. Experimental study in dogs. Cardiovasc Res 3:37, 1969.
18. Nuutinen L, Hollmén A: Cardiopulmonary bypass time and renal function. Ann Chir Gynaecologiae 65:191, 1976.
19. Senning Å, Andres J, Bornstein P, Norberg B, Andersen MN: Renal function during extracorporeal circulation at high and low flow rates: Experimental studies in dogs. Ann Surg 151:63, 1960.
20. Selmonosky CA: Studies on urinary urea concentration after cardiopulmonary bypass: A sensitive index of altered renal hemodynamics. Ann Surg 172(2): 226, 1970.
21. Selmonosky CA: Early detection of renal failure after cardiopulmonary bypass. Arch Surg 99:64, 1969.
22. Landes RG, Lillehei RC, Lindsay WG, Nicoloff DM: Free-water clearance and the early recognition of

acute renal insufficiency after cardiopulmonary bypass. Ann Thorac Surg 22(1):41, 1976.
23. Heimann T, Brau S, Sakurai H, Peirce EC, II: Urinary osmolal changes in renal dysfunction following open-heart operations. Ann Thorac Surg 22(1):44, 1976.
24. Holper K, Struck E, Sebening F: The diagnosis of acute renal failure (ARF) following cardiac surgery with cardio-pulmonary bypass. Thorac Cardiovasc Surg 27(1):231, 1979.
25. Tan C-K, Glisson SN, El-Etr AA, Ramakrishnaiah KB: Levels of circulating norepinephrine and epinephrine before, during, and after cardiopulmonary bypass in man. J Thorac Cardiovasc Surg 71:928, 1976.
26. Balasaraswathi K, Glisson SN, El-Etr AA, Azad C: Effect of priming volume on serum catecholamines during cardiopulmonary bypass. Can Anaesth Soc J 27:135, 1980.
27. Taylor KM, Jones JV, Walker MS, Rao S, Bain WH: The cortisol response during heart-lung bypass. Circulation 54:20, 1976.
28. Nonoyama A, Katsuda H, Nakahashi M, Uchiyama S, Kubo S, Kagawa T: Studies on the massive administration of corticosteroid during open heart surgery. Its effect to renal function. Jpn Circ J 34:711, 1970.
29. Engelman RM, Gouge TH, Smith SJ, Stahl WM, Gombos EA, Boyd AD: The effect of diuretics on renal hemodynamics during cardiopulmonary bypass. J Surg Res 16:268, 1974.
30. Nuutinen L, Hollmén A: The effect of prophylactic use of furosemide on renal function during open heart surgery. Ann Chir Gynaecol 65:258, 1976.
31. Nuutinen LS: The effect of nitrous oxide on renal function in open heart surgery. Ann Chir Gynaecol 65:200, 1976.
32. Reed CC, Romagnoli A, Taylor DE, Clark DK: Particulate matter in bubble oxygenators. J Thorac Cardiovasc Surg 68(6):971, 1974.
33. Clark RE, Dietz DR, Miller JG: Continuous detection of microemboli during cardiopulmonary bypass in animals and man. Circulation 54(III):74, 1976.
34. Kessler J, Patterson RH Jr: The production of microemboli by various blood oxygenators. Ann Thorac Surg 9:221, 1970.
35. Dutton RC, Edmunds LH, Jr.: Measurement of emboli in extracorporeal perfusion systems. J Thorac Cardiovasc Surg 65(4):523, 1973.
36. Utley JR, Wachtel C, Cain RB, Spaw EA, Collins JC, Stephens DB: Effects of hypothermia, hemodilution, and pump oxygenation on organ water content, blood flow and oxygen delivery, and renal function. Ann Thorac Surg 31:121, 1981.
37. Utley JR, Marshall WG, Boatman GB, Dickerson G, Ernst CB, Daugherty ME: Trapping, nontrapping, and release of nine and fifteen micron spheres in dog kidneys. Surgery 87:222, 1980.
38. Thompson RB: The haemolytic anaemias. In *Disorders of the Blood,* edited by RB Thompson. New York, Churchill Livingstone, 1977, p. 305.
39. Clyne DH, Kant KS, Pesce AJ, Pollak VE: Nephrotoxicity of low molecular weight serum proteins: Physicochemical interactions between myoglobin, hemoglobin, Bence Jones proteins and Tamm-Horsfall mucoprotein. Curr Prob Clin Biochem 9:299, 1979.
40. Andersen MN, Mouritzen CV, Gabrieli E: Mechanisms of plasma hemoglobin clearance after acute hemolysis: Studies in open-heart surgical patients. A comparative study of five different units. Ann Surg 163(4), 529, 1966.
41. Andersen MN, Kuchiba K: Blood trauma produced by pump oxygenators. J Thorac Cardiovasc Surg 57: 238, 1969.
42. Osborn JJ, Cohn K, Hait M, Russi M, Salel A, Harkins G, Gerbode F: Hemolysis during perfusion: Sources and means of reduction. J Thorac Cardiovasc Surg 43:459, 1962.
43. Lindberg EF, Berghuis J, Theye RA, Kirklin JW: Plasma hemoglobin levels associated with use of a vertical-sheet pump-oxygenator (Mayo-Gibbon type). Surgery 55:665, 1964.
44. McCaughan JS Jr, McMichael H, Schuder JC, Kirby CK: The use of a totally occlusive pump as a flowmeter with observations on hemolysis caused by occlusive and nonocclusive pumps and other pump-oxygenator components. Surgery 44(1):210, 1958.
45. Yarborough KA, Mockros LF, Lewis FJ: Hydrodynamic hemolysis in extracorporeal machines. J Thorac Cardiovasc Surg 52(4):550, 1966.
46. Roe BB, Swenson EE, Hepps SA, Bruns DL: Total body perfusion in cardiac operations. Use of perfusate of balanced electrolytes and low molecular weight dextran. Archa Surg 88:128, 1964.
47. Mielke JE, Hunt JC, Maher FT, Kirklin JW: Renal performance during clinical cardiopulmonary bypass with and without hemodilution. J Thorac Cardiovasc Surg 51:229, 1966.
48. Lilleaasen P, Stokke O: Moderate and extreme hemodilution in open-heart surgery: Fluid balance and acid-base studies. Ann Thorac Surg 25(2):127, 1978.
49. Verska JJ, Ludington LG, Brewer LA III: A comparative study of cardiopulmonary bypass with nonblood and blood prime. Ann Thorac Surg 18:72, 1974.
50. Kanter GS: Renal clearance of sodium and potassium in hypothermia. Can J Biochem Physiol 40:113, 1962.
51. Terblanche J, Isaacson LC, Eales L, Barnard CN: Renal function during and immediately after profound hypothermia. Surgery 50:869, 1961.
52. Karim F, Reza H: Effect of induced hypothermia and rewarming on renal hemodynamics in anesthetized dogs. Life Sci 9(1):1153, 1970.
53. Paton BC, Rosenkrantz J: Non-hemic priming fluids for extracorporeal circulation. Dis Chest 48:311, 1965.
54. Etheredge EE, Levitin H, Nakamura K, Glenn WWL: Effect of mannitol on renal function during open-heart surgery. Ann Surg 161(1):53, 1965.
55. Utley JR, Stephens DB, Wachtel C, Cain RB, Collins JC, Spaw EA, Moores WY: Effect of albumin and mannitol on organ blood flow, oxygen delivery water content, and renal function during hypothermic, hemodilution cardiopulmonary bypass, Ann Thorac Surg, 1981.
56. Long DM Jr, Sanchez L, Varco RL, Lillehei CW: The use of low molecular weight dextran and serum

albumin as plasma expanders in extracorporeal circulation. Surgery 50:12, 1961.
57. Schüpbach P, Pappova E, Schilt W, Kollar J, Kollar M, Sipos P, Vucic D: Perfusate oncotic pressure during cardiopulmonary bypass. Optimum levels as determined by metabolic acidosis, tissue edema, and renal function. Vox Sang 35:332, 1978.
58. Tucker BJ, Blantz RC: An analysis of the determinants of nephron filtration rate. Am J Physiol 232: F477, 1977.
59. Brenner BM, Falchuk KH, Keimowitz RI, Berliner RW, Troy JL, Green N: The relationship between peritubular capillary protein concentration and fluid reabsorption by the renal proximal tubule. J Clin Invest 48:1519, 1969.
60. Falchuk KH, Brenner BM, Tadokoro M, Berliner RW: Oncotic and hydrostatic pressures in peritubular capillaries and fluid reabsorption by proximal tubule. Am J Physiol 220(5):1427, 1971.
61. Philbin DM, Levine FH, Emerson CW, Coggins CH, Buckley MJ, Austen WG: Plasma vasopressin levels and urinary flow during cardiopulmonary bypass in patients with valvular heart disease. Effects of pulsatile flow. J Thorac Cardiovasc Surg 78:779, 1979.
62. Philbin DM, Coggins CH, Wilson N, Sokoloski J: Antidiuretic hormone levels during cardiopulmonary bypass. J Thorac Cardiovasc Surg 73(1):145, 1977.
63. Many M, Giron F, Birtwell WC, Deterling RA, Jr, Soroff HS: Effects of depulsation of renal blood flow upon renal function and renin secretion. Surgery 66: 242, 1969.
64. Goodman TA, Gerard DF, Bernstein EF, Dilley RB: The effects of pulseless perfusion on the distribution of renal cortical blood flow and renin release. Surgery 80:31, 1976.
65. Taylor KM, Morton IJ, Brown JJ, Bain WH, Caves PK: Hypertension and the renin-angiotensin system following open-heart surgery. J Thorac Cardiovasc Surg 74(6):840, 1977.
66. Bondoli A, Sabato A, Petrozzi U, Schiavello R, Oddi N, Villani A: Plasma cortisol in open-heart surgery. Resuscitation 5:183, 1976.
67. McLeish KR, Luft FC, Kleit SA: Factors affecting prognosis in acute renal failure following cardiac operations. Surg Gynecol Obstet 145:28, 1977.

CHAPTER 6

CARDIOPULMONARY BYPASS IN CHRONIC RENAL DISEASE

JOHN P. CONNORS, M.D.

A small but steadily growing experience with cardiac surgical procedures requiring cardiopulmonary bypass in patients with chronic renal disease has developed during the past 10 years. Factors responsible for this include the increasing number of individuals enrolled in chronic dialysis programs, the obvious prolongation of life provided by dialysis, the propensity for individuals with chronic renal failure to develop life-threatening complications involving the central circulation, and the evidence that these patients, when managed properly, tolerate major surgical procedures with an acceptable risk.

At present, over 50,000 uremic patients are enrolled in dialysis programs, with this number expected to double over the next two decades.[1] More importantly, prolongation of life in this group has been impressively achieved, with yearly mortality reduced to approximately 10%.[2]

During the early history of chronic renal dialysis, it became apparent that successfully managed patients tolerated elective and emergent major surgical procedures.[3, 4] The hallmark of this success consisted of close cooperation between surgeons and nephrologists in the management of problems unique to this group. The latter include fluid, electrolyte, and acid-base imbalance, anemia, coagulopathy, hypertension, myocardiopathy, lowered immunity to infection, and delayed wound healing.

Major cardiovascular complications have been recognized as responsible for death in 50% or more of patients on long-term hemodialysis.[5, 6] Central circulatory problems resulting from accelerated atherosclerotic vascular changes, hypertrophic cardiomyopathy, and subacute bacterial endocarditis (SBE) represent common and life-threatening complications in this disease.[7–12] Initially, the role of the cardiothoracic surgeon in the care of such patients was prompted by their tendency to develop a distinct form of pericardial inflammation. Relatively large series of patients with uremic pericarditis have been reported to date, and although the majority can be managed conservatively, incipient or obvious cardiac tamponade requires surgical intervention.[13, 14] Again, with proper and coordinated care, the experience with varied pericardial drainage procedures has proved most gratifying.

Most of the cardiac surgical procedures in patients on chronic dialysis involve coronary revascularization or valvular replacement following the ravages of endocarditis (Fig. 6.1). Rapidly progressive coronary artery disease in the group has been recognized and poorly understood. Their tendency toward hypertension, hypertriglyceridemia, early vascular calcification and glucose intolerance play a significant role in the early development of coronary artery obstructive disease.[5] As a result, myocardial infarction represents the cause of death in approximately one-third of patients on hemodialysis.[7] In addition, the symptoms of ischemic myocardial disease are often exacerbated by the anemia of chronic

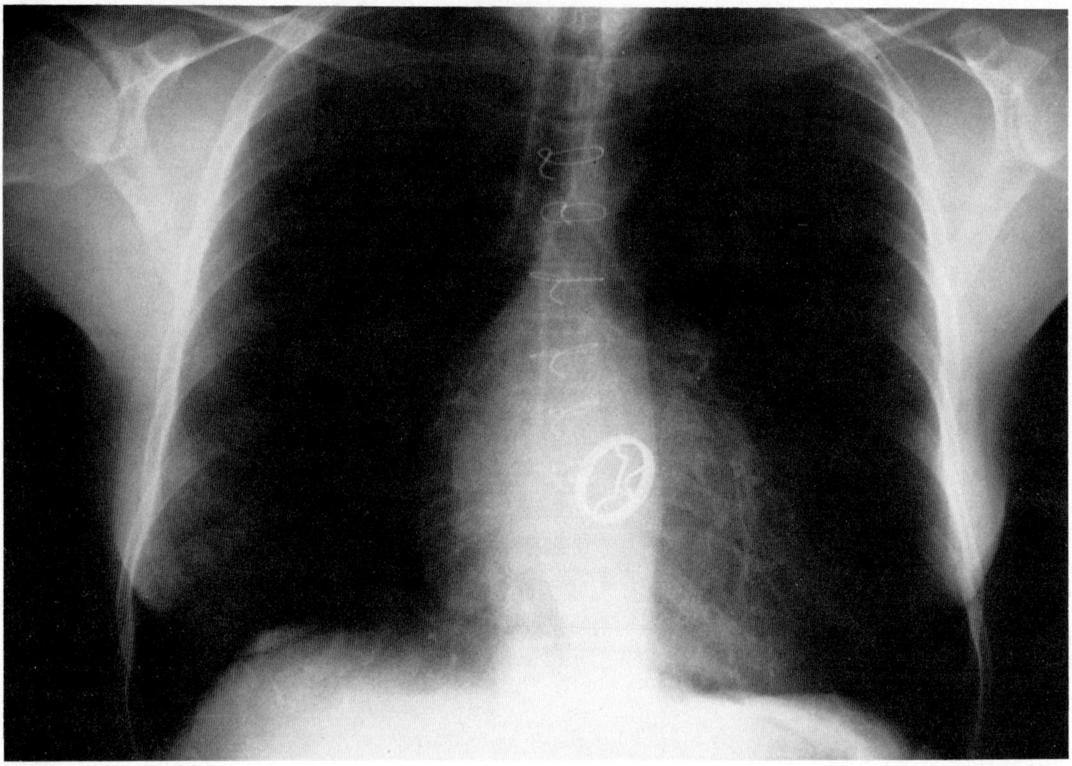

Figure 6.1. The chest x-ray of a 51-year-old female 7 years after mitral valve replacement and tricuspid annuloplasty. She remains on thrice weekly dialysis and sodium warfarin anticoagulation.

renal failure, the presence of an arteriovenous fistula, and the hemodynamic stress of repeated dialysis. Severe and disabling angina pectoris may necessitate changes from home to in hospital dialysis and even chronic peritoneal dialysis. Minimizing the stress for renal transplantation has also been utilized as an indication for bypass surgery in some of these patients.[15] By and large, the limited results with coronary revascularization in this group indicate that the procedures are well tolerated and that the risks approach those with normal renal function. Consequently, medical management associated with intractable symptomatology or the presence of life-threatening left main coronary artery obstructive disease represent appropriate indications for bypass surgery in the patients with chronic renal failure.

Advanced cardiac valvular lesions requiring surgical replacement or reconstruction are largely related to ongoing or healed endocarditis. Bacterial endocarditis occurs with increased frequency in patients with chronic renal disease, the reported incidence varying from 2.7 to 6.6%.[12, 16, 17] Factors contributing to the development of valvular infections include depressed immunity, the presence of an arteriovenous fistula (whether infected or sterile), cardiomegaly resulting in valvular deformity, and transient episodes of bacteremia during dialysis. Furthermore, various reviews have emphasized the particularly disappointing results with antibiotic therapy in individuals with endocarditis and chronic renal disease. Leonard et al.[12] described the development of SBE in 9 patients, seven of whom died following antibiotic specific therapy. Among the two survivors, one had an aortic valve replacement. A review by Cross et al.[18] including all reported cases of SBE in patients requiring long-term dialysis noted that 14 of 19 individuals treated with organism specific antibiotics died. The ten patients in this report who underwent valve replacement survived. It therefore seems appropriate to recommend cardiac valvular surgery in the setting of SBE and dialysis dependence when the valvular incompetence is associated with progressive cardiac decompensation. Additionally, the virtual uncontrollability of endocarditis in these patients, coexistent with myocardiopathy, has prompted some to recommend early valve replacement.[19]

Less commonly, other forms of cardiac valvular disease, including rheumatic valvulitis, have represented indications for replacement.[1] The potential for prosthetic valvular infection resulting from bacteremias during ensuing dialysis must influence such considerations. However, instability during dialysis and advanced cardiac decompensation seem appropriate reasons for valvular surgery.

PREOPERATIVE EVALUATION AND MANAGEMENT

Peculiarities involving the management of chronically dialysed patients faced with a potential cardiac surgical procedure and cardiopulmonary bypass must be addressed in the preoperative period. For example, cardiac catheterization, unless properly approached, could represent a life-threatening experience for these patients. Sudden shifts in intravascular volume during and immediately following catheterization can result in severe hypertensive and hypotensive crises. Additionally, optimum cardiac function and the avoidance of severe arrhythmias during catheterization require that acid-base balance and normal potassium levels be achieved by precatheterization dialysis. (Accordingly, we have recommended dialysis the morning prior to surgery cardiac catheterization thereafter, and dialysis again the evening before the procedure.[19]) The length of dialysis can be variable, with the runs made against low potassium baths to ensure control of total body potassium levels. In anticipation of volume overload at surgery, the preoperative dialysis regime should include an attempt to remove as much excess fluid as possible, the goal being to send these individuals to operation close to dry weight.

Patients with chronic renal failure invariably exhibit significant anemias for a variety of reasons, including depressed erythropoietin production, decreased red blood cell survival, nutritional factors, and a uremic toxic depression of the bone marrow.[20–23] Their hematocrits often range between 25 and 30% raising a question regarding the necessity for preoperative transfusion in order to maximize oxygen-carrying capacity during the procedure and wound healing thereafter. There is no evidence that transfusions presensitize these patients prior to renal transplantation.[24] Our experience and that of others suggests that patients with hematocrits over 25% tolerate major operations without the necessity of being exposed to the risks of preoperative transfusion. Similarly, a host of factors, including thrombocytopenia, prolongation of the prothrombin time, and hypofibrinogenemia, contribute to the well-recognized coagulopathy of uremia.[25, 26] Again, the preoperative administration of blood coagulating elements appears unwarranted since the coagulopathy is usually mild. Bleeding problems rarely develop in well dialysed patients, particularly when the surgeon maintains meticulous attention to hemostasis.

The risk of infection represents a major concern in any patient undergoing cardiac surgery. Depressed immunity to infection and transient episodes of bacteremia during dialysis enhance the hazard in patients with chronic renal failure.[27–29] The administration of broad spectrum antibiotics, therefore, seems justified, particularly when the operation involves valve replacement.

Uremic patients tolerate anesthetic premedications well, since the majority of these agents are metabolized by the liver. The regime recommended by Posner et al.[30] seems appropriate and includes 0.6 mg of atropine, 15 mg of diazepam, and 15 mg of morphine intramuscularly 90 minutes prior to the anesthetic. A variety of general anesthetics, including ketamine with nitrous oxide supplementation, halothane, and morphine, have been utilized safely in these patients. Muscle relaxation can be achieved with standard doses of pancuronium bromide.

CARDIOPULMONARY BYPASS AND OPERATIVE MANAGEMENT

Although there are several theoretical considerations regarding the techniques of extracorporeal circulation employed in patients with chronic renal failure, a review of the reported experience with cardiac surgery in these patients confirms that a variety of oxygenators, pump primes, and medication protocols can be used successfully. Nevertheless, the unique problems posed by cardiopulmonary bypass in the uremic patient prompt the establishment of certain guidelines. The choice of an oxygenator (that is, a bubble *vs.* membrane device) would seem to be largely academic. We and most other teams experienced in this area have used bubble oxygenators, due to a preference for standard equipment and the anticipation of a relatively brief run on cardiopulmonary bypass. Membrane oxygenators may be preferable if the complexity of the procedure demands a longer perfusion time, although conflicting data exist regarding their preservation of coagulation elements.

The composition of the pump prime merits more specific consideration. Components of the prime should be determined by the nature of the coronary obstructive disease, the severity of the anemia, the anticipated length of the procedure, and the availability of dialysis immediately postoperatively. Fresh whole blood (to minimize potassium concentration) has been used in amounts varying between 500 and 1500 ml, the latter dependent upon the levels of the preoperative hematocrit. The balance of the prime solution can include most standard electrolyte solutions, provided they contain less than 5 mEq per liter of potassium. Additives such as heparin, Tham (Abbot Laboratories, North Chicago, Ill.), glucose, and colloidal solutions have had no adverse effects. With the extraction of substantial fluid via dialysis preoperatively and a protocol that provides for immediate postoperative dialysis, we chose to use standard hemodilution with a 2000-ml dextrose and 0.9% saline prime.

Parameters monitored during the operation should include central venous, pulmonary, and systemic arterial pressures. Some have cautioned against the use of the upper extremity arteries and veins since new dialysis access sites might be required postoperatively.[30] Accordingly, they suggest that femoral rather than radial artery pressures be monitored and that the arteriovenous fistula site be particularly protected during the course of the operative procedure. Systemic heparinization with 3 mg per kilogram precedes cardiopulmonary bypass; appropriate additions of anticoagulant are made according to the accelerated clotting time or measured heparin levels. Flows during perfusion should be standard at 2.4 liters per minute per meter squared. The perfusion pressure may have to be adjusted according to the severity of coronary or extracardiac atherosclerotic disease. Potassium levels must be monitored at least hourly on bypass with levels above 6.0 mEq per liter treated with the administration of sodium bicarbonate, insulin, and glucose, or the instillation of Kayexalate (Winthrop Laboratories, New York, New York) through a nasogastric tube. Interestingly, hemodialysis during cardiopulmonary bypass has been reported recently as an alternative method to control potassium levels and fluid volume.[31]

Cardiac arrest, cardioplegia, and myocardial hypothermic protection can be achieved without the need for intracoronary potassium containing solutions. Myocardial hypothermia may be enhanced by surface cooling, particularly during valvular procedures. Obviously, the parenteral administration of intravenous fluids must be minimized. The return of the residual pump fluid to the patient after the completion of bypass should be guided by the hemodynamic status. Centrifugation of the remaining pump contents and the administration of packed red blood cells limits the volume load in these patients. Autologous blood extracted preoperatively or fresh whole blood may be used to optimize the cardiac filling pressures. Most vasopressors and antiarrhythmic agents are metabolized by the liver. The doses of these agents should be concentrated in the intravenous solutions.

POSTOPERATIVE MANAGEMENT

The successful management of these patients following cardiac surgery requires attention to predictable and often very early abnormalities involving fluid and electrolyte balance. The maintenance of acceptable hemodynamics and serum potassium levels may require bedside dialysis support within the first few hours after the procedure. In order to minimize the amount of parenteral fluid administered, all but the necessary pressure monitoring lines should be withdrawn after the patient returns to the intensive care unit.[32] Serum potassium levels must be followed at least every 4 hours during the first postoperative day.

Our suggestions regarding dialysis originally included daily runs for 3 to 4 days following operation; however, recent experience demonstrates that a rigid dialysis schedule is probably unnecessary and that the judicious use of intermittent dialysis constitutes safe and acceptable management.[1, 19, 32] The mobilization of fluid with gradual improvement in cardiac function and the catabolic effects of surgery resulting in the extracellular flux of potassium ion often demand at least short runs of dialysis during the first few days of recovery. Again, fluid and electrolyte restriction combined with prophylactic Kayexalate may obviate the need for frequent dialysis. Both peritoneal and hemodialysis techniques have been proposed and used without difficulty.[1, 19, 32] Those supporting the peritoneal approach cite the potential for arrhythmias, the need for local heparinization, and the possibility of hemodynamic instability as contraindications to hemodialysis. On the other hand, the disadvantages of peritoneal dialysis in this setting include rapid shifts in vascular volume and electrolytes, lower potassium clearance, and compromise of ventilation. We have experienced no major problems with regional heparinization and hemodialysis during the early postoperative period.

Daily fluid administration should match insensible volume losses with the total infusion consisting of no more than 750 ml of a dextrose-containing solution every 24 hours. We have replaced mediastinal drainage on a ml per ml basis with fresh whole blood. Hematocrits should be maintained over 25% with transfusions of packed fresh red blood cells. The routine administration of platelet concentrates and fresh frozen plasma have been recommended by some, but unless it is indicated by the amount of traumatic suctioning during the procedure with an appropriate level of thrombocytopenia (platelet count less than 75,000) and continued bleeding, we consider it an unnecessary risk.[33]

Broad spectrum antibiotics should be continued in appropriate doses for 7 days postoperatively with digitalis preparations re-

Table 6.1
Reported Cardiac Surgical Procedures in Patients with Chronic Renal Failure

Procedure	Patients
Coronary artery bypass	33
Cardiac valve replacement	33
Ascending aortic grafts for dissection	2
Pericardiectomy with cardiopulmonary bypass	1
Repair false aneurysm left ventricle	1

Table 6.2
Results of Coronary Bypass in Patients with Chronic Renal Failure

Date of Report	Author	Patients	Outcome
1974	Menzoian[35]	1	Transplanted 15 months later, well 5 months post transplant
1974	Sakurai[36]	1	Well 6 months postop
1975	Lansing[37]	1	Well 1 year postop
1976	Kuehnel[38]	6	All well 5–31 months postop
1977	Crawford[39]	2	Survived, no follow-up
1977	Chawla[40]	2	1 patient died 50 months postop (noncardiac), 1 patient well 4 months postop
1977	Siegel[41]	1	Survived, no follow-up
1978	Cheng[42]	1	Survived, no follow-up
1980	Monson[1]	14	2 early deaths (arrhythmia, sepsis), 12 well 4–55 months postop
1981	Garcia-Rinaldi[32]	4	1 death 35 days postop (pulmonary embolus), 3 well 15–28 months postop

duced to half the maintenance dose.[1] Slowed wound healing requires that the skin sutures remain intact for 2 to 3 weeks after the procedure.[34]

THE RESULTS OF SURGERY

A review of the English literature reveals that 70 dialysis-dependent patients have undergone a variety of cardiac surgical procedures [1, 12, 19, 29–32, 35–48] (Table 6.1). The majority of these cases have been reported during the past 5 years, with the latter probably related to improvements in dialysis, extracorporeal equipment, and operative techniques. The efficacy and safety of coronary artery bypass surgery has likewise contributed to the recently expanded experience. An assessment of early mortality from the literature seems meaningless since the number of cases to date has been so small and the tendency

Table 6.3
Results of Cardiac Valve Replacements in Patients with Chronic Renal Failure

Date of Report	Author	Procedure (Disease)	Outcome
1968	Lansing[43]	AVR* (SBE) MVR (Rheumatic)	Survived 4 yrs death unrelated to AVR Survived 7 mos death unrelated to MVR
1972	Ribot[44]	2 MVRs (SBE)	1 pt survived 3 yrs + well, other no follow-up
1972	Manhas[45]	2 AVRs (1 SBE)	1 pt survived 2 yrs + well, other no follow-up
1972	Saldanha[29]	AVR (SBE)	Survived 1 yr, death unrelated to AVR
1972	Glabman[46]	4 AVRs (SBE)	All survived with no follow-up
1973	Leonard[12]	AVR (SBE)	Kidney transplant 6 mos postop; well 1 yr after transplant
1975	Neptune[48]	AVR (SBE)	Kidney transplant 3 mos later, died 2½ yrs post transplant with cryptococcal septicemia
1975	Posner[30]	AVR	Survived, no follow-up
1975	Wilcox[47]	AVR	Well 1 yr postop
1977	Chawla[40]	6 AVRs AVR, MVR	1 AVR died 1 day postop with bleeding AVR, MVR died 7 mos postop, death unrelated to AVR, MVR 5 AVRs well 3–69 mos postop
1978	Connors[19]	AVR (SBE)	Died 3 yrs postop with prosthetic SBE
		MVR, tricuspid annuloplasty	Well 7 yrs postop
1978	Lansing (personal communication)	2 valve replacements	Both well 3 yrs postop
1979	Soffer[31]	AVR	Well 6 wks postop
1980	Monson[1]	2 MVRs, CAB 1 MVR (SBE) 1 MVR (rheumatic) 2 AVRs (SBE)	Both survived, no follow-up Well 3 mos postop Died 39 mos postop with CVA 1 AVR died 2 mos post transplantation 14 mos post AVR; other AVR well 49 mos postop

* AVR, aortic valve replacement; MVR, mitral valve replacement; CAB, coronary artery bypass; CVA, cerebral vascular accident; pt, patient.

toward reporting successful results has been so obvious. However, one gains the general impression that uremic patients tolerate cardiac surgery with a higher, but acceptable, risk level than the population with unimpaired renal function. There were two early deaths among the 33 patients undergoing coronary artery bypass (Table 6.2) and one operative death in 33 patients submitted to cardiac valve replacements (Table 6.3).

A significant number of complications occur postoperatively despite optimal management. An impressive list of these was outlined by Monson,[1] whose group recently reviewed an experience involving 22 patients (Table 6.4). Uncertainty regarding the long-term benefits of cardiac surgery in this group should further temper the recommendations for procedures of this magnitude. Follow-up remains limited for patients who underwent coronary artery bypass and valve replacements, with isolated reports substantiating survival beyond 4 years in both groups.[1, 19, 40] Unfortunately, there is little reason to believe that coronary revascularization will significantly affect those factors accelerating the atherosclerotic process in individuals on chronic dialysis. Indeed, long-term follow-up may well demonstrate decreased graft patency when compared to other groups with normal renal function. As a consequence, the indications for revascularization should remain strict and include symptoms truly refractory to medical management or the presence of advanced and life-threatening obstructions in the left main coronary circulation. Successful renal transplantation following coronary artery bypass has been reported.[35, 40, 49, 50] The implications regarding an arrest in vascular atherogenesis following transplantation make the recommendation for prior revascularization more appealing.

Similar caution must be employed in dialysis-dependent patients with advanced valve disease. Their follow-up has been likewise brief but generally encouraging despite a requirement for anticoagulation in many and the risk of prosthetic infection in those continuing on dialysis. The presence of an arteriovenous fistula, possible bacteremic episodes related to dialysis, and decreased immunity to infection resulted in the death of one of our patients with prosthetic endocarditis 3 years after aortic valve replacement. We had elected not to treat our patients with continuous antibiotics following discharge in order to minimize infections with opportunistic and antibiotic-resistant organisms. These patients should be covered with prophylactic antibiotics at the time of dental or other surgical procedures, as well as during respiratory tract or other infections. Lengthy antiseptic preparation of the fistula site should be performed before each dialysis. Despite continued anticoagulation with sodium warfarin (Coumadin) and maintenance on dialysis, one of our patients remains well 7 years after mitral valve replacement and tricuspid annuloplasty (Fig. 6.1). Two patients have been transplanted after aortic valve replacement.[12, 48] One remained well 1 year thereafter, while the other died with cryptococcal septicemia 2½ years following transplantation.

Table 6.4
Intraoperative and Postoperative Complications in 17 of 22 Patients with End-Stage Renal Disease[1]

Complication	No. of Patients
Pericarditis	4
Atrial arrhythmia	3
Dialysis-related mental changes	3
Postoperative bleeding	2
Perioperative myocardial infarction	2
Prolonged respiratory support	2
Pneumonia	2
Cytomegalovirus pneumonitis	1
Sternal wound infection	1
Leg wound infection	1
Pulmonary edema	1
Ketoacidosis	1
Left ventricular false aneurysm	1
Digitalis toxicity	1
Pleural effusion requiring drainage	1
Pneumothorax	1
Gastrointestinal bleeding	1
Splenic abscess	1
Spontaneous splenic rupture	1
Acute brain syndrome	1
Total	31

(Reproduced with permission from B. K. Monson et al.[1])

SUMMARY

A limited experience with cardiopulmonary bypass in dialysis-dependent patients suggests that with proper selection and management, associated risks can be reduced to acceptable levels. A recommendation for open heart surgery in this group should be influenced by the realization that a continued requirement for postoperative dialysis jeopardizes long-term benefits of the procedure. As a consequence, only those individuals in this group with truly advanced and life-threatening cardiovascular disease should be considered candidates for cardiac surgery.

References

1. Monson BK, Wickstrom PH, Haglin JJ, Francis G, Comty CM, Helseth HK: Cardiac operation and end-stage renal disease. Ann Thor Surg 30:267, 1980.
2. de Wardener HE: The natriuretic hormone. In: *European Dialysis and Transplant Association—Proceedings of the Conference*, edited by JF Morehead, C Mion, and RA Baillod. London, Pitman Medical, 1973, p. 11.
3. Hampers CL, Bailey GL, Hager EB, Vandam LD, Merrill JP: Major surgery in patients on maintainance hemodialysis. Am J Surg 115:747, 1968.
4. Haimov M, Glabman S, Schupak E, Neff M, Burrows L: General surgery in patients on maintainance hemodialysis. Ann Surg 179:863, 1974.
5. Merrill JP: Cardiovascular problems in patients on long-term hemodialysis. JAMA 228:1149, 1974.
6. Gurland HJ, Brunner FP, Dehn HV, Härlen H, Parsons FM, Schörer K: Combined report on regular dialysis and transplantation in Europe, III, 1972. In: European Dialysis and Transplant Association—Proceedings of the Conference, edited by JF Morehead, C Mion, and RA Baillod. London, Pitman Medical, 1973, p. xvii.
7. Lindner A, Charra B, Sherrard DJ, Scribner BH: Accelerated atherosclerosis in prolonged maintenance hemodialysis. N Engl J Med 290:697, 1974.
8. Hook EW Jr, Wainer HS, McGee TJ, Sellers TF Jr: Acquired arteriovenous fistula with bacterial endarteritis and endocarditis. JAMA 164:1450, 1957.
9. Kurtz DM: Endocarditis after chronic hemodialysis. N Engl J Med 280:1302, 1969.
10. Smith CM, Morton JD, Thompson RD: Bacterial endarteritis. A probable case in an arteriovenous fistula used for long-term hemodialysis. JAMA 210: 131, 1969.
11. Goodman JS, Crews HD, Ginn HE, Koenig MG: Bacterial endocarditis as a possible complication of chronic dialysis. NEJM 280:876, 1969.
12. Leonard A, Raij L, Shapiro FL: Bacterial endocarditis in regularly dialyzed patients. Kidney Int 4:407, 1973.
13. Collins HA, Killen DA, Gobbel WG Jr, Ginn HE: Pericardiectomy for uremic pericardial tamponade. Ann Thorac Surg 9:327, 1970.
14. Connors JP, Kleiger RE, Shaw RC, Voiles JD, Clard RE, Harter H, Roper CL: The indications for pericardiectomy in the uremic pericardial effusion. Surgery 80:689, 1976.
15. Kuehnel E, Lundh H, Bennett W, Porter G: Aortocoronary bypass surgery in patients with end-stage renal disease. Trans Am Soc Artif Int Organs 22:14, 1976.
16. King LH Jr, Bradly KP, Shires DL Jr, Donohue JP, Glover JL: Bacterial endocarditis in chronic hemodialysis patients. A complication more common than previously suspected. Surgery 69:554, 1971.
17. Verierstraeten P: La survie du Brightique traite par l'hemodialyse. J Sci Med (Lille) 88:491, 1970.
18. Cross AS, Steigbigel RT: Infective endocarditis and access site infections in patients on hemodialysis. Medicine 55:453, 1976.
19. Connors JP, Shaw RC: Considerations in the management of open-heart surgery in uremic patients. J Thorac and Cardiovascular Surg 75:400, 1978.
20. Naets J-P: Disappearance of the erythropoietic factor from plasma of anemic dogs after nephrectomy. Nature 184:371, 1959.
21. Joske RA, McAlister JM, Prankerd TAJ: Isotope investigations of red cell production and destruction in chronic renal disease. Clin Sci 15:511, 1956.
22. Hampers CL, Streiff R, Nathan DG, Snyder D, Merrill JP: Megaloblastic hematopoiesis in uremia and in patients on long-term hemodialysis. NEJM 276: 551, 1967.
23. Nathan DG, Schupak E, Stohlman F Jr, Merrill JP: Erythropoiesis in anephric man. J Clin Invest 43: 2158, 1964.
24. Hume DM: Kidney transplantation. In: *Human Transplantation*, edited by FT Rapaport, and J Dausset. New York, Grune & Stratton 1968, p. 131.
25. Rath CE, Mailliard JA, Schreiner GE: Bleeding tendency in uremia. NEJM 257:808, 1957.
26. Lewis JH, Zucker MB, Ferguson JH: Bleeding tendency in uremia. Blood 11:1073, 1956.
27. Montgomerie JZ, Kalmanson GM, Guze LB: Renal failure and infection. Medicine 47:1, 1968.
28. Cossart YE, Gillespie EH, Jones DM, Kelsey JC, Moore B, Murray IG, Polakoff S, Turner GC, Burbridge DHD, Coleman JC, Stirland RM: Infection risks of haemodialysis—some preventive aspects. Report to Public Health Laboratory Service by the Working Party on Haemodialysis Units. Br Med J 3: 454, 1968.
29. Saldanha LF, Goldman R, Adashek K, Mulder DG: Treatment of bacterial endocarditis complicating haemodialysis. Br J Med 3:92, 1972.
30. Posner MA, Reves JG, Lell WA: Aortic valve replacement in a hemodialysis dependent patient: Anesthetic considerations—a case report. Anesth Anal (Paris) 54:24, 1975.
31. Soffer O, MacDonell RC Jr, Finlayson DC, Difulco TJ, Bradley JK, Jones EL, Clements SD, Rigatti R, Clark EC: Intraoperative hemodialysis during cardiopulmonary bypass in chronic renal failure. J Thorac Cardiovas Surg 77:789, 1979.
32. Garcia-Rinaldi R, Rea JE, Callagher MW, Byrum MS, Crumb CK, Knight WP: Cardiac Surgery in the patient with end-stage renal disease: Principles of

perioperative management. Contemp Dialysis 2:55, 1981.
33. Collins JJ: Discussion, cardiac operation and end-stage renal disease. Ann Thor Surg 30:267, 1980.
34. Stein AA, Wiersum J: The role of renal dysfunction in abdominal wound dehiscence. J Urol 82:271, 1959.
35. Menzoian JO, Davis RC, Idelson BA, Mannick JA, Berger RL: Coronary artery by-pass surgery and renal transplantation: A case report. Ann Surg 179: 63, 1974.
36. Sakurai H, Ackad A, Friedman HS, Lajam F, Haft JI, and Stein RM: Aortocoronary bypass graft surgery in a patient on home dialysis. Clin Nephrol 2:208, 1974.
37. Lansing AM, Masri ZH, Karalakulasingam R, Martin DG: Angina during hemodialysis: Treatment by coronary bypass graft. JAMA 232:736, 1975.
38. Kuehnel E, Lundh H, Bennett W, Porter G: Aortocoronary bypass surgery in patients with end-stage renal disease. Trans Am Soc Artif Intern Organs 22: 14, 1976.
39. Crawford FA Jr, Selby JH Jr, Bower JD, Lehan PH: Coronary revascularization in patients maintained on chronic hemodialysis. Circulation 56:684, 1977.
40. Chawla R, Gailiunas P Jr, Lazarus JM, Gottlieb MN, Lowrie EG, Collins JJ, Merrill JP: Cardiopulmonary bypass surgery in chronic hemodialysis and transplant patients. Trans Am Soc Artif Intern Organs 23: 694, 1977.
41. Siegel MS, Norfleet EA, Gitelman HJ: Coronary artery bypass surgery in a patient receiving hemodialysis. Arch Int Med 137:83, 1977.
42. Cheng PC, Brown AH: Aortocoronary bypass surgery and chronic renal failure: Case report. NZ Med J 87:319, 1978.
43. Lansing AM, Leb DE, Berman LB: Cardiovascular surgery in end-stage renal failure. JAMA 204:682, 1968.
44. Ribot S, Rothfeld D, Frankel HJ: Infections endocarditis in maintainance hemodialysis patients. A report of four episodes among three patients. Am J Med Sci 264:183, 1972.
45. Manhas DR, Merendino KA: The management of cardiac surgery in patients with chronic renal failure. A report of three cases. J Thorac Cardiovasc Surg 63:235, 1972.
46. Glabman SL, Lukhan S, Litwak R, Juraldo R: Bacterial endocarditis leading to aortic valve destruction and open heart surgery in chronic dialysis patients (abstr.). Program of the Fifth International Congress of Nephrology, Mexico City, Mexico, October 1972, p. 16.
47. Wilcox BR, Asaph JW, Brown DR: Aortic valve replacement in the anephric patient. Ann Thorac Surg 20:282, 1975.
48. Neptune WB: Discussion of aortic valve replacement in the anephric patient. Ann Thorac Surg 20:287, 1975.
49. Nakhjavan FK, Kahn D, Rosenbaum J, Ablaza S, Goldberg H: Aortocoronary vein graft surgery in a cadaver kidney transplant recipient. Arch Intern Med 135:1511, 1975.
50. Beauchamp GD, Sharma JN, Crouch T, Reed W, Killen DA, McCallister BD, Crockett JE, Bell HH: Coronary bypass surgery after renal transplantation. Am J Cardiol 37:1107, 1976.

CHAPTER 7

CEREBRAL DYSFUNCTION FOLLOWING CARDIOPULMONARY BYPASS

ROBERT J. ELLIS, M.D.

Cerebral dysfunction remains a hazard to patients undergoing cardiac surgery. Since Bjork and Hulquist[1] first reported massive cerebral damage following cardiac surgery, several clinical studies[2, 3] were undertaken to elucidate the factors responsible for this complication.

Cerebral dysfunction is assumed to result generally because of either inadequate perfusion or embolism, or a combination of these. Based on these two causes of dysfunction, certain criteria regarding flow rate, perfusion pressure, and the need for filtration were recommended for the maintenance of cardiopulmonary bypass (CPB) flow and pressure to prevent cerebral dysfunction.

Historically, prior to the use of blood filters in the cardiopulmonary bypass system, many studies appeared to support the need for filtration and filters became a part of cardiopulmonary bypass without any randomized studies performed to prove the need. It is possible that inadequate perfusion as well as inadequate defoaming agents were used to filter the air bubbles the blood which accounted for such a high incidence of cerebral damage the implicating factor was hypothermia, while today cardiac surgeons use some form of hypothermia as a routine part of cardiopulmonary bypass. However, Javid et al.[4] and Gilman[3] described a 30% incidence of cerebral dysfunction occurring in their patients when cardiopulmonary bypass was conducted at normothermia. There has been a significant reduction in the incidence of cerebral dysfunction accounted for by the generalized improvement and refinements in the overall technique of cardiopulmonary bypass. In fact, in the most recent report regarding cerebral dysfunction the incidence was less than 3% in a series of 450 patients.[5]

Prior to discussing the factors which are necessary for adequate perfusion while on cardiopulmonary bypass, it is important to review what is currently understood regarding cerebral blood flow and the factors which are important in its regulation.[6, 7]

AUTOREGULATION

It has been calculated that the human brain requires 0.5 ml/minute/gm to maintain metabolic function with normal carbon dioxide level. Cerebral blood flow was considered dependent on arterial pressure and metabolic function prior to 1950. In 1945 the concept of autoregulation was investigated with the Kety and Schmidt[8] technique to measure cerebral blood flow. Various studies by Symon et al.,[9] Harper,[10] and Haggendal[11] substantiated the principal of autoregulation. Data from Harper demonstrated that in dogs cerebral blood flow is constant over a wide range of mean arterial pressures and begins to be pressure dependent after it falls below 50 torr. More recently, studies conducted by Selkoe and Myers[12] in monkeys have demonstrated that cerebral damage is avoided at mean arterial pressures as low as 25 torr. In 13 of 14 monkeys, only when the pressure fell to 20 torr was there isolectrical activity and cerebral damage.[12] When the pressure was 25 or greater, 1 of 15 monkeys developed brain damage, and no monkeys developed brain damage at pressures greater than 35 torr (Table 7.1). This experiment, however, was conducted under Nembutal anesthesia. It is well known that Nembutal anesthesia has a protective effect on cerebral function during ischemic periods. This data would suggest that while at normothermia, extremely low pressures can be present without compromise to cerebral blood flow.

Perfusion pressure is defined as the difference between cerebral arterial pressure and venous pressure; however, as alluded to earlier, the cerebral blood flow remains normal throughout a wide range of pressure changes. For example, in hypertensive patients cerebral blood flow remains normal. This is important to appreciate because stump pressure or the degree to which back flow varies with peripheral vascular resistance cannot be equated with cerebral blood flow in patients undergoing carotid surgery. It is assumed based on these studies that cerebral blood flow in man is maintained until mean arterial pressure (MAP) falls below 50 torr at normothermia. This is only valid when the autoregulatory system is intact. In a patient who has suffered a stroke, the autoregulatory system in this area of the brain may not be responsive and, therefore, may be dependent on higher perfusion pressures than the normal areas of the brain.

The current theories regarding which factors are thought to be responsible for autoregulation are classified as either myogenic or metabolic in origin. The myogenic theory (Bayliss[13]) states that the smooth muscle of the blood vessel changes in relation to the external pressure. Evidence has accumulated to demonstrate that this change is not rapid and requires from 30 seconds to 2 minutes. Although the myogenic theory has many proponents, the concept of autoregulation is thought to be principally governed by the metabolic state. Evidence has accumulated that specifically the level of carbon dioxide in arterial blood is reponsible for the changes in blood flow. Sherrington as early as 1890 suggested that cerebral blood flow was related to the pH of the brain. Whether it is lactic acid accounting for changes in pH or rising carbon dioxide producing changes in pH is not essential. It is clear that blood flow is regulated predominately by these two factors carbon dioxide and pH. It is also possible that the Bayliss effect is controlled by the autonomic nervous system, but little data is available to support this concept.

Table 7.1

MABP (mm Hg)	No. of Animals	Brain Lesioned	Brain Intact
≤25	14	13	1
26–34	12	1	11
>35	4	0	4

(Reproduced with permission from D. J. Selkoe and R. E. Myers.[12])

Oxygen Tension. From the data available, moderate fluctuations in arterial PO_2 do not affect cerebral blood flow, but hypoxia is associated with changes in cerebral blood flow. This is more a result of anerobic metabolism and lactic acid production.

Carbon Dioxide Tension. It has been established that carbon dioxide is a potent vasodilator. A change in carbon dioxide torr of 1 increases cerebral blood flow 1 ml/100 gm/minute within the range of 20–60 torr carbon dioxide level. The effect of carbon dioxide is mostly secondary to the extracellular pH.

Lactic Acid and Extra Cellular pH. Cerebral blood flow is coupled to neural metabolism and is predominantly controlled by lactic acid. As extracellular pH falls, vascular dilatation occurs.

The above factors are the most effective during cardiopulmonary bypass. Others factors such as neuronal reflexes and coupling agents are less well understood and cannot be controlled during cardiopulmonary bypass. The factors such as flow rate, pressure, carbon dioxide, and oxygen content can all be varied to improve cerebral blood flow.

EFFECT OF HYPOTHERMIA

Currently, some degree of hypothermia is utilized by the majority of cardiac surgeons during the cardiopulmonary bypass. Bjork suggested that the use of hypothermia caused brain damage. In reviewing his experience, it appears that the damage was more related to increased viscosity. Histological examination of the brain demonstrated congested cerebral vessels with platelet aggregations. Hemodilution was not used. Presently, hemodilution lowers viscosity during cardiopulmonary bypass. Hypothermia is defined as mild between temperatures of 32 and 37°C, moderate between temperatures of 28 and 32°C, and deep between temperatures of 20 and 28°C. Deep hypothermia is commonly used in the repair of congenital heart defects when cardiopulmonary bypass is used, whereas temperatures below 20°C are used for procedures requiring circulatory arrest. Recent work supports hypothermic temperatures of 26°C during the performance of adult cardiac surgery to prevent rewarming of the subendocardium of the heart during cardioplegic arrest.

For each degree of fall in temperature, oxygen consumption is reduced 10%. This was studied in experimental animals by Hagerdal and others[14] and demonstrated that the metabolic rate decreases linearly in a temperature range between 22 and 37°C (Table 7.2). Between the temperatures of 22 and 37°C the cerebral blood flow is not altered or reduced, but when temperatures fall below 22°C the cerebral blood flow is 15% of the level at normothermia. In spite of this reduction of cerebral blood flow at temperatures below 22°C, there was no reduction in the metabolic energy substrates. White,[15] in his experiments of selective cooling of the brain, demonstrated that autoregulation was not altered until the brain temperature fell to 13°C. During moderate or deep hypothermia, the cerebral blood flow is maintained near normal in spite of reduced temperatures. There was no vasoconstriction observed in these studies.

Table 7.2

Temperature (°C)	Oxygen Consumption (%)	Circulatory Arrest (min)
37	100	4–5
29	50	8–10
22	25	16–20
16	12	32–40
10	6	64–80

(Reproduced with permission from Meijne: Archivum Chirurgicum Neerlandicum, 25:227, 1973.)

The partial pressure of carbon dioxide continues to be important at hypothermic temperatures as well as at normothermia. Although hypercapnia produces an increase in cerebral blood flow up to levels of 80 mm Hg, data has been collected to indicate that there is no difference in the role carbon dioxide plays in the effect of cerebral blood in cortical blood flow at 30°C temperature. At temperatures below 22°C when carbon dioxide pressure fell to 15 mm Hg, cerebral blood flow did fall to 15% of normal. Currently, methods of cardiopulmonary bypass attempt to maintain carbon dioxide pressure at normal levels during hypothermia and, therefore, cerebral blood flow is maintained near normal. The flow rate can be reduced to 30 ml/kg/minute during periods of moderate hypothermia without brain damage. This has been documented by both Ellis et al.[16] and Kolkka[5] in a prospective and retrospective study. Hypothermia is certainly an adjunct to cerebral protection during cardiopulmonary bypass and permits reduction in both pressure and flow without any impairment to cerebral function.

RISK FACTORS FOR PERIOPERATIVE CEREBRAL DYSFUNCTION

Review of the literature reveals several types of etiologic risk factors which appear related to the development of CPB-related cerebral dysfunction. These factors can be divided into three broad categories: patient factors, operative factors, and postoperative factors.

Age. Investigation of adult patient-related factors demonstrated advanced age to be important in assessing risk of post-CPB CNS dysfunction. Some authors describe age greater than 50 years as significantly increasing risk of cerebral abnormality while others find age greater than 60 years to be the critical level for age-related risk. A few investigators have failed to find significant increases in CNS risk associated with age. Some studies suggest that age-related risk factors may differ significantly, depending upon the type of cardiac disorder the patient manifests and the type of surgical procedure undertaken. Advanced age increased risk of CNS disorders only in patients with aortic valve lesions. Kolkka and Hilberman[5] reported that age appeared to be compounded with type and complexity of surgical procedure. Older patients have valve replacement alone or associated with other repairs (including coronary revascularization) were at greater risk than older patients having coronary artery bypass grafting (CABG) alone. Both groups of older patients were at greater risk than younger patients.

Past Medical History. A history of cerebrovascular disease or other neurologic disorders has been associated with increased risk of postoperative CNS dysfunction. Sotaniemi,[17] in a more detailed analysis of type of preexisting cerebrovascular neurologic disease, found that the presence of a preoperative history of cerebrovascular accident (CVA) or a tendency to syncopal attacks doubled the risk of postoperative brain damage. This increased risk was manifested whether or not clinical neurologic signs were still present on preoperative examination of the CVA patients. This finding was also reported by Branthwaite,[18] but others have reported that a history of CVA is a significant risk factor only if clinical neurologic signs are still present preoperatively. On the other hand, Sotaniemi[17] found that preoperative history of transient ischemic attacks (TIAs) did not make those patients more vulnerable to postoperative CNS disorder. He concluded that cerebrovascular disease cannot be regarded as a homogeneous entity for predicting neurologic outcome of cardiac surgery and extracorporeal inculation. Further, this is one of the few studies that has examined the prognostic significance of a history of syncopal attacks (as opposed to CVAs or TIAs). Further exploration of the varying risks of different types of preexisting cerebrovascular disease and of other nonvascular neurologic disease remains to be done.

Lee et al.[19] reported that the type of cardiac disease, as well as the duration of severity of heart disease, were all important in determining risk of postoperative CNS dysfunction. Lee found that patients with significant cardiac symptomatology of greater than 6 months duration had a 73% incidence of CNS defects post CPB.

Patients with valvular heart disease were noted to be at greater risk than those with atherosclerotic or other cardiac disorders. Sotaniemi found that degree of valvular calcification was important in influencing neurologic risk only when the calcification was considered as heavy or when abundant fragmentation of this debris occurred.

History of myocardial infarction prior to open heart surgery has also been reported to substantially increase the probability of postoperative cerebral dysfunction.

Other patient-related variables that have been investigated regarding association with increased risk post CPB neurologic impairment include preoperative blood urea nitrogen values, patient weight, history of hypertension, and history of diabetes. Kolkka reported that higher preoperative blood urea nitrogen values were associated with higher incidence of prolonged neurologic impairment.

Operative Factors. Intraoperative risk factors are those occurring during the surgical procedure, including those occurring during cardiopulmonary bypass. Cardiopulmonary bypass appears to be very important in increasing risk of neuropathologic complications. Aguilar et al.[20] observed significantly more (85% of cases) neuropathology in autopsies of open heart patients who died postoperatively than in non-CPB patients (70%). Others found that CPB patients, when compared to general surgery patients, manifested significantly more impairment of concentration and slowing in cognitive processing when both groups were evaluated on the 5th or 6th postsurgical day. By the 6th or 7th postoperative week all differences in cognitive functions between the two groups disappeared, suggesting that mild nonfocal post CPB cerebral dysfunction may be a temporary rather than permanent effect.

Type of Oxygenator. In a few studies, type of oxygenator used during CPB has been reported to influence risk of cerebral complications, but the results have not been consistent. Types of oxygenators compared are bubble oxygenators and membrane oxygenators. It has been demonstrated that use of the membrane type resulted in better postsurgical visual motor performance than did use of the bubble type. Sotaniemi also noted in his series that use of the membrane oxygenator was associated with lower incidence (20%) of neurologic dysfunction than that seen overall in his patient population (37%). Ninety percent (90 of 100 people) of his patients were perfused with a bubble device, and only 10% (10 of 100) utilized a membrane device. While the proportion of patients perfused with membrane oxygenators is low, the findings are suggestive and worthy of further exploration.

Perfusion Pressure and Flow Rate. The vital importance of maintaining adequate perfusion pressure during CPB has been reported in the literature. However, disagreement exists about which perfusion pressure is adequate.

Many investigators reported that low arterial pressure increases postoperative neurologic dysfunction. Stockard et al.[21] reported that the risk and severity of CNS dysfunction was related to the magnitude and duration of operative hypotension. They concluded, using a combined index of duration and magnitude of low pressure (TM less than 50 or torr × minutes below 50 mm Hg), that maintenance of pressure above 50 torr resulted in reduced risk for CNS dysfunction. Several recent studies, however, have failed to find low arterial pressure to be significantly related to neurologic risk.[5, 16] Sotaniemi found no correlation between brain damage and hypotension in his series, even in patients of advanced age.[17] Kolkka found neither MAP (mean arterial pressure) nor the TM less than 50 index of value in predicting risk of neurologic dysfunction at discharge (Table 7.3). In fact, their patients with higher MAP had a higher incidence of neurologic sequelae than did the lower pressure group (Table 7.4). This finding was confounded by the fact that the high pressure group also was significantly older than the low pressure group. Ellis et al.[16] demonstrated in a prospective study that there was no correlation between psychological dysfunction and perfusion pressure, flow rate (30 ml/kg) and length of time each was reduced. This was because flow rate was reduced during a period of moderate hypothermia (<28°C) when was different from both Javid and Lee's earlier observation at normothermia.

Table 7.3
Summary Data from 8-Month Prospective Study

No. of patients	204
MAP	
Mean	49 ± 7
Range	(29–66)
TM < 50 (torr × min)	
Mean	560 ± 498
Range	(0–3.135)
Flow (ml/kg/min)	
Mean	42 ± 7
Range	(26–64)

(Reproduced with permission from R. Kolkka and M. Hilberman.[5])

Embolism. A literature review suggests two major proximal or direct causes of neurologic damage and neuropsychologic or behavioral dysfunction: (1) embolization and (2) inadequate cerebral perfusion. Macroemboli of air and particulate matter from the heart introduced during open heart procedures have been implicated by some authors. More frequently, microembolization from pump bubble oxygenators or stored blood has been reported as a proximal cause of CNS dysfunctions. Microemboli have been described as air, foreign particles, antifoaming agents, and microaggregates of platelets and fibrin.

MONITORING ADEQUACY OF CEREBRAL BLOOD FLOW

Electroencephalogram

There is no ideal way of monitoring cerebral blood flow during cardiopulmonary bypass. Many authors have studied the use of electroencephalography during the operation.[22–24] There appears to be a high correlation between the EEG and cortical blood flow. Hypoxia and air embolism will alter EEG activity. Inadequate cerebral perfusion may be predicted during the electroencephalogram. Findings consistent with inadequate cerebral blood flow are: suppression of background rhythm activity and slow waves seen in the record. These findings all occur with

Table 7.4
Comparison of Characteristics of Those Patients Exhibiting Some Neurologic or Neuropsychological Dysfunction at Discharge with Those Patients without Evident Residual Dysfunction

	No Deficit at Discharge	Some Deficit at Discharge	*p* Value
No of patients	169	35	
CABG only (%)	55	29	<0.01
Cardiopulmonary			
Bypass duration (Min)	107 ± 38	140 ± 45	<0.001
Flow (ml/kg/min)	42 ± 7	45 ± 9	0.4
MAP (torr)	49 ± 7	51 ± 7	<0.1
TM < 50 (torr X min)	554 ± 478	589 ± 591	<0.1

(Reproduced with permission from R. Kolkka and M. Hilberman.[5])

both hypothermia and anesthesia with normal cerebral blood flow. Several studies have determined the effectiveness of EEG monitoring, and there appears to be no correlation between changes in the electroencephalogram and pressure or flow during cardiopulmonary bypass.

The presence of slow electroencephalographic activity does not imply cerebral damage from anoxia. As an example, in 53 children undergoing cardiac surgery where electroencephalograms were analyzed, slow activity was observed in the immediate postoperative period.[25] This slowing of activity was probably secondary to water loading, as documented in experimental studies performed in rabbits. A reduction in voltage and a reduced responsiveness of animal was directly related to the reduction in serum osmolarity. In this group of children, the EEG changes paralleled physiological response to operative trauma. The EEG became normal after the electrolyte levels returned to normal. Their findings add to the difficulty in interpreting EEG during cardiopulmonary bypass because of the definite hemodilution.

Cerebral Function Monitor

This is a device which records electrical activity of the brain at frequencies between 2 and 15 Hz. The advantage of this device compared to the EEG is that it is smaller and is easier to use in the operating room. It requires placement of silver chloride electrodes on the parietal region of the head. The device records activity of the brain and can identify poor perfusion by the reduced electrical activity. This device has the same limitations as the EEG because it demonstrates a reduction in brain activity with both hypothermia and anesthesia.

Biochemical

Another method of monitoring cerebral perfusion is the determination of arterial-jugular venous oxygen differences as suggested by Wollman et al.[26] This method also demonstrates a reduction in the arterial-jugular oxygen difference with both hypothermia and anesthesia. In conclusion, there is no ideal method for determining the adequacy of cerebral blood flow during cardiopulmonary bypass.

FILTERS

Microembolism was not appreciated in the early years of cardiac surgery until Ehrenhaft and Claman[27] suggested it as a possible cause of cerebral injury.[27] Swank and Porter[28] demonstrated that particulate material could be filtered from banked blood with a Dacron wool filter. He postulated that such a filter should be used during cardiopulmonary bypass because whole blood was used in the priming solution. It was during this period that the homologous blood syndrome was described, which in retrospect appears to be caused by pulmonary microembolism of the particulate material in stored blood.

In a detailed study by Hill et al.,[29] the type of emboli in the brain of patients dying following cardiac surgery was described. The emboli appeared to be composed of either fat or platelet aggregation Hill suggested that a filter of 40 μm or less would be effective in decreasing microemboli. Solis and Patterson[30, 31] in separate investigations attempted through both clinical and animal experiments to quantify the amount of particulate material occurring during cardiopulmonary bypass. Solis used a Coulter counter in clinical studies and measured microaggregates returning through the cardiotomy return line. Solis used Swank's Dacron wool filter during the studies. The highest number of microemboli occurred from the cardiotomy line when there was greatest use of the cardiotomy suction (Table 7.5). The filter reduced the number of particles from the cardiotomy suction. The Dacron wool filter filtered 86% of the large particles up to 32 μm, and 90% of those 13 to 25 μm. Solis concluded that the number of particulate microemboli from bubble oxygenators was small and occurred mainly during the initial 10 minutes of cardiopulmonary bypass whereas the cardiotomy suction continued to have particulate material throughout the procedure.

Prior to this data, the only filter used to defoam was a filter capable of removing particles 120 μm in size. Solis concluded that the placement of the filter should be after the cardiotomy reservoir and it would eliminate 90% of all particulate microemboli. Although microemboli are reduced with the use of filter, data demonstrating a real difference in clinical outcome was lacking. The work by Taguchi et al.[32] on autofiltration appears to be the only prospective study available and supports the use of filtration (Table 7.6). The retrospective data appear to support their use because prior to filtration the incidence of

Table 7.5

Site of Blood Sample	Volume of Particles ($\times 10^3\ \mu m^3/mm^3$)	
	Coronary Suction	Sump
Venous line to oxygenator	26.2 ± 7.4	19.7 ± 6.5
Cardiotomy return line	493 ± 139	62.3 ± 15.9
Defoaming column of oxygenator	18.4 ± 4.3	24.9 ± 5.9

(Reproduced with permission from R. T. Solis.[30])

cerebral dysfunction was as high as 35% and today approaches 2%.

Patterson et al.[33] attempted to correlate the incidence and type of neurological dysfunction without filtration in dogs undergoing 2 hours of cardiopulmonary bypass (Table 7.7). They postulated that the transient neurological syndromes observed clinically were related to a transient microvascular blockade by such particulate material. Using a technique in which a suspension of lamp black material could be injected in dogs following cardiopulmonary bypass when no filtration was used, a quantitative demonstration of blockade could be determined by gross examination of the brain at timed intervals following cardiopulmonary bypass. Animals were sacrificed immediately following cardiopulmonary bypass, and 50% of the vascular bed of the brain was determined to be abnormal. With sequential studies at 7 days there was no microvascular blockade observed, and the blockade fell to 50% on the 3rd day. Correlation between neurological deficit and days following cardiopulmonary bypass was compared. Gait problems cleared in direct relation to the disappearance of the microvascular blockade. This was further confirmed by Hallenbeck et al.,[34] who demonstrated in dogs that neuronal function was preserved when filtration was used during cardiopulmonary bypass. Using autoradiographs, they demonstrated that filtration reduced the area of nonperfusion. In the group in which filtration was used, the percent of recovery was 69%, as compared to only 14% in the nonfiltered group ($p < 0.0004$). EEG activity and evoked cortical potential bear a direct relationship to the rate of cerebral blood flow. Flow rates between 12 and 16 ml/100 gm are acceptable. Above 16 ml/100 gm, the cortical evoked response is normal, and when the flow rate is reduced to 12 ml/100 gm, there is no response. Filtration in these experiments preserved nutrient cerebral blood flow at the normal level. In the unfiltered experiments, what occurred was a progressive shutdown of the nutrient flow to levels less than 12 ml/100 gm, at which point the cortical evoked response was abolished. They concluded that Dacron wool filtration prevented microvascular blockade and pre-

Table 7.6
Incidence of Low Cardiac Output Syndrome, Brain Damage and Psychiatric Manifestations in Patients in Whom Autofiltration Was Used or Not Used

Complications	Use of Autofiltration	Total No. of Patients	No. of Patients with Complications	
			No.	%
Low cardiac output syndrome*	Used	100	4	4.0
	Not used	100	18	18.0
Brain damage	Used	100	0	0
	Not used	100	5	5.0
Psychiatric manifestations	Used	100	5	5.0
	Not used	100	14	5.0
				14.0

(Reproduced with permission from: K. Taguchi et al.[32])
* $\chi^2 = 10.01, p < 0.01$.
† $\chi^2 = 5.14, p < 0.025$.
‡ $\chi^2 = 4.71, p < 0.05$.

Table 7.7
Degree of Blockade of the Cerebral Vascular Bed

Dog No.	No Filter	25 × 36 μm	36 × 36 μm	Dual Dacron Filters
1	4.0+	0.2	1.4	0.4
2	4.0+	1.3	3.5	1.9
3	2.3+	1.3	1.1	1.7
4	3.9+	1.3	2.6	1.4
5	3.8+	0.8	3.7	1.4
Mean	3.6+	1.0+	2.5+	1.4+

(Reproduced with permission from R. H. Patterson Jr. et al.[33])

served neuronal function and supported their use in cardiopulmonary bypass.

It is interesting that there was a significant reduction in the overall incidence of cerebral dysfunction since filters were added to the cardiopulmonary bypass system. In comparing the data where the incidence of cerebral dysfunction is known, there is a reduction in the number of motor deficits to less than 2%. It is clear that improvements in the manufacture of oxygenators has occurred. The use of hemodilution has also helped in the reduction of cerebral dysfunction. In spite of the lack of prospective studies documenting the need for such filtration, the experiment work by the authors quoted and the retrospective studies performed by Hill clearly support the need for such filters. The need for filters in the arterial line is less clear, and certain centers have not accepted their use in the arterial line. Current planning by the manufacturers of oxygenators is a modification of the cardiotomy reservoir to incorporate the 40-μm filter in the reservoir itself.

PROFOUND HYPOTHERMIA AND CIRCULATORY ARREST

It is clear that for certain complex congenital heart defects the technique of profound hypothermia and circulatory arrest first introduced by the Mohri is necessary for successful repair in infancy. Although hypothermia protects the brain during periods of nonpulsatile perfusion such as that during cardiopulmonary bypass, the limits of total circulatory arrest at a temperature of 18°C for periods of 30 minutes or greater are not well known. Certain neurological sequela such as seizures, paresis, and chorea type movements have all been reported with the technique of profound hypothermia and circulatory arrest. In an attempt to determine what the limits of the technique are, a review of the literature has not determined a safe period. Series of patients requiring greater than 60 minutes of profound hypothermia and circulatory arrest have been reported to have neurological sequelae. The majority of surgeons using this technique are attempting to limit its use to certain defects, such as those requiring repair through the atria, transposition of the great vessels and atrioventricular canal defects. These surgeons are now advocating cardiopulmonary bypass for the repair of the other congenital heart defects.

Weiss et al.[24] attempted to judge the tolerance of the brain to hypothermia and circulatory arrest by defining criteria of the electroencephalogram latency period and survival during various temperatures. The techniques used by their groups, as well as others, cooled the infant to 25°C, either by placing ice bags around the patient or by cold water immersion. This technique allows for a more even cooling of the patient or by cold water immersion. This technique allows for a more even cooling of the patient and his vital organs and minimizes the thermal gradients seen with immediate core cooling from perfusion. The time to achieve 25°C varies with the weight of the child and may take as long as 90 minutes. After this temperature is achieved, the child is placed on cardiopulmonary bypass and is cooled to 18°C. The patient, after the period of arrest required for surgical correction, is rewarmed by restarting extracorporeal bypass to return the core temperature to 36°C. Various changes in the EEG were observed, such as disappearance of rapid rhythms, inversion of delta waves, and dedifferentiation of anterior and posterior patterns. None of these patterns could be used to indicate the short-term prognosis from the EEG interpretation. There was concern earlier that the latency period of return of the EEG after circulatory arrest was related to cerebral injury. The data from Weiss demonstrated that a flat EEG for up to 30 or 40 minutes after the end of circulatory arrest may be a normal occurrence and may not be related to a specific neurologic injury. The EEG did not universally become flat at 20°C, but activity was still present at temperatures of 11°C. Further data on latency and survival of EEG demonstrated that there was no correlation between late function and the EEG. Essentially, the EEG of the infants followed the patterns seen in the older children for whom cardiopulmonary bypass was used for surgical correction. The question as to the limit of profound hypothermia and cardiovascular circulatory arrest was not identified by the EEG. Latency time for EEG recovery can not be used as a determination of metabolic insult.

Postoperative neurological sequela, such as seizures, altered consciousness, hypotonia, paresis, rigidity, and deficits in higher learning all suggest that this technique is associated with either focal or generalized lesions. The causes of cerebral dysfunction with this technique are postulated to occur secondary to reflow phenomenon, which was described by Norwood et al.[35] Uneven brain cooling due to inadequate perfusion and microembolism factors may still be the predominant causes of cerebral dysfunction with this technique. Support for uneven brain cooling was demonstrated by Aoyagi et al.[36] He attempted to study in baboons the blood flow to various regions of the brain before and after circulatory arrest. Animals were surface cooled to a brain temperature of 32°C and then systemically perfused to a temperature of 18°C. Circulatory arrest lasted 30 minutes, after which the animals were rewarmed with cardiopulmonary bypass to 35°C. The cerebral metabolic rate was reduced to 13% of control from 1.59 ml/100 gm/minute to 0.20 ml/100 gm/minute. The authors observed a discrepancy between the brain temperature and nasopharyngeal temperature during both cooling and rewarming and demonstrated an increase in cerebral vascular resistance occurring during the cooling. The microsphere technique to calculate blood flow documented considerable paradoxical alteration. The cerebral microcirculation was shown to have various flow patterns for different areas of the brain. The hypothermic vasoconstrictive response was initially more predominant in the subcortical white matter. During rewarming, ischemic areas were distributed equally throughout the brain area. It appeared from their study that the assertion that the rewarming period was associated with focal areas of damage again is supported by the reflow data of Norwood.

Little information is available regarding late dysfunction and psychomotor function. According to Messmer et al.,[37] there were no problems related to deep hypothermia and circulatory arrest up to 43 minutes when patients were psychologically tested in a prospective manner. There were no differences in global intellectual function. However, another study in which parents and physicians were asked to describe their children's function, indicated that the children who required this technique appeared to have only 41% assessment of normality, as compared to children who underwent cardiopulmonary bypass who had an 80% assessment of normality.[38] Their physical assessment demonstrated slow growth, easy fatigability, and poor coordination. When the technique of profound hypothermia and circulatory arrest was utilized, this was very difficult to analyze because of the lack of objective criteria and was based solely on subjective factors. It is apparent that profound hypothermia and circulatory arrest are associated with cerebral ischemia which may not result in any behavioral signs in the late follow-up of these children. Clearly, more studies need to be performed to determine the status of this technique on cerebral metabolism.

NEUROPATHOLOGY STUDIES

Hill et al.,[29] in an extensive study of 215 patients dying following either cardiac surgery or cardiac bypass, described the pathological findings. A high incidence of fat emboli occurred (70%), as compared to only 50% in nonoperated deaths, suggesting that the use of blood was indirectly responsible for this finding. Eighty-two of the patients who died following cardiopulmonary bypass had fat emboli, and only 20 patients had no fat emboli. Of the 82 patients who had fat emboli, it was of a diffuse nature. The source of fat was considered to be the blood used in the prime of the pump. Of all the variables investigated, the duration of bypass was the most significant. In perfusion times less than 90 minutes, there were no fat emboli identified. Thirty-one percent of the patients who died had nonfat emboli, and these were composed of fibrin and platelets. Hill believed these to be emboli related to the use of coronary suction.

Aguilar et al.[20] examined 206 patients who died following cardiac surgery. Neuropathologic examination demonstrated the following findings: emboli in small vessels, acute petechial perivascular and focal subarachnoid hemorrhages, and acute ischemic neuronal damage. Widely scattered, small fresh subarachnoid and intracerebral hemorrhages were commonly found in brains of patients following cardiopulmonary bypass. Neuronal degeneration was prevalent in the hippocampus and calcarine cortex of the occipital lobes.

Since 1969 when filters were used, there was a disappearance of nonfat emboli. Fat emboli were present in 130 of 166 patients or 78% of this series, while other series have noted 100% fat emboli occurring prior to the use of filtration. Other materials, such as silicone or antifoam A, were observed in the early period of cardiac surgery but have not been seen in the last 10 years because they are not incorporated into the oxyenator. In this series of patients, 12% had polarizable bodies seen in the brain which were presumed to be platelet aggregates, and since the use of the Dacron wool filter there has been a sharp reduction in these polarizable bodies.

In the identification of factors responsible for the high degree of embolization, the only factor which was significantly related was the duration of greater than 90 minutes. Patients who had cardiopulmonary bypass for less than 90 minutes. Patients who had cardiopulmonary bypass for less than 90 minutes had no emboli. Various authors have focused on the diffuse nature of the pathological picture caused by cerebral anoxia secondary to hypotension whereas others have stressed the focal nature of neurological damage or embolism as the major factor in the neuropathological finding. In conclusion, the pathological picture is one of multiple factors contributing to brain damage. It is impossible to determine which of the two broad groups of factors are predominant.

PROBLEM OF COEXISTENT CAROTID AND CORONARY ARTERY DISEASE

There exists controversy regarding the timing of surgery in patients with both carotid and coronary artery disease. Although clinical judgment argues for doing the procedure which is at high risk first, the data to support this judgment are lacking. There is no prospective study to indicate which procedure, carotid endarectomy, CABG, or both, should be performed initially. Data from various centers indicate that patients with carotid disease who have undergone carotid endarectomy are at high risk of developing a myocardial infarction. Myocardial infarction is the most frequent noncerebral cause of both early and late mortality. Twenty-five percent of the patients who died in the immediate postoperative period following carotid endarectomy suffered a myocardial infarction. Prophylactic carotid endarectomy was suggested as the initial procedure prior to any surgical procedure which may be associated with hypotension. There is no data to support this opinion, which is based on anecdotal information.

It is clear from this review of the literature that the incidence of cerebral complications including neurological psychological averages 17% and that of pure motor deficits averages 2% in all patients undergoing cardiac surgery. There is no data which describe the incidence of cerebral dysfunction occurring in patients with coexistent extracranial disease. Bernhard et al. first approached the problem of coexistent disease by doing carotid endarectomy first. Their immediate postoperative mortality was 20%, with the three deaths occurring directly from myocardial failure. This led their colleagues to do a series of 15 patients in which simultaneous procedures were done. Only one patient developed a cerebrovascular accident while no patient died from either brain or cardiac problems. The authors concluded that both procedures should be performed in patients who were at high risk for developing a stroke or myocardial infarction. Another study by Urschel and associates[40] demonstrated that when three groups were compared (carotid initially, coronary artery surgery initially, or both procedures combined), only one patient suffered a stroke. This was secondary to hypoxia related to problems with the ventilator. These data did not support combined procedures initially because there was an increased morbidity in this group. The authors suggested that each situation should be assessed individually and that a rigid approach should not be utilized.

Mehigan et al.[41] suggested that a planned approach should exist based on the findings of severe extracranial disease. If the patient has severe angina at rest or left main disease, a combined approach is in order. If the patient has stable angina, carotid surgery should be performed initially. All other patients should have the *primary* system corrected which is consistently causing problems associated with the highest risk to the patient. It appears that at least 6% of patients undergoing cardiac surgery have coexistent disease. In Mehigan's series of 23 patients who had carotid surgery, only 2 patients developed unstable angina and underwent cardiac surgery. No patient had either a stroke or myocardial infarction in this group. In 29 patients where simultaneous procedures were performed, four deaths occurred (14%) which were deemed poor risks. However, there is no statement made regarding the duration of the procedure and whether this high mortality rate in this series of patients was related to the duration of the anesthetic procedure. Comparing this figure of 14% for simultaneous procedure to their own mortality of 1.4% for CABG alone would argue against combined procedures.

A similar view was shared by Hertzer et al.[42] of the Cleveland Clinic in 1978 where, in a series of 59 patients who underwent staged procedures, a mortality of 1.7% secondary to myocardial failure was observed. In 115 patients where the combined procedures were performed, 4.3% died (five patients). The incidence of myocardial infarction in the staged group was 10% with evidence of new Q waves which was similar to that of the staged group. Neurological complications occurred in 3.1% of patients with the staged procedure whereas in the combined procedure, 8.7% had neurological complications. Five patients in this group had permanent strokes.

Their data argues against combined procedures because the mortality rate of 2.2% and stroke incidence of 1.8% between 1969 and 1976 for all cases were similar to a mortality rate of 1.7% and stroke rate of 1.5% when the procedures were staged. These authors concluded that the incidence of stroke was less with staged procedures than with combined procedures, and recommendations were that all patients should have staged procedures, except those with left main coronary artery disease, those with diffuse disease without collateral circulation, and those with unstable angina. These three groups should undergo simultaneous procedures.

When a critical review of these papers is made, there is no support for simultaneous procedures. In Table 7.8 the number of patients in each group is listed with the incidence of death, stroke, and myocardial infarction with each of the three modalities. If one considers stroke to be prevented during cardiac surgery, then when comparing the results with staged procedures *vs.* combined procedure there is no statistical difference using Chi square analysis. This would indicate that stroke will not be prevented by a simultaneous procedure. If one considers myocardial failure to be life threatening, then this procedure should be performed first. If the carotid is at high risk, then that should be performed first. Most authors agree to staging procedures where the risk of one system is greater than the risk of the other system. There is general confusion about what to do with the patient with left main disease and significant carotid disease, and there is no support to do the carotid surgery first to prevent a stroke. If one assumes that strokes from carotid disease are related to decrease in blood flow, then logic would argue for a combined approach. On the other hand, when strokes are related to embolic phenomena, then the incidence of stroke would be the same whether the staged or simultaneous procedure is advocated. This latter idea is supported by the published data from the series of papers reviewed. If the patient has severe unstable angina, he should undergo cardiac surgery. If the patient has unstable carotid disease, he should undergo carotid surgery first. No other conclusion can be drawn from the data published.

Table 7.8
Combined Carotid + CABG

	Patients	Death (5%)	Myocardial infarction (7%)	Stroke (7%)
Bernard	15	0	0	1
Urshel	8			
Mehigan	29	4	0	0
Hertler	115	5	12	10
	167	9	12	11

* $\frac{\text{Stroke}}{\chi^2}$ = probability not significant (pns) when combined *vs.* staged.

References

1. Björk VO, Hultquist G: Brain damage in children after deep hypothermia for open-heart surgery. Thorax 15:284, 1960.
2. Brierley JB: Neuropathological findings in patients dying after open-heart surgery. Thorax 18:291, 1963.
3. Gilman S: Cerebral disorders after open-heart operations. NEJM 272:489, 1965.
4. Javid H, Tufo HM, Najafi H, Dye WS, Hunter JA, Julian OC: Neurological abnormalities following open-heart surgery. J Thorac Cardiovasc Surg 58: 502, 1969.
5. Kolkka R, Hilberman M: Neurologic dysfunction following cardiac operation with low-flow, low-pressure cardiopulmonary bypass. J Thorac Cardiovasc Surg 79:432, 1980.
6. McDowall DG: Cerebral blood flow. In *General Anesthesia*, edited by T Gray, JE Utting, and JF Nunn. London, Butterworth, 1980, pp. 657–684.
7. Mchedlishvili G: Physiological mechanisms controlling cerebral blood flow. Stroke 11:240, 1980.
8. Kety SS, Schmidt CF: The determination of cerebral blood flow in man by the use of nitrous oxide in low concentrations. Am J Physiol 143:53, 1945.
9. Symon L, Held K, Dorsch NWC: A study of regional autoregulation in the cerebral circulation to increased perfusion pressure in normocapnia and hypercapnia. Stroke 4:139, 1973.
10. Harper AM: Autoregulation of cerebral blood flow: Influence of the arterial blood pressure on the blood flow through the cerebral cortex. J Neurol Neurosurg Psychiastry 29:398, 1966.
11. Häggendal E: Blood flow autoregulation of the cerebral grey matter with comments on its mechanism. Acta Neurol Scan 14 (Suppl):104, 1965.
12. Selkoe DJ, Myers RE: Neurologic and cardiovascular effects on hypotension in the monkey. Stroke 10: 147, 1979.
13. Bayliss WM: On the local reaction of the arterial wall to changes of internal pressure. J Physiol (Lond.) 28:220, 1902.
14. Hagerdal M, Harp J, Nilsson L, Siesjo BK: The effect of induced hypothermia upon oxygen consumption in the rat brain. J Neurochem 24:311, 1975.
15. White RJ: Cerebral hypothermia and circulatory arrest: Review and commentary. Mayo Clin Proc 53: 450, 1978.
16. Ellis RJ, Wisniewski A, Potts R, Calhoun C, Loucks P, Wells MR: Reduction of flow rate and arterial pressure at moderate hypothermia does not result in cerebral dysfunction. J Thorac Cardiovasc Surg 79: 173, 1980.
17. Sotaniemi KA: Brain damage and neurological outcome after open-heart surgery. J Neurol Neurosurg Psychiatry, 43:127, 1980.
18. Branthwaite MA: Detection of neurological damage during open-heart surgery. Thorax 28:464, 1973.
19. Lee WH Jr, Brady MP, Rowe JM, Miller JWC Jr: Effects of extracorporeal circulation upon behavior,

personality, and brain function. Part II. Hemodynamic, metabolic, and psychometric correlations. Ann Surg 173:1013, 1971.
20. Aguilar MJ, Gerbode F, Hill JD: Neuropathologic complications of cardiac surgery. J Thorac Cardiovasc Surg 61:676, 1971.
21. Stockard JJ, Bickford RG, Myers RR, Aung MH, Dilley RB, Schauble JF: Hypotension-induced changes in cerebral function during cardiac surgery. Stroke 5:730, 1974.
22. Salerno TA, Lynn RB, White DN, Charrette EJP: Cerebral surveillance during cardiac surgery. Canadian J Surg 22:325, 1979.
23. Salerno TA, Lince DP, White DN, Lynn RB, Charrette EJP: Monitoring of electroencephalogram during open heart surgery: A prospective analysis of 118 cases. J Thorac Cardiovasc Surg 76:97, 1978.
24. Weiss M, Weiss J, Cotton J, Nicolas F, Binet JP: A study of the electroencephalogram during surgery with deep hypothermic and circulation arrest in infants. J Thorac Cardiovasc Surg 70:316, 1975.
25. Harden AR, Glaser G, Damiglione G: Electroencephalographic and plasma electrolyte changes after cardiac surgery in children. Br Med J 4:210, 1968.
26. Wollman H, Stephen GW, Clement AJ, Danielson GK: Cerebral blood flow in man during extracorporeal circulation. J Thorac Cardiovasc Surg 52:558, 1966.
27. Ehrenhaft JL, Claman, MA: Cerebral complications of open heart surgery. J Thor Cardiovasc Surg 41: 503, 1961.
28. Swank RL, Porter GA: Disappearance of micro-emboli transfused into patients during cardiopulmonary bypass. Transfusion 3:192, 1963.
29. Hill JD, Aguilar MJ, Baranco A, de Lanerolle P, Gerbode F: Neurological manifestations of cardiac surgery. Ann Thorac Surg 7:409, 1969.
30. Solis RT, Noon GP, Beall AC Jr, DeBakey ME: Particulate microembolism during cardiac surgery. Ann Thorac Surg 17:332, 1974.
31. Patterson RH Jr, Rosenfeld L, Porro RS: Transitory cerebral microvascular blockade after cardiopulmonary bypass. Thorax 31:736, 1976.
32. Taguchi K, Washizu T, Hirao M, et al.: Alleviation of post-perfusion complications by autoregulation of cardiotomy blood return in 100 patients: A comparison with sequential controls. Hiroshima J Med Sci 21:65, 1972.
33. Patterson RH Jr, Wasser JS, Porro RS: The effect of various filters on microemboli cerebrovascular blockade following cardiopulmonary bypass. Ann Thorac Surg 17:464, 1974.
34. Hallenbeck JM, Furlow TW Jr, Ruel TA, and Greenbaum LJ Jr: Extracorporeal glass-wool filtration of whole blood enhances post-ischemic recovery of the cortical sensory evoked response. Stroke 10:158, 1979.
35. Norwood WI, Norwood CR, Castaneda AR: Cerebral axoria: Effect of deep hypothermia and pH. Surgery 86:203, 1979.
36. Aoyagi M, Flasterstein AH, Barnette J, Von Koch L, Ross JN Jr, Kennedy JH: Cerebral effects of profound hypothermia (18°C) and circulatory arrest. Circulation 51(Suppl 1):52, 1974.
37. Messmer B, Schallberger U, Gattiker R, Senning Å: Psychomotor and intellectual development after deep hypothermia and circulatory arrest in early infancy. J Thorac Cardiovasc Surgery 72:495, 1976.
38. Wright JS, Hicks RG, Newman DC: Deep hypothermia arrest: Observations on later development in children. J Thorac Cardiovasc Surg 77:466, 1979.
39. Bernhard VM, Johnson WD, Peterson JJ: Carotid artery stenosis: Association with surgery for coronary artery disease. Arch Surg 105:837, 1972.
40. Urschel HC, Razzuk MA, Gardner MA: Management of concomitant occlusive disease of the carotid and coronary arteries. J Thorac Cardiovasc Surg 72: 829, 1976.
41. Mehigan JG, Buch WS, Pipkin RD, Fogarty TJ: A planned approach to coexistent cerebrovascular disease in coronary artery bypass candidates. Arch Surg 112:1403, 1977.
42. Hertzer NR, Loop FD, Taylor PC, Beven EG: Staged and combined surgical approach to simultaneous carotid and coronary vascular disease. Surgery 84: 803, 1978.

CHAPTER 8

CENTRAL NERVOUS SYSTEM INJURY DURING SURGERY OF THE DESCENDING AORTA

WALTER P. DEMBITSKY, M.D.

One of the most feared complications of surgery on the descending aorta is injury to the central nervous system. This usually is manifested by the appearance of paraplegia in the postoperative period.[1] Although cord damage is more common, brain injury can also occur. The surgeon may observe problems of spinal cord function and also the interesting and increasingly more common problem of worsening a preexisting cerebral injury during the surgery upon trauma patients with combined aortic tears and brain contusions. Neurovascular physiologic mechanisms are important in these relationships.

NEUROVASCULAR PHYSIOLOGY

The central nervous system is encased in a rigid compartment comprised of the skull and spinal column. About 150 ml of cerebral spinal fluid circulates freely through the interstices of the brain at a pressure of 7.5 to 15 mm Hg. This fluid is produced in the cerebral ventricles and is finally absorbed by the venous system, primarily in the sagittal sinus. The absorption is passive and is facilitated by the negative pressure present in the sagittal sinus in the erect position. Absorption is impaired by increases in central venous pressure. The arterial inflow to the brain is autoregulated in response to pressure changes. Under normal circumstances the flow increases only in response to metabolic demand; as the metabolic rate of central nervous tissue increases, the blood flow increases. The flow is autoregulated between the pressures of 60 and 160 mm Hg. As seen in Figure 8.1, as the pressure falls below 60, the flow becomes linearly related to pressure producing brain ischemia; similarly, as the pressure rises above 160, flow again becomes linear and brain edema may develop.[2]

The central nervous system perfusion pressure (CNSPP) is equal to the difference between the mean blood pressure ($\overline{BP}$) and the intracranial pressure (ICP). The minimum CNSPP needed to sustain central nervous system function varies with the metabolic rate of the brain but is usually between 40 and 50 mm Hg. As an example, with a mean blood pressure of 60 and an intracranial pressure of 7.5 to 15 mm Hg, the perfusion pressure is 60-15 or 45 mm Hg. The intracranial pressure is buffered by having a displaceable intracranial volume, is demonstrated in Figure 8.2. Since the central nervous system tissue is nearly incompressible, any increase in the intracranial volume must be met by a decrease in either of the displaceable components of the intracranial volume: blood or cerebral spinal fluid. If these cannot be displaced from the skull to the spinal column and then into the recesses of the spinal nerve roots, the intracranial pressure will rise. As seen in Figure 8.3, if the arterial blood pressure rises or vasoparalysis due to hypercapnia or drugs such as Halothane or Nitroprusside occurs, the increased intracranial arterial blood volume must be met with a decrease in cerebral spinal fluid or venous blood volume for the intracranial pressure to remain low.

When the aorta is occluded, the intracranial arterial pressure rises. The normal brain is protected with acute hypertension by the autoregulatory vasoconstrictor response, which maintains a constant flow. If the pressure acutely exceeds 160 mm Hg or the vasoconstrictor response is abolished, brain edema may develop.[3] This produces an increase in nondisplaceable volume. The increased intracranial volume of blood and edema fluid may be well tolerated by the normal brain. In patients with an elevated intracranial pressure due to a brain injury, the additional rise in intracranial pressure can compromise the central nervous system perfusion pressure and increase brain damage.

In the spinal cord during aortic occlusion, the perfusion pressure may not be maintained. If the arterial flow to the cord originates distal to the aortic occlusion, the mean arterial blood pressure supplying the distal spinal cord can fall to 15 mm Hg. During clamping the cerebral spinal fluid pressure temporarily rises and then stabilizes at 15 mm Hg, thereby nullifying the perfusion pressure in the spinal cord and causing ischemic cord damage (i.e., CNSPP = 15 − 15 = 0).[4]

The difficulty relating spinal cord paralysis to aortic clamping is that the experimental evidence linking cord damage to aortic occlusion differs from the clinical experience re-

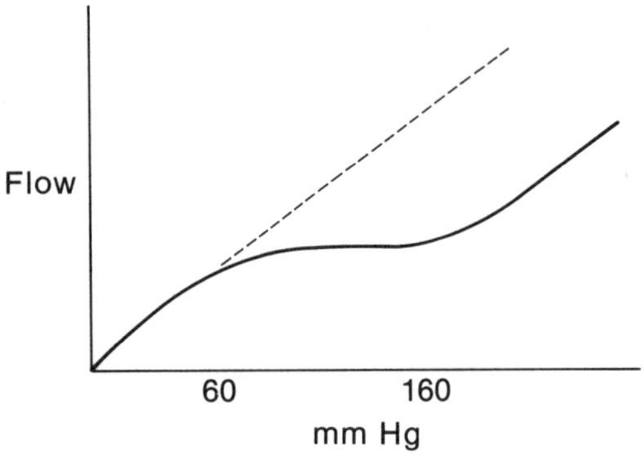

Figure 8.1. Autoregulation of central venous system flow is represented by the *solid curve.* Below a systolic pressure of 60 and above a pressure of 160 flow becomes linearly related to pressure. The *dashed line* represents the flow-pressure relationship when autoregulation has been abolished.

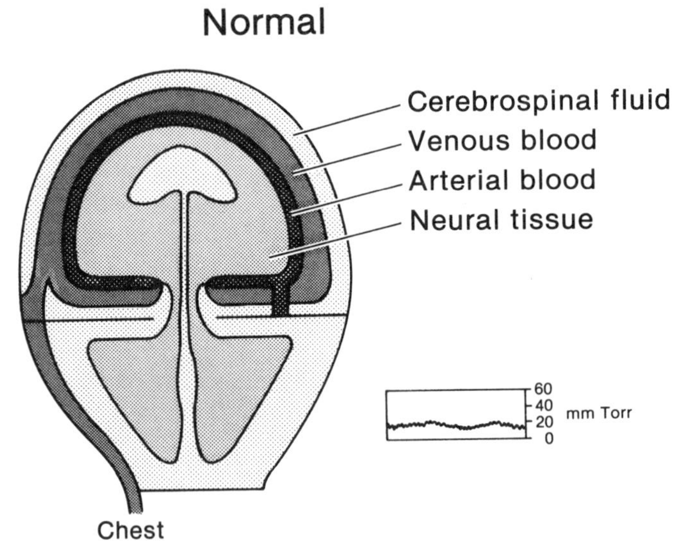

Figure 8.2. The various components of the intracranial portion of the central nervous system are represented. The displaceable components of the cranium are the blood and cerebrospinal fluid.

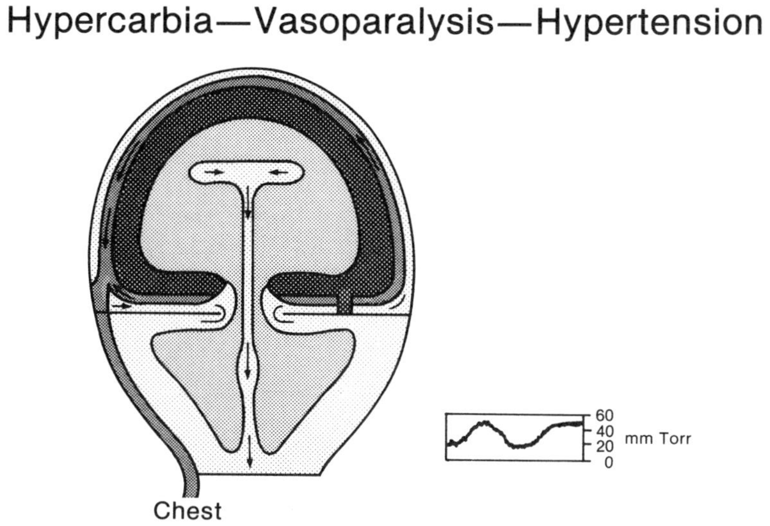

Figure 8.3. An increase in the arterial portion of the intracranial volume can produce a rise in the intracranial pressure.

ported in the literature. Clinically, some surgical groups have stated that up to 45 minutes of aortic occlusion is well tolerated,[5] although reports of cord damage following as little as 10 minutes of aortic occlusion and cases of longer than 60 minutes without injury have been reported.

Experimentally, paraplegia in animals is progressive after 30 minutes.[4, 6] It is lessened with maneuvers which reduce the oxygen consumption of the cord, such as hypothermia[6] and barbiturate administration.[7] It is also lessened by maneuvers which reduce the cerebral spinal fluid pressure, such as inferior vena caval occlusion,[8] which lowers cardiac output, cerebral intracranial pressure, and cerebral spinal fluid pressure. Removal or cerebral spinal fluid[9] thereby reduces cerebral spinal fluid pressure and increasing perfusion pressure.[4] The metabolic rate of the central nervous system tissue measured in flow metabolism units is reduced significantly by phenobarbital or hypothermia. Both these interventions are synergistic in reducing the metabolism of the central nervous tissue.[10]

SPINAL CORD DYSFUNCTION

A major reason for the discrepancy between experimental and clinical results may be species differences, but at least as significant is the variability in the blood supply to the spinal cord. There are three main regions of blood supply to the spinal cord. The cervical cord is supplied by vertebral branches of the subclavian artery. These are occluded in the subclavian artery as a temporary shunt. The midthoracic cord is supplied by arteries arising from T7. The lower cord is supplied by a large unpaired artery described by Kadyi and Adamkiewicz[11] in the late 19th century. In 85% of patients this large unpaired artery arises from the level of T9-L2 or L1-L2. In 15% of the cases, this artery arises from the level of T5-T8. This artery contributes blood flow to the anterior spinal artery, which can provide for collateral circulation throughout the spinal cord. The anterior spinal artery may be a continuous blood vessel along the entire spinal cord. As seen in Figure 8.4, the artery can be discontinuous.[1] In these instances occlusion of the blood supply which originates in the distal aorta can create cord ischemia in the area of the anterior spinal artery.

Anterior spinal artery occlusion produces paraplegia, incontinence, decreased deep tendon reflexes, loss of superficial sensation and loss of light touch, and superficial pain sensation. Deep pain, vibratory motion, or position sense are preserved. These sensations are transmitted from peripheral receptors to the brain via the dorsal vertebral columns and can be spared during an episode of anterior spinal artery ischemia which compromises the ventral cord (see Fig. 8.5). The anterior portion of the spinal cord contains rapid transit nerve fibers having high metabolic rate making them more susceptible to hypoxic damage.

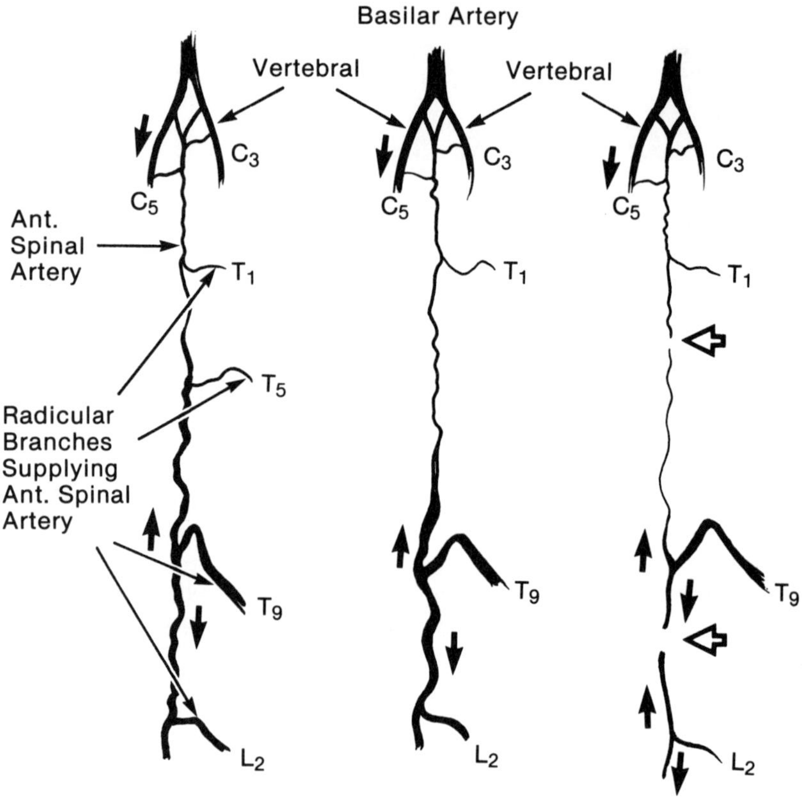

Figure 8.4. Blood supply variation to the spinal cord adapted from Brewer. Diagram on the right demonstrates a discontinuous anterior spinal artery with the distal cord supply originating from the descending aorta. Occlusion of the descending aorta might not produce paraplegia in the situation represented on the left but would in the situation on the right.

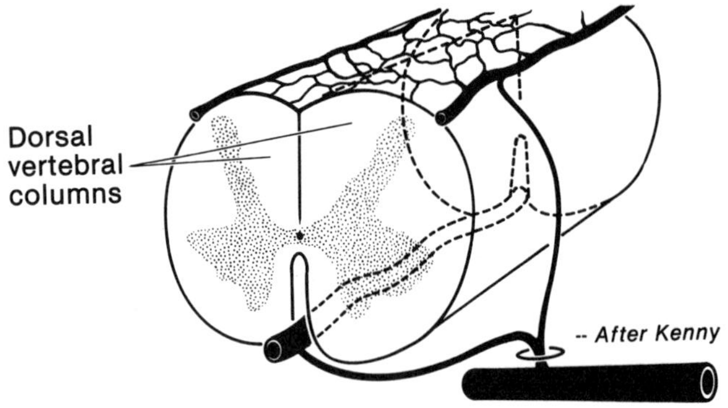

Figure 8.5. The dorsal vertebral volumes may be spared during an episode of anterior spinal artery ischemia.

Historically, the first approach to descending aortic surgery was simple aortic clamping for the repair. Later, hypothermia was added to diminish the incidence of cord paralysis. Because of cardiac, metabolic, and pulmonary problems created by hypothermia, it was largely abandoned. More recently, the surgical techniques which attempt to reduce cord damage have been designed to limit ischemia by maintaining a distal aortic pressure of 50 mm Hg[12] and by anastomosing large vessels which may be the source of spinal cord blood in the graft.[5] Occasionally, diseases of the descending aorta cannot be treated without a high risk of creating paraplegia.[13] Following insertion of a graft in the descending aorta, distal aortic pressure must be preserved by avoiding declamping shock. If no provision for distal flow is made during aortic clamping, the cross clamp must be slowly released—allowing the dilated peripheral vessels to regain tone. This technique also allows for slow washout of the acid metabolites which accumulate peripherally during clamping.

As seen in Figures 8.6 and 8.7, paraplegia is prevented by preservation of large intercostal arteries which may possibly supply blood to the spinal cord. This is particularly important in patients whose spinal cord is supplied by a discontinuous anterior spinal artery. Preoperative identification of the spinal cord blood supply would be optimal. Although anatomic definition of cord blood flow is less feasible in patients with degenerative aortic disease, careful study of the descending aortogram may reveal the location of large radicular arteries supplying the cord. Specific spinal cord angiography is improving. With current techniques, the risk of spinal cord injury during spinal cord angiography is in the range of 2–3%. Therefore,

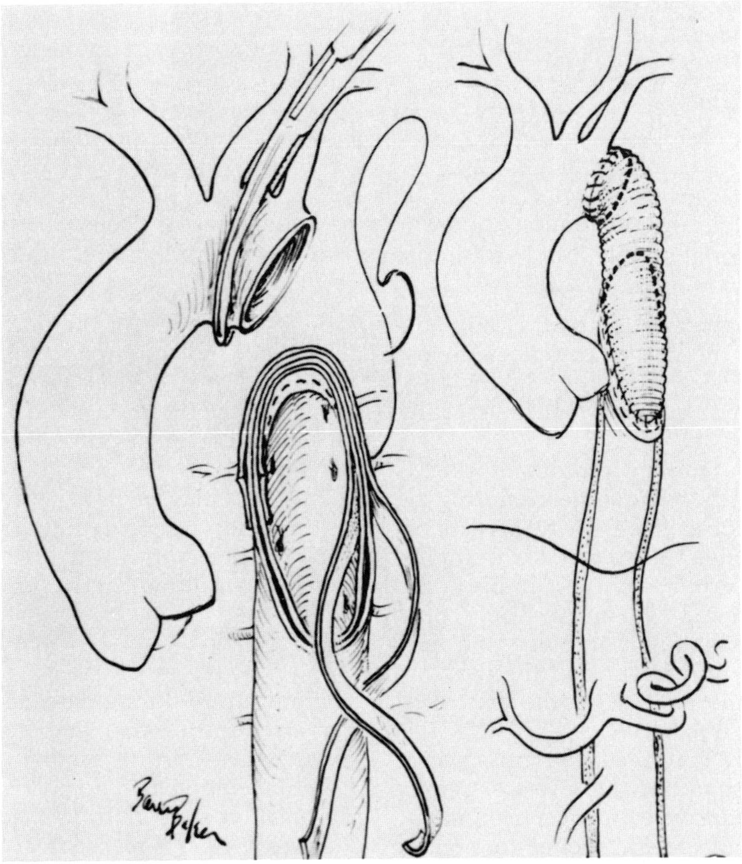

Figure 8.6. Intraoperative technique which may be used to preserve the integrity of the spinal cord arterial supply. Large intercostal arteries are not ligated.

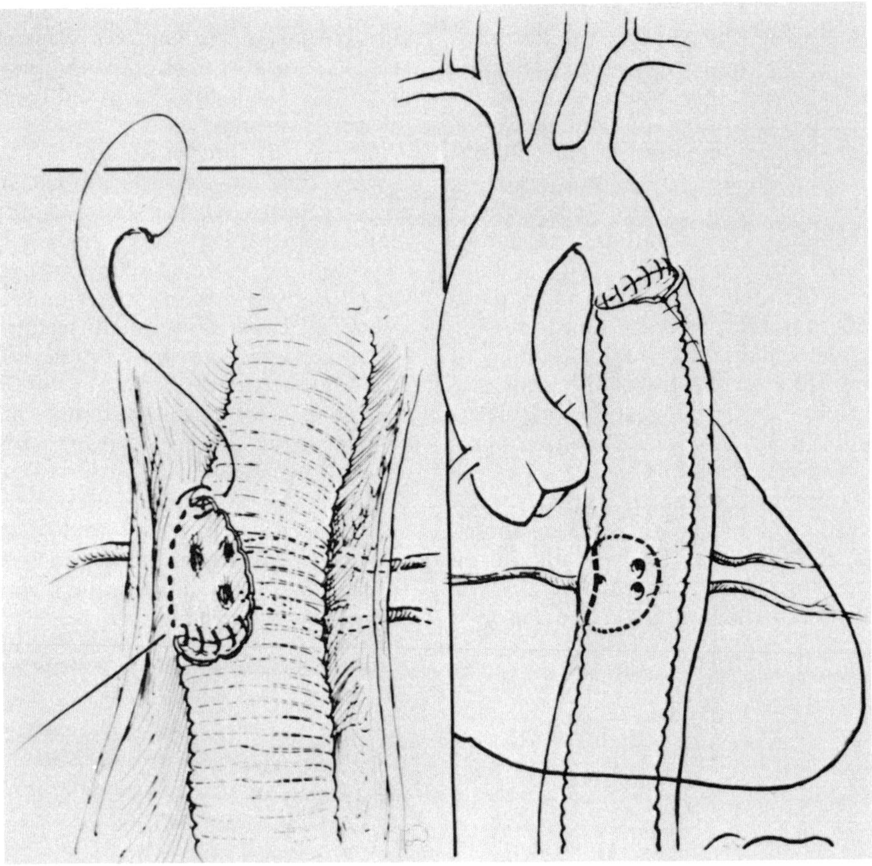

Figure 8.7. Intraoperative technique which may be used to preserve the integrity of the spinal cord arterial supply. Large intercostal arteries are not ligated.

routine angiography of the cord is not warranted because the risk of paraplegia is less than 2% with surgery. Other noninvasive methods have not been helpful in assessing cord blood flow.

Intraoperative spinal cord monitoring is used by some orthopedic surgeons during the surgery of kyphoscoliosis. In these patients stimuli are applied to the distal extremities, and potentials evoked by the stimuli in the brain are monitored with an electroencephalogram. Abnormalities in impulse transmission generated by pressure on the cord are reflected as abnormalities in the electroencephalographic tracing.

As previously described, the gross sensations used to stimulate the lower extremity which then produce electroencephalographic potentials are not specific enough to monitor anterior spinal cord function. Since gross sensations are carried in the dorsal columns of the spinal cord, anterior spinal cord ischemia could go undetected using the current techniques. In the future, specific peripheral stimuli simulating light or superficial touch which are carried in the anterior portion of the spinal cord may be used to evoke brain potentials and, therefore, may be used to monitor anterior spinal cord ischemic events which occur intraoperatively.

CEREBRAL DYSFUNCTION

Brain injury during descending aortic surgery is due to either embolization, arterial hypotension, or intracranial hypertension. Cerebral emboli may originate from proximal cannulation sites or from the atheroma dislodged by clamps placed near the left carotid artery. Palpation of the left superficial temporal pulse can detect inadvertent occlusion of the left carotid artery. Systemic air emboli may occur during left ventricular or ascending aortic cannulation. Arterial hypotension can occur during rapid release of the cross clamp of the aorta. Greater than 10 minutes may be necessary during the release of the clamp to preserve systemic pressure.[14] Rapid resumption of distal flow often produces arterial hypotension which, combined with acute acid washout from the periphery, can produce cardiac arrest.

Patients who require careful anesthetic and surgical management are those with associated aortic and brain injury. This combination of injuries is increasing in frequency in trauma centers. Currently, between 500 and 1000 patients are treated for it yearly in the United States. The hypertension associated with aortic injury in these patients can contribute to the brain injury. During surgical repair, proximal hypertension is often exacerbated by aortic clamping. Systemic heparinization is an additional risk in the presence of cerebral contusion. Additionally, patient position on the operating room table may compromise venous drainage from the brain and raise intracranial pressure (Fig. 8.8) and increase brain ischemia.

In the normal brain, the acute arterial hypertension associated with aortic occlusion is well tolerated. In patients with an aortic injury associated with a brain injury, acute aortic occlusion can cause a precipitous rise in the intracranial pressure. As seen in Figure 8.9, gradually increasing increments of intracranial volume are well tolerated until a critical value is reached. When this critical value is reached and displaceable fluid no longer exists inside the central nervous system compartment, any additional increase in volume causes a dramatic rise in the intracranial pressure. To maintain normal cerebral perfusion pressure (CNSPP = BP − ICP), it is essential to monitor the intracranial pressure. This can

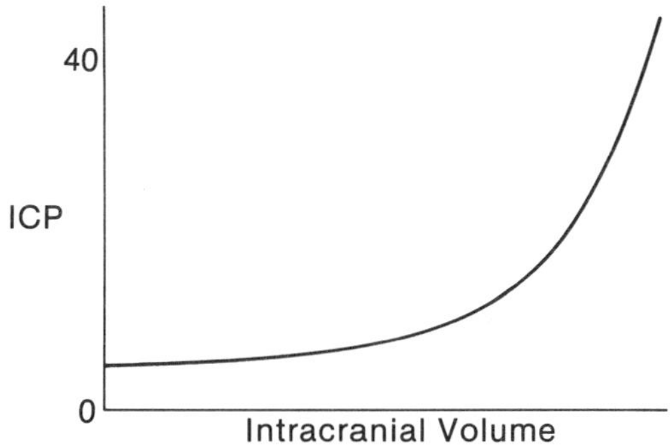

Figure 8.9. Intracranial volume can increase with only a small rise in the intracranial pressure until the buffering capacity of the displaceable intracranial volume is spent. Then a small increment in volume will produce a dramatic rise in pressure.

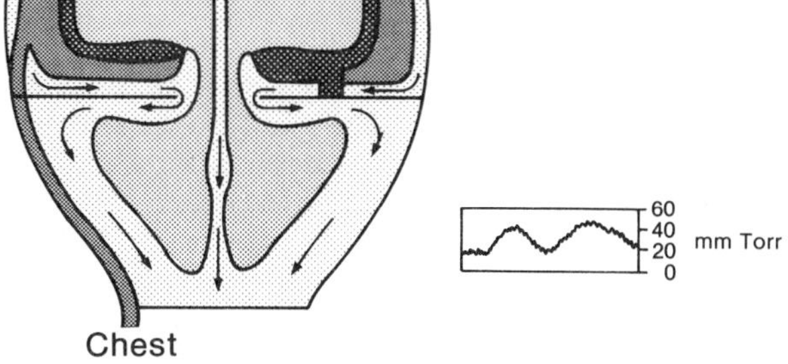

Figure 8.8. Impairment of cerebral venous drainage by improper head positioning and use of positive end-expiratory pressure can increase intracranial pressure.

be easily done with a subdural bolt, an epidural transducer, or a ventriculostomy needle or catheter.[15] The ventriculostomy needle provides a means to remove cerebrospinal fluid to reduce intracranial pressure. Maintenance of a central nervous system perfusion pressure of 50 mm Hg or greater is essential if cerebral ischemia is to be avoided. Intracranial hypertension can usually be reduced by hyperventilating the patient and maintaining a pCO_2 of 25–40 mm Hg. The simultaneous intravenous administration of mannitol and dexamethasone is also beneficial. Barbiturate administration reduces the metabolic rate of the brain and hence reduces cerebral blood flow requirements and may prevent cerebral ischemic injury. Venous pressure can be lowered by keeping the patient's head in a nondependent position and avoiding positive end expiratory pressure.[16] It is important to recognize that the venous pressure in the right atrium may be normal, but the jugular veins may be kinked at the neck due to improper head positioning. The small increase in intracranial volume produced by increased venous pressure in a patient with intracranial hypertension can cause an abrupt rise in intracranial pressure. It is also important in these patients to avoid systolic pressure greater than 160 mm Hg. As the pressure exceeds 160 mm Hg, the autoregulation of cerebral flow ceases and the blood flow becomes linearly related to presssure. At high arterial pressures, the brain is no longer protected from edema formation, and the small increment in nondisplaceable intracranial volume in the form of edema fluid can produce large increases in intracranial pressure, causing cerebral ischemia.[2] Other goals in managing these patients should be to avoid hypoxemia, to keep the arterial oxygen saturation greater than 85%, and to avoid systemic acidosis. Maintenance of a pH between 7.4 and 7.5 is optimal.

Cerebral vasodilators should not be used in patients with a cerebral injury and upper extremity hypertension. Halothane,[16] nitroprusside,[17] and hydralazine[18] are potent cerebral vasodilators and predispose the brain to edema formation. Use of these drugs in patients with brain injury can be harmful. Some systemic antihypertensives which can be used are propranolol (Inderal) and trimethaphan camsylate (Arfonad). When general anesthesia is required, the agents used should be those that have a minimal effect on the brain. Thiopental acts favorably by reducing the oxygen consumption of neural tissue and is an ideal drug in this situation. Nitrous oxide is an excellent inhalant amnestic agent for use with brain injury but is not a sufficiently potent anesthetic agent to use for general purposes. Since it must be used at high partial pressure and, therefore, with low inspired oxygen partial pressure, its use in hypoxic trauma patients may be contraindicated. Muscle relaxants may be used as needed. Another excellent group of drugs to use in these patients is opiates. Both morphine and fentanyl have a minimal effect on cerebral vasculature.

Since pharmacologic manipulation of blood pressure may represent a liability to the brain, another method of reducing upper extremity hypertension associated with aortic occlusion which can be safely used is some form of extravascular conduit. The three techniques used to reduce the hemodynamic impact of acute aortic occlusion are: left heart bypass, femoral-femoral bypass, and passive shunt (Fig. 8.10). Using left heart bypass, the cannula is usually inserted into the left atrium and the drainage is infused into the femoral artery. This offers the advantage of having immediate control of the blood pressure and eliminates the necessity for using an oxygenator. This technique has been applied using nonthrombogenic tubing, thereby avoiding systemic heparinization and making it ideal for use in trauma patients with cerebral injuries.[19] The right ventricular outflow tract can be cannulated and left heart bypass can be effected in this manner. The advantage of cannulating the right ventricular outflow tract is that total cardiopulmonary bypass can be readily instituted if needed. The primary liability is that an oxygenator and, hence, heparin must be used. Femoral-femoral bypass has been used clinically in large series. It provides the advantage of being a good means of closed chest resuscitation of a patient in hypovolemic shock. One group used nonthrombogenic tubing and drained blood from the right atrium and reinfused it into the femoral artery with good results in 10 patients.[20] With the patient ventilated with

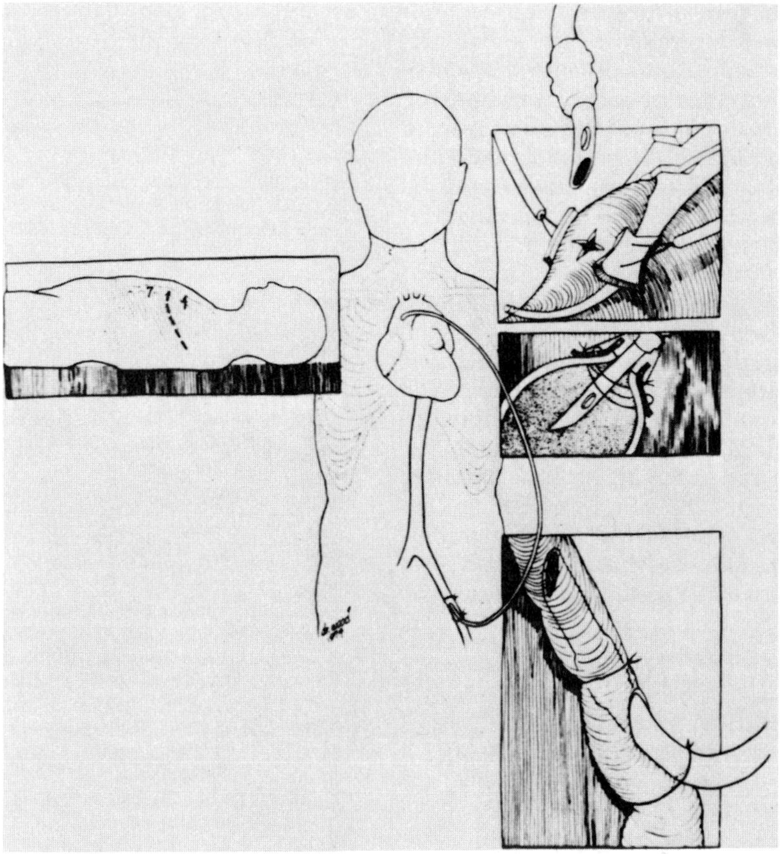

Figure 8.10. A technique for inserting a large passive extravascular shunt. (Reproduced with permission from: W. Nylander et al.[7])

100% oxygen, saturation of the infused arterial blood was 70%. An additional advantage of femoral-femoral bypass is that it is easily converted to total cardiopulmonary bypass.

The most popular technique is the use of heparin-embedded passive shunt.[21–27] The mean distal aortic blood pressure can be kept near normal with the properly placed large internal diameter shunt.[28] Two sizes are available. The smaller 7.5-mm internal diameter shunt should not be used to repair the descending aorta because the transmitted flow is too low. During descending aortic surgery, the larger 9.5-mm internal diameter shunt should always be used. Proximal cannulation can be the apex of the left ventricle, the ascending aorta, or the left subclavian artery. Cannulation of the left subclavian artery may cause an iatrogenic subclavian steal to occur. Since the anterior spinal artery often is a branch of the vertebral artery which originates from the subclavian artery, the steal may create spinal cord ischemia in the cervical region. It is therefore not advisable to use the subclavian artery in these patients. Furthermore, the subclavian artery is often close to the site of aortic disease and therefore must be excluded from the arterial circulation by the vascular clamp. The apex to the left ventricle is easily cannulated. Because the passive shunt has no valve in it, a hemodynamic state similar to aortic insufficiency is produced. The regurgitant fraction from the large shunt has been shown to be about 15%. Occasionally, in patients with metabolic abnormalities, cannulation of the ventricular apex can produce ventricular fibrillation. The third proximal cannulation site is the ascending aorta. This offers the advantages of providing a higher diastolic pressure and avoiding the 15% regurgitant flow into the ventricle. Because of these two phenomena, the flow is 30% greater in shunts originating from the ascending aorta.[29] The advantage of the shunt is that no systemic heparinization is needed and aortic decompression is effective. Blood loss during surgery using a shunt can be recovered using autotransfusion techniques.

Distal insertion sites for the shunts are the femoral arteries or the supradiaphragmatic descending aorta. If the supradiaphragmatic aorta is used, one should not be tempted to use the similar diameter shunt. Mean pressure drop across the large caliber passive shunt is 35 mm Hg, with a large range between 5 and 70.[28] Because of this large range, it is important to monitor a distal aortic pressure to be sure that a mean distal pressure 50 mm Hg is maintained.

CONCLUSION

Surgery in the descending aorta was initially performed using simple aortic occlusion. Because of the high incidence of paraplegia, the technique changed gradually to include mechanical manipulation of the vascular system. Recently, a trend toward simple aortic occlusion became again evident.[14, 30, 31] Because no conclusion can be drawn from the available literature regarding the relationship of paraplegia to aortic occlusion, one must attempt to avoid spinal cord ischemia by applying current anatomic and physiologic knowledge to the care of the patient. Today these considerations should prompt the surgeon to mechanically support the distal circulation during aortic occlusion if the distal aortic pressure is less than 50 mm Hg. In the cases of combined brain and aortic injuries, careful monitoring of the central nervous system perfusion pressure is essential.

Avoidance of cerebral edema by careful attention to the types of drugs used during surgery and the maintenance of a normal systemic arterial pressure while maintaining a normal cerebral perfusion pressure are critical. By using the described principles during the care of patients with descending aortic disease, the incidence and severity of central nervous system injury can be minimized.

References

1. Brewer LA, III, Fosburg RG, Mulder GA, Verska JJ: Spinal cord complications following surgery for coarctation of the aorta. A study of 66 cases. J Thorac and Cardiovasc Surg 64:368, 1972.
2. Marshall WJS, Jackson JLF, Langfitt TW: Brain swelling caused by trauma and arterial hypertension. Arch Neurol 21:545, 1969.
3. Forster A, Horn KV, Marshall LF, Shapiro HM: Influence of anesthetic agents on blood-brain barrier function during acute hypertension. Acta Neurol 56 (64):60–61, 1977.
4. Blaisdell FW, Cooley DA: The mechanism of paraplegia after temporary thoracic aortic occlusion and its relationship to spinal fluid pressure. Surgery 51: 351, 1962.
5. Crawford ES, Palamara AE, Saleh SA, Roehm JOF Jr: Aortic aneurysm: Current status of surgical treatment. Surg Clin North Am 59:597, 1979.
6. Owens JC, Prevedel AE, Swan H: Prolonged experimental occlusion of the thoracic aorta during hypothermia. Arch Surg 70:95, 1955.
7. Nylander W, Hammon J, Oldfield E, Plunkett R, Meacham W: Pharmacologic Modification of Spinal Cord Ischemia in the Dog. (Abstract presented at The Society of Thoracic Surgeons Meeting January 27, 1981).
8. Gobbel WG Jr, Dalton JB, Taylor WL, Scott HW Jr, Carlson RI: Beneficial effects of inferior vena caval occlusion when the thoracic aorta is occluded. Surg Forum 8:406, 1957.
9. Myamoto K, Ueno A, Wada T, Kimoto S: A new and simple method of preventing spinal cord damage following temporary occlusion of the thoracic aorta by draining the cerebrospinal fluid. J Cardiovasc Surg 1:188, 1960.
10. Hägerdal M, Welsh FA, Keykhah MM, Perez E, Harp JR: Protective effectives of combinations of hypothermia and barbiturates in cerebral hypoxia in the rat. Anesthesiology 49:165, 1978.
11. Adamkiewicz A: Die blutgefasse des mensch lichen ruckenmarkes. I. Teil. Die gefasse der ruckenmarksubstanz. II. Tiel. Die gefasse der Ruckenmarkoberflache. Sitz Akad Wissenshaften Wien Math Natur Klass 84:469, 1882; 85:101, 1882.
12. Hughes RK, Reemtsma K: Correction of coarctation of the aorta. Manometric determination of safety during test occlusion. J Thorac Cardiovasc Surg 62: 31, 1971.
13. Harrington DP, Barth KH, White RI Jr, Brawley RK: Traumatic pseudonaneurysm of the thoracic aorta in close proximity to the anterior spinal artery: A therapeutic dilemma. Surgery 87:153, 1980.
14. Najafi H, Javid H, Hunter J, Serry C, Monson D: Descending aortic aneurysmectomy without adjuncts to avoid ischemia. Ann Thorac Surg 30:326, 1980.
15. James HE, Bruno L, Shapiro H, Levitt JD, Aidinis S, Langfitt TW, Shalna E: Methodology for intraven-

tricular and subarachnoid continuous recording of intracranial pressure in clinical practice. Acta Neurochir 33:45, 1976.
16. Aidinis SJ, Lafferty J, Shapiro HM: Intracranial responses to PEEP. Anesthesiology 45:275, 1976.
17. Gagnon RL, Marsh ML, Smith RW, Shapiro HM: Intracranial hypertension caused by nitroglycerin. Anesthesiology 51:86–87, 1979.
18. Overgaard J, Shinhøj E: A paradoxical cerebral hemodynamic effect of hydralazine. Stroke 6:402–404, 1975.
19. Connolly JE, Wakabayashi A, German JC, Stemmer, EA, Serres, EJ: Clinical experience with pulsatile left heart bypass without anticoagulation for thoracic aneurysms. J Thorac Cardiovasc Surg 62:568, 1971.
20. May IA, Ecker RR, Iverson LIG: Heparinless femoral venoarterial bypass with an oxygenator for surgery on the descending thoracic aorta. J Thorac Cardiovasc Surg 73:387, 1977.
21. Krause AH, Ferguson TB, Weldon CS: Thoracic aneurysmectomy utilizing the TDMAC-heparin shunt. Ann Thorac Surg 14:123, 1972.
22. Donahoo JS, Brawley RK, Gott VL: The heparin-coated vascular shunt for thoracic aortic and great vessel procedures: A ten-year experience. Ann Thorac Surg 23:507, 1977.
23. Gott VL: Heparinized shunts for thoracic vascular operations. Ann Thorac Surg 14:219, 1972.
24. Valiathan MS, Weldon CS, Bender HW Jr, Topaz SR, Gott VL: Resection of aneurysms of the descending thoracic aorta using a GBH-coated shunt bypass. J Surg Res 8:197, 1968.
25. Lawrence GH, Hessel EA, Sauvage LR, Krause AH: Results of the use of the TDMAC-heparin shunt in the surgery of aneurysms of the descending thoracic aorta. J Thorac Cardiovasc Surg 73:393, 1977.
26. Cukingnan RA, Fee HJ, Carey JS: Repair of lesions of the descending thoracic aorta with the TDMAC-heparin shunt. J Thorac Cardiovasc Surg 75:227, 1978.
27. Lawrence GH, Hessel EA, Sauvage LR, Krause AH: Results of the use of the TDMAC heparin shunt in the surgery of aneurysms of the descending thoracic aorta. J Thorac Cardiovasc Surg 73:393, 1977.
28. Kouchoukos NT, Lell WA, Karp RB, Samuelson PN: Hemodynamic effects of aortic clamping and decompression with a temporary shunt for resection of the descending thoracic aorta. Surgery 85:25, 1979.
29. Wechsler AS, Wolfe WG: Heparinless shunting during cross-clamping of the thoracic aorta. Ann Thorac Surg 23:497, 1977.
30. Crawford ES, Rubio PA: Reappraisal to avoid ischemia in the treatment of aneurysms of descending thoracic aorta. J Thorac Cardiovasc Surg 66:693, 1973.
31. Appelbaum A, Karp RB, Kirklin JW: Surgical treatment for closed thoracic aortic injuries. J Thorac Cardiovasc Surg 71:458, 1976.

CHAPTER 9

COAGULATION ABNORMALITIES WITH CARDIOPULMONARY BYPASS

JOHN A. YOUNG, M.D.

The severe hematologic and coagulation abnormalities associated with cardiopulmonary bypass[1-3] have become less frequent and severe. Factors which have contributed to this improvement include: better oxygenator and perfusion equipment, the improved training of clinical perfusionists, use of moderate hypothermia, hemodilution, reduced flow rates, frequent monitoring of metabolic parameters, and a more rational use of heparin and protamine. The purpose of this review is to review the effects of cardiopulmonary bypass on normal coagulation mechanisms by emphasizing how the coagulation system reacts to contact with the thrombogenic surface of the extracorporeal circuit.

THE COAGULATION SYSTEM

Although many aspects of the coagulation system are interdependent, coagulation is best understood by reviewing the components of it, as well as the commonly used tests for evaluating its integrity. These components and tests are summarized in Figure 9.1.

Clot Formation

The chemical events leading to a fibrin clot begin with the surface activation of Factor 12 by any nonendothelial surface, such as exposed collagen following vascular trauma, or the extracorporeal circuit during cardiopulmonary bypass. Activated Factor 12 is the enzyme for the substrate procoagulant of Factor 11, converting it to its enzymatically active form. This process continues with the sequential enzymatic conversion of each of the procoagulant substrates into the enzyme necessary for the activation of the next procoagulant substrate. Factor 12 activates Factor 11, which activates Factor 9; Factor 9 activates Factor 8, which activates Factor 10, the first step in the final, or common pathway of coagulation. This part of the coagulation system is referred to as the slow pathway, the intrinsic or intravascular system.[4, 5]

Activation of Factor 10, can also be accomplished by a shorter pathway, referred to as the extrinsic or extravascular system.[5] It depends on the activation of Factor 7 by tissue thromboplastins, including tissue factor and tissue phospholipid.

Factor 10, which can be activated by both Factor 8 of the intrinsic system and Factor 7 of the extrinsic system, activates Factor 5 to the prothrombin converting principle which catalyzes the conversion of prothrombin to thrombin. Thrombin (Factor 2) catalyzes the enzymatic cleavage of the fibrinopeptide side arms of the fibrinogen molecule, leaving behind soluble fibrin monomer, which polymerizes and is stabilized by Factor 13, the fibrin stabilizing factor, forming an insoluble fibrin clot.

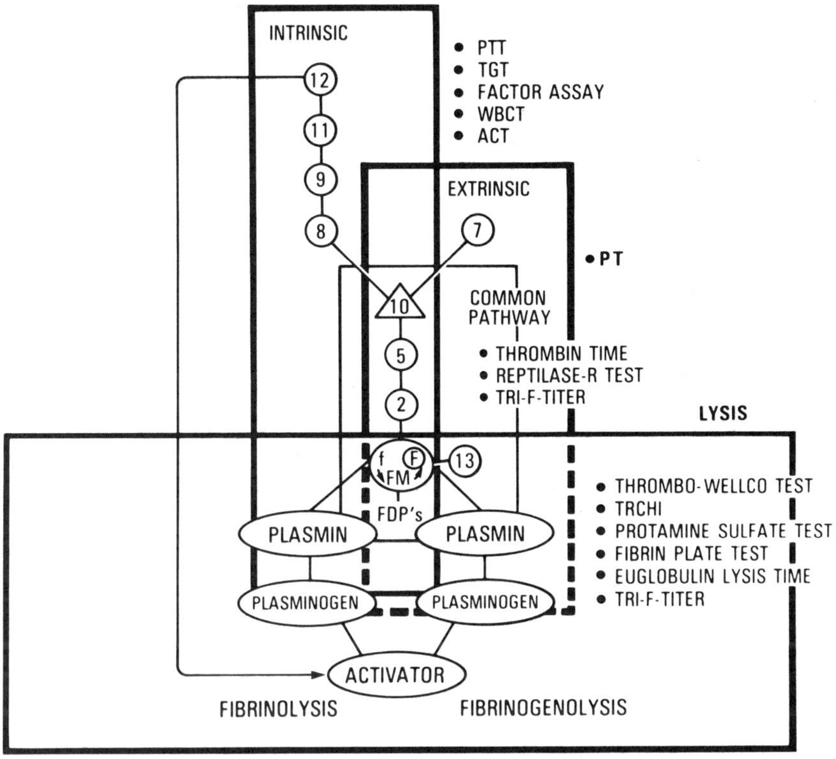

Figure 9.1. Schematic representation of coagulation lysis and coagulation function studies. *f*, fibrinogen; *FM*, fibrin monomer; *F*, fibrin; *FDP*, fibrin degradation products. The rapid and specific evaluation of postperfusion coagulation abnormalities requires the selection and evaluation, usually of a combination of some of these commonly used tests.

Clot Lysis

Clot lysis occurs when the enzymatically inert plasminogen molecule is activated to its proteolytically active form, plasmin, by plasminogen activator substances.[6] Plasmin is an enzyme capable of digesting not only fibrin, but also fibrinogen, the procoagulant forms of Factors 2, 5, 8, and several other proteins, including glucagon, ACTH, and growth hormones.[7–9] The mechanisms controlling plasminogen activation are either coagulation dependent, for which the term secondary fibrinolysis is used, or coagulation independent, for which the term primary fibrinogenolysis is used.[10] Fibrinolysis and fibrinogenolysis may be compensated or uncompensated. Hyperfibrinolysis and fibrinogenolysis refer to uncompensated lysis and imply that a pathologic imbalance exists between lysis and coagulation.

Secondary Fibrinolysis

Fibrinolysis commences with the activation of Factor 12, which activates the Fletcher Factor activator (prekellikrein activator). It in turn activates Hageman cofactor (Factor 12 cofactor, more recently name the plasminogen proactivator) to become the plasminogen activator.[8] Plasminogen, which is enzymatically inert, has a high affinity for fibrin. When a fibrin clot forms, circulating plasminogen attaches to fibrin polymer, where it is in position to digest fibrin when activated to plasmin (Fig. 9.2). Fibrinolysis may be localized intravascularly, as in venous thrombosis, or disseminated intravascularly, as in disseminated intravascular coagulation (DIC). Fibrinolysis may also occur extravascularly at the site of an undrained clot, such as the bladder following prostate surgery, the hemithorax if blood is not evacuated follow-

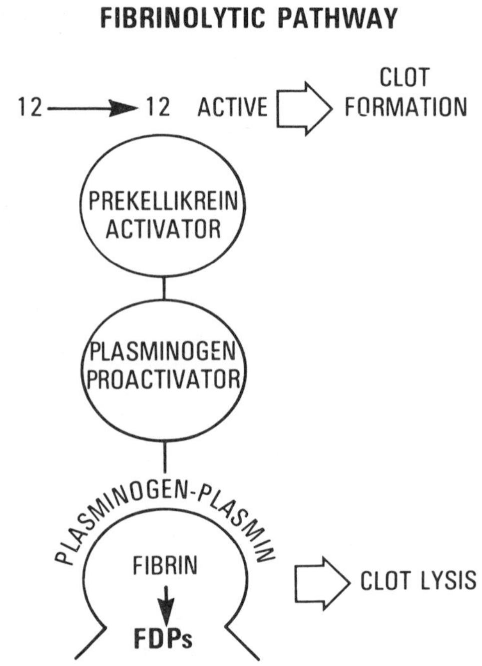

Figure 9.2. Schematic representation of coagulation-dependent fibrinolytic pathway.

ing trauma or surgery, and around the heart in the pericardial sac following open heart surgery. If the clot forms intravascularly, fibrinolysis results in the liberation of fibrin degradation products into the circulation. If the clot forms extravascularly, fibrin degradation products are not liberated freely into the circulation. In both intravascular fibrinolysis, coagulation factors are consumed and circulating plasminogen levels decrease since plasminogen is absorbed by clot. Circulating plasmin levels should be normal or only slightly elevated, since the site of plasminogen activation and conversion to plasmin occurs within the fibrin clot.[7, 10] High circulating plasmin activity is not characteristic of fibrinolysis.

When clot lysis exceeds clot formation, an uncompensated or hyperfibrinolytic state exists. An example of this is the hemophiliac, who begins to bleed. The fibrinolytic system is normal in the hemophiliac, but a hyperfibrinolytic state exists, compared with the feeble ability to form clots. Clotting and clot lysis are not balanced. Treatment involves the administration of missing coagulation factors to improve the ability to form clots, as well as an antifibrinolytic agent, such as ϵ- aminocaproic acid to suppress fibrinolysis and bring into balance clotting and clot lysis.[11] The hemophilia analogy may apply to some patients following cardiopulmonary bypass if clotting factors have been consumed or depleted by excessive coagulation at the blood-pump interface due to inadequate heparinization. As the clotting system is being depleted, the fibrinolytic system is being activated by coagulation, and a potentially imbalanced or hyperfibrinolytic state may result. Restoration of a normal balance depends on the elimination of the thrombogenic stimulus, the extracorporeal circuit, and the replacement of coagulation factors. In more severe cases, antifibrinolytic agents may also be indicated to bring clotting and clot lysis into balance.[11, 12]

DIC is a coagulopathy frequently referred to in the perfusion literature.[13–15] The primary pathophysiology in DIC is intravascular hypercoaguability, although hypocoaguability and bleeding result from factor consumption and secondary fibrinolysis. Bleeding, the end result of factor consumption and clot lysis is further exacerbated by the presence of circulating fibrin degradation products, which have anticoagulant properties.

The temporary treatment of DIC involves the administration of heparin and fresh clotting factors; however, survival depends on the elimination of the primary stimulus for clotting. Antibibrinolytic drugs, such as ϵ-aminocaproic acid, are contraindicated during active DIC before the elimination of the stimulus for clotting.

Despite frequent references to its existence, there has never been a well-documented case of DIC resulting directly from cardiopulmonary bypass. Inadequate anticoagulation during cardiopulmonary bypass (extracorporeal intravascular hypercoagulability) associated with active coagulation, factor consumption, and secondary fibrinolysis, however, may occur, producing a coagulopathy similar to DIC.[16–18]

Primary Fibrinogenolysis

Fibrinogenolysis involves the primary activation of circulating plasminogen to plasmin. The mechanisms involved in the direct activation of plasminogen are less well understood than for fibrinolysis but may include release of thromboplastic tissue substances into the circulation and disruption of vascular endothelium rich in plasminogen activator substances. Ischemia is thought to be a particularly potent stimulator of plasminogen activation; however, shivering and peripheral vasoconstriction, as well as vigorous exercise, are also strong nonspecific activators of the plasminogen-plasmin system.[8] Fibrinogenolysis is not dependent on coagulation for activation. The most extreme example of fibrinogenolysis is the defibrinogenation that occurs following electrocution. Circulating plasminogen is completely and instantaneously activated, and no fibrinogen can be detected in the blood. Compensated fibrinogenolysis, as well as uncompensated hyperfibrinogenolysis, occur.[10]

Whether or not fibrinolysis and/or fibrinogenolysis occur during and following cardiopulmonary bypass has been debated.[13, 19] It seems clear, however, that both can and do occur in both compensated and uncompensated forms.[10, 12, 20–28] The perfusion circuit, as well as alterations of peripheral vascular physiology during cardiopulmonary bypass, represent mechanisms responsible for the activation of fibrinolysis and fibrinogenolysis (Fig. 9.3), although the relative frequency and importance of each during and following cardiopulmonary bypass remain to be determined.[27–29] It is important to recognize that anticoagulation during cardiopulmonary bypass will be either adequate or inadequate. When anticoagulation is adequate, primary fibrinogenolysis may occur depending on the release of activator substances into the circulation. Active coagulation and substantial factor consumption should not occur, and secondary fibrinolysis will not be stimulated. When anticoagulation is inadequate, coagulation occurs at the blood-pump interface, resulting in coagulation factor consumption and secondary fibrinolysis. A severe coagulopathy can result if primary fibrinogenolysis by mechanisms other than coagulation has also been strongly stimulated.[10, 26] Adequate anticoagulation during cardiopulmonary bypass is therefore, essential and should be defined as the point at which the coagulation time is sufficiently prolonged so as to eliminate the activation of coagulation when the blood comes in contact with the inherently thrombogenic surface of extracorporeal circuit.

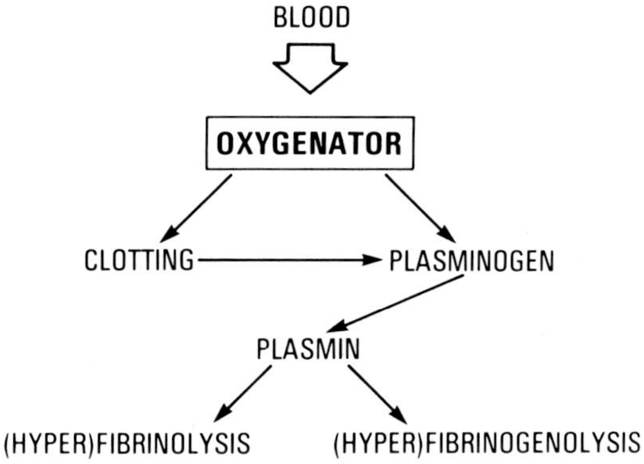

Figure 9.3. Fibrinolysis and fibrinogenolysis may be stimulated by the interface of blood with the extracorporeal circuit and the physiologic alterations associated with bypass. Hyperlysis implies an imbalance between the ability to form clots and the strength of the lytic process. *FDP*, fibrin degradation products.

COAGULATION FUNCTION TESTS

A rudimentary knowledge of the currently used and frequently referred to methods for evaluating the coagulation system in the pre- and postoperative period is helpful (Fig. 9.1).

Coagulation Times: Whole Blood Coagulation Time (WBCT) and Activated Clotting Time (ACT)

The whole blood coagulation time, or Lee-White method, was one of the first tests used to assess the integrity of the coagulation system.[30, 31] All subsequent tests of coagulation involving surface contact with a glass surface are a variation of this test. Technique is important and care must be taken not to aspirate tissue thromboplastin at the time of venipuncture. Clotting begins with the activation of Factor 12 by the glass surface of the test tube. It is not a particularly sensitive test, but it will detect severe defects involving Factors 12, 11, 9, and 8, as well as defects of the common pathway. Abnormal coagulation time is 10–15 minutes. The whole blood coagulation time will also be prolonged in the presence of circulating anticoagulants such as heparin and fibrin degradation products.

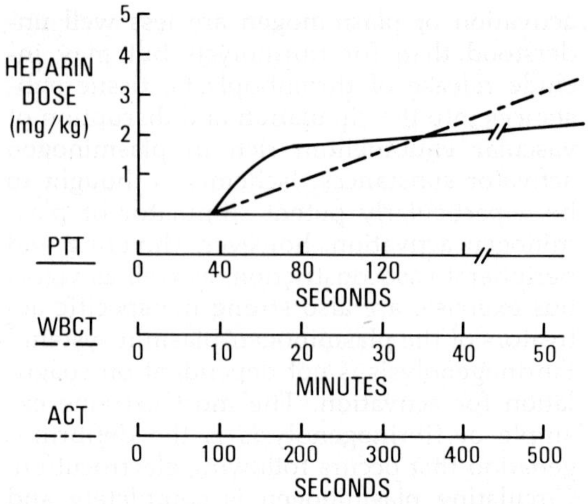

Figure 9.4. The graph represents the difference between the heparin dose-response curves using the parital thromboplastin time (*PTT, solid line*), the whole blood coagulaton time and the activated coagulation time (*WBCT, dashed line*). The disadvantage of the *PTT* for measuring heparin effect is the exponential dose-response. The advantage of activated clotting time (*ACT*) is that a straight line dose-response exists that is similar to the WBCT but the time is measured in seconds rather than minutes. Heparin half-life can be measured from both the *WBCT* and *ACT*, but not from the *PTT*.

Historically, the WBCT has been used to monitor heparin effect, since a straight line dose-response relation exists between the heparin concentration and the coagulation time.[32–34] Its use during open heart surgery is limited by the time required to ensure that the coagulation time is sufficiently prolonged—about four times normal or between 40 and 50 minutes. The activated clotting time (ACT), developed by Hattersley, is a variation of the whole blood coagulation time. Clotting is accelerated about 10 times by the addition of diatomaceous earth.[35] A straight line dose-response relation also exists between the amount of heparin administered and the prolongation of the ACT.[36] Heparin half-life, necessary to calculate supplemental heparin dosage with time, can also be computed from the dose-response curves of the WBCT and the ACT.[36] This is not true of any of the other heparin-sensitive coagulation tests which will be discussed[37] (Fig. 9.4).

Partial Thromboplastin Time

The partial thromboplastin time (PTT) was developed to identify abnormalities existing in the intrinsic system.[38, 39] Since the end point for the PTT is a fibrin clot, it also depends on an intact common pathway. The PTT is performed in a glass tube by combining citrated plasma with calcium (to reverse the citrate effect) and a procoagulant, which completely activates Factor 12. If the test is normal, then it can be assumed that there are no significant abnormalities that exist in the intrinsic and the common pathways. If the PTT is abnormal, other tests are necesssary to identify the specific defect, which may exist either in the intrinsic system or the common pathway. The PTT is very sensitive to heparin, as well as other circulating anticoagulants, such as fibrin degradation products. Although the PTT is commonly used to monitor heparin therapy, it is not a good test for this purpose since the heparin dose-PTT response curve is exponential and accurate in a semilinear fashion only at heparin levels far below those required for cardiopulmonary bypass.[32] At higher doses corresponding to a coagulation time 4 times that which is normal, the partial thromboplastin time is always infinite. Even at lower doses corresponding to the semilinear portion of the PTT heparin dose-response curve, the prolongation of the PTT does not correspond with either the whole blood coagulation time or the ACT[32] (Fig. 9.4). The PTT, however, is an important method for diagnosing coagulation defects preoperatively and provides essential information in combination with other tests for evaluating the postoperative coagulation status.[10, 12]

Prothrombin Time

The one-stage prothrombin time (PT), or "Quick" test (40), is used to measure the integrity of the extrinsic system, which involves only Factor 7.[41] It also depends on the integrity of the common pathway since, as in the PTT, the end point measured by the prothrombin time is fibrin clot formation.

The PT is performed in a manner similar to that of the PTT, except that a tissue thromboplastin is combined with citrated plasma and calcium. The tissue thromboplastin activates Factor 7 bypassing the intrinsic system. The PT is also very sensitive to heparin and other circulating anticoagulants which affect the common pathway.

If either the PT or the PTT is normal, then it follows that the common pathway is intact. If the PT alone is abnormal, then Factor 7 is deficient. If the PTT alone is abnormal, then Factors 12, 11, 9, or 8 may be deficient.

Thromboplastin Generation Time

The expanded partial thromboplastin time or thromboplastin generation time (TGT) should be done if the PT is normal, but the PTT is abnormal. This test was designed to identify specific abnormalities in the intrinsic system involving Factors 8 and 9.[42] The test is performed with two samples of the patient's citrated plasma. Aged serum (missing Factors 1, 5, and 8) is added to the first tube, and absorbed plasma (missing Factors, 2, 7, 9, and 10) is added to the second tube. Calcium is added to both tubes. If the aged serum corrects the clotting abnormality, then Factor 9 is deficient. If absorbed plasma results in normal clotting, and the PT is normal, then Factor 8 is deficient. Since Factors 11 and 12 are added to each of the tubes, this test will not identify deficiencies in these factors. The TGT, like the PT and PTT, is sensitive to circulating anticoagulants. Although this test is important in the preoperative evaluation of patients with an abnormal coagulation profile, it is of little value in the postoperfusion assessment of coagulation defects when the question to be answered is rarely whether Factor 8 or Factor 9 specifically is deficient.

Thrombin Time

If both the PT and the PTT are abnormal, the thrombin time (TT) may be used to identify quantitative as well as qualitative fibrinogen defects.[43] The TT is performed by adding calcium and purified thrombin to citrated plasma. Both the intrinsic and extrinsic pathways are bypassed, as well as the upper portion of the common pathway. In the absence of an anticoagulant, the thrombin time will be prolonged in proportion to decreasing amounts of fibrinogen substrate. A normal TT indicates the absence of significant hypofibrinogenemia, dysfibrinogenemia (as can occur in polycythemic conditions), fibrinolysis, and fibrin degradation products. The TT will be prolonged by circulating anticoagulants such as heparin, which blocks the effect of thrombin on fibrinogen, and by fibrin degradation products, which inhibit the polymerization of fibrin monomers. The Reptilase-R time and protamine corrected thrombin time are both variations of the TT developed to improve the specificity of this test.

Purifed snake venom is substituted for thrombin in the Reptilase-R (Abbott Laboratories, North Chicago, Ill.). The Reptilase-R time is not affected by heparin but will be prolonged by significant hypofibrinogenemia or elevated fibrin degradation products. An abnormal TT and a normal Reptilase-R time means that heparin is the most likely circulating anticoagulant, that fibrin degradation products are not significantly elevated, and that the fibrinogen level is not severely depressed.

The protamine corrected thrombin time, in which protamine sulfate is added to reverse heparin effect, can be used in place of the Reptilase-R time test. While normalization of the TT by the addition of protamine is presumptive evidence that significance circulating heparin is present, it shoudl be noted that protamine sulfate inhibits the anticoagulant effects of fibrin degradation products and may obscure the effect of significant levels of fibrin degradation products, which can result in a prolonged TT. If either the PT or the PTT are normal, then there is probably no need to perform a TT since both the PT and PTT depend on an intact common pathway.

TEST OF LYSIS

Although there are many tests for measuring plasmin activity either directly or indirectly, circumspection is necesssary for their use in the assessment of open heart patients. Interpretation of the significance of these tests, one or more of which are frequently positive during and following cardiopulmonary bypass, is difficult since little or no correlation exists between a positive test and postoperative bleeding.[12, 18, 29, 44] Furthermore, each test measures highly specific aspects of the fibrinolytic process, and virtually no comparison can be made between the results of one test and another.[12, 45]

Thrombo-Wellcotest

The Thrombo-Wellco Test Kit (Latex Agglutination Kit, Burroughs-Wellcome Laboratory, Research Triangle Park, N. C.), or latex agglutination method, is the most popular method for assaying the presence of circulating fibrin degradation products. It is, therefore, a measure of the end results on intravascular plasmin activity but does not distinguish between fibrinolysis and fibrinogenolysis. Fibrin degradation products in excess of 10 μg/ml are evidence of significant lysis.[46] The tanned red cell hemagglutination inhibition test (TRCHI), using commercially available reagents, correlates closely with the latex fixation method and is also frequently used to measure fibrin degradation products following open heart surgery.[47] Although the Thrombo-Wellco and TRCHI are often positive during and following cardiopulmonary bypass, no correlation exists between bleeding and a positive test.[12, 26, 44] These tests are very sensitive for circulating fibrin degradation products and can also be elevated in a variety of general surgical procedures not involving cardiopulmonary bypass. The significance of elevated fibrin degradation products following cardiopulmonary bypass is uncertain.

Fibrin Plate Test

The fibrin plate test assesses the presence of circulating plasminogen, plasminogen activator, and plasmin and distinguishes between fibrinolysis and fibrinogenolysis.[48] In fibrinogenolysis, circulating plasminogen is decreased, and plasminogen activator and plasmin activity are increased. In fibrinolysis, plasminogen is decreased. A positive fibrin plate test is good evidence for fibrinogenolysis. The test can be interpreted in 6 hours; however, its sensitivity is increased at 24 hours. Because of the time required to perform the test, it is not of practical value in the immediate perioperative diagnosis and decision to treat fibrinogenolysis. Although the fibrin plate test is frequently abnormal in patients following cardiopulmonary bypass,[25, 49] a poor correlation exists between a positive test and postoperative bleeding.[25] On the other hand, the implication of a positive fibrin plate test in the absence of hypofibrinogenemia and factor consumption is that a primary fibrinogenolytic process can occur during and following even adequately anticoagulated cardiopulmonary bypass.

Protamine Sulfate Test for Soluble Fibrin Monomer

The protamine sulfate test for soluble fibrin monomer detects the presence of fibrin monomer and fibrin degradation product complexes.[50] When protamine sulfate is added to plasma containing soluble fibrin monomer and fibrin degradation product complexes, it cleaves the fibrin monomer from the degradation products, allowing fibrin monomer to polymerize and form fibrin strands. The protamine sulfate test for fibrin monomer (fibrin degradation products are not measured) is thought to be more specific for fibrinolysis stimulated by intravascular coagulation than either the Thrombo-Wellco or TRCHI tests (the fibrin degradation products are measured, but not soluble fibrin monomer). Call et al.[44] reported that in 69 of 255 open heart patients the protamine sulfate test for fibrin monomer was positive, indicating that active intravascular coagulation was occurring. On the other hand, Bick et al. (26) reported that while fibrin degradation products were elevated in 36% (11/30) of patients following cardiopulmonary bypass, in no case was there a positive protamine sulfate test for fibrin monomer (0/30). This discrepancy may reflect the small number in Bick's series, but more importantly may relate to the relatively high plasma heparin levels achieved in Beck's series during bypass (average plasma heparin concentration of 9.01 μg/ml), ensuring adequate anticoagulation and eliminating surface-induced coagulation by the perfusion circuit. Call did not indicate how much heparin was administered. If it was low, as suggested by the frequency of hyperfibrinolysis in his series, then a positive protamine test is not surprising. Kalter et al.,[23] using a 3 mg/kg heparin dose protocol maintaining the ACT at greater than 250 seconds (twice normal), observed increased fibrin degradation products in five of nine patients using the Thrombo-Wellco Test Kit. One of these patients also had a positive protamine sulfate test for fibrinmonomer.

PHARMACOLOGY OF COAGULATION MODIFYING DRUGS

Heparin

Heparin is an acid mucopolysaccharide with a strong negative charge. It has the unique ability of stopping the coagulation process in the presence of antithrombin III or heparin cofactor.[51] Antithrombin III inhibits the effect of thrombin on fibrinogen. Its activity is low in the absence of heparin. However, in the presence of heparin, its activity is increased as much as 100-fold. Although originally thought to only inhibit the effect of thrombin on fibrinogen, antithrombin III is now recognized to have an inhibitory effect on other serine protease factors, including Factors 11, 10, 9, and possibily Factor 12 (Fig. 9.5).[51, 52] Interestingly, during periods of active intravascular coagulation such as DIC, the level of antithrombin III drops significantly.[53] A drop in antithrombin III has also been documented during cardiopulmonary bypass with inadequate anticoagulation but remains at normal or near normal levels when anticoagulation is adequate.[10, 26, 54, 55] To what level a drop in antithrombin III will result in significant heparin insensitivity is not definitely known.

Considerable differences exist between the commercially available heparin preparations.[56, 57] Bovine lung and swine gut are the two most common sources of commercial heparin. Swine gut heparin is significantly more antigenic than bovine lung heparin. It may also be a strong plasminogen activator resulting in hemorrhage after protamine reversal by inducing fibrinogenolysis.[56] For this reason bovine lung heparin is usually preferred for open heart surgery.

Previously it was assumed that 1 mg of heparin was equivalent to 100 units of heparin activity. In fact, the activity of heparin may vary between 70 and 140 units per mg when heparin activity is actually tested for.[57, 58] The fact that heparin batch potency may vary, as well as the fact that the patient's sensitivity to heparin differs, means that during cardiopulmonary bypass the methods used to monitor heparin administration should measure the effect of heparin on the coagulation time rather than assume that a specific amount of heparin administered to all patients will be adequate to prevent coagulation during bypass.[36, 54, 59–61]

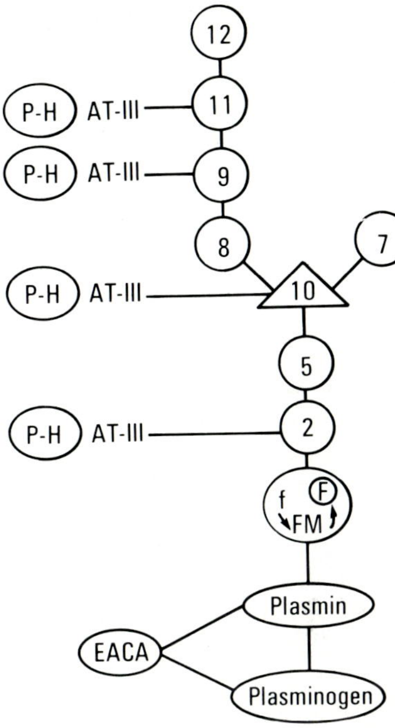

Figure 9.5. Coagulation pathway with sites of action of protamine sulfate (*P*), heparin (*H*), and ϵ-aminocaproic acid (*EACA*). In absence of protamine, heparin increases the natural anticoagulant effect of antithrombin III (*AT-III*) on the serine proteases 100-fold. *EACA* primarily inhibits plasminogen activation and, to a lesser extent, inhibits the enzymatic effect of plasmin on fibrinogen (*f*), fibrin monomer (*FM*), and Fibrin (*F*).

Protamine Sulfate

Protamine sulfate is a strong organic base which binds heparine in a 1:1 ratio, preventing it from enhancing the anticoagulant effect of antithrombin III on the serine protease coagulation factors[52] (Fig. 9.5). It is effective only on circulating heparin, and for that reason a 1.3:1 protamine to heparin ratio is recommended[62] to effectively reverse circulating heparin, as well as prevent heparin rebound, which may occur with the reentry of heparin from tissues into the circulation. This dose also takes into account the somewhat shorter half-life of protamine sulfate than heparin.[52, 64]

Two other effects of protamine sulfate should be mentioned. First, protamine sulfate in excess of heparin can itself be a weak anticoagulant. This effect, however, becomes significantly only in doses in excess of 3–4 mg/kg.[65] It is not a clinically significant anticoagulant following heparin reversal unless inordinately high doses of protamine are administered. Second, protamine is able to inhibit the anticoagulant effect of fibrin split products by cleaving soluble fibrin monomer from the degradation products. This property is the basis for its use in the protamine sulfate test for fibrin monomer previously described, as well as the Tri-F titer. The significance of this effect of protamine sulfate *in vivo* is not known, and inhbition of the effects of fibrin degradation products with large doses of protamine sulfate is not recommended.

ε-Aminocaproic Acid

ε-aminocaproic acid binds plasminogen in a 1:1 stoichiometric complex, blocking plasminogen activation. To a lesser extent it also binds plasmin itself, altering its molecular configuration and inhibiting its proteolytic activity (Fig. 9.5).[64] ε-aminocaproic acid is not recommended in secondary hyperfibrinolysis if the stimulus for thrombosis is ongoing, as in active DIC[8], or during cardiopulmonary bypass with inadequate anticoagulation. It can, however, be very effective when the mechanism for hypercoagulation and secondary fibrinolysis has been eliminated from the circulation.[10, 12] ε-aminocaproic acid is also effective in cases of primary hyperfibrinogenolysis associated with adequately anticoagulated cardiopulmonary bypass when it is associated with significant bleeding.[10, 12]

PREOPERATIVE ASSESSMENT OF COAGULATION SYSTEM

The preoperative evaluation of patients undergoing open heart surgery should include a careful history and physical examination. The history should include a complete review of current medications and a personal as well as a family history of bleeding tendencies. A coagulation test profile including a partial thromboplastin time, prothrombin time, fibrinogen level, platelet count, and thermogram should be evaluated preoperatively. This coagulation profile will uncover most coagulation abnormalities, even in the absence of significant clinical signs or symptoms. In some cases a thrombin time, expanded partial thromboplastin time, and bleeding time may also be indicated. A positive history for bleeding or an abnormal coagulation profile is a good indication to consult a coagulation specialist preoperatively.

Although most patients undergoing cardiopulmonary bypass will have a normal preoperative coagulation profile, if coagulopathies association with cardiopulmonary bypass can occur in patients without preexisting coagulation defects, the effect of an obscure but significant preoperative coagulation defect will be magnified in the postoperative period. On the other hand, many patients with existing coagulation defects can have open heart surgery performed safely when the problem is recognized and treated prospectively.

MANAGEMENT OF THE COAGULATION SYSTEM DURING CARDIOPULMONARY BYPASS

Differing opinions exist regarding the pharmacologic management of the coagulation system during and after cardiopulmonary bypass. These include: the use of low,[3, 22, 24, 27, 66–68], high,[13, 16, 54, 59, 61, 69] and middle dose heparin[12, 20, 21, 23, 62, 71, 72]; the administration of ε-aminocaproic or other antifibrinolytic agents before, during, and after cardiopulmonary bypass,[22, 27, 49, 66, 68, 72] during and after cardiopulmonary bypass,[20] always or frequently after cardiopulmonary bypass,[12, 49] and virtually never. High[69] and low dose protamine reversal,[73] 1.3:1 protamine-heparin reversal,[21, 22, 62] and even no protamine reversal at all have been recommended.[66, 68] Although it is recognized that the effects of cardiopulmonary bypass on the coagulation system are multiple, including quantitative and qualitative changes in platelets, coagulation factor depletion through dilution and/or consumption, stimulation of fibrinolysis and/or fibrinogenolysis, as well as, the appearance of a variety of circulating anticoagulants and clotting inhibitors, there is little agreement as to their relative frequency and importance. It is noteworthy, however, that investigations using high dose heparin protocols for bypass (greater than 3 mg/kg) tend to emphasize defects in the preoperative coagulation status and the effect of cardiopulmonary bypass on platelet numbers and function, though not to the exclusion of fibrinolysis.[10, 13, 26, 55, 72] Conversely, when a low dose heparin protocol (3 mg/kg or less) is used routinely, fibrinolysis and coagulation factor depletion have been emphasized.[3, 12, 20, 23, 24, 27, 54, 66, 68, 73] Unfortunately, many reports on the effects of cardiopulmonary bypass on the coagulation mechanisms do not indicate how much heparin is used or how heparin effect was monitored. This is important since the adequacy of heparinization during cardiopulmonary bypass affects the function of the coagulation system during bypass and is relevant to the incidence and character of coagulopathies following heparin reversal. The relation between the adequacy of heparinization during cardiopulmonary bypass and decreased postoperative bleeding was recognized by Senning[59] and lead him in 1959 to increase the heparin dose routinely used for cardiopulmonary bypass from 2.5 mg/kg to 4.0 mg/kg. Subsequently, Blomback et al.[16] documented that, with increasing heparinization, fibrinolysis decreased. They also demonstrated that pediatric patients were relatively heparin resistent and required more heparin to achieve the same plasma level and anticoagulation effect as adults. Douglas et al.,[69] reporting an initial experience with open heart surgery in 1966, identified fibrinolysis as a major postoperative coagulopathy, relating it to inadequate heparinization (3 mg/kg). They recommended increasing the initial heparin dose to 4.5 mg/kg.

The problem with all heparin administration protocols, however, was pointed out by Bull et al.[36] when they showed that there was no satisfactory protocol which does not measure the effect of heparin on the coagulation time, taking into account patient sensitivity to heparin and variable heparin potency. The only test suitable for measuring heparin effect on the coagulation time of whole blood in the open heart room is the ACT.35, 36, 61 A semiautomated version of the ACT is particularly suitable for heparin administration and calculation of the protamine reversal dose in the operating room.[74] The automated activated coagulation time (A-ACT) can be performed by the perfusionist and does not require any special reagents or involve complicated serial dilution techniques.

Bull et al.[36] used the ACT to evaluate the heparin sensitivity of patients preoperatively and then calculated what the ACT would have been using one of several standard protocol methods for heparin administration. He found that a significant number of their patients, using any one of the protocol methods, would have been either underheparinized or overheparinized if the "safe" range for the ACT was between 300 and 600 seconds, or 3–6 times normal.[36, 61] He also showed that no method for monitoring heparin effect other than the whole blood clotting time or the activated clotting time can be used to monitor heparin half-life, necessary for the determination of additional heparin.[36]

The lower limit of the "safe" range recommended by Bull et al. was 300 seconds, or 3 times normal. This was determined by the clinical observation that when the coagulation time was prolonged to at least 3 times normal, no clots formed in the operative field or in the oxygenator.[36] The "safe" range, however, should be defined as a coagulation time prolonged sufficiently to completely inhibit coagulation when blood interfaces with the perfusion circuit. In order to define this point, Young et al.[54] reported a series of experimental perfusions in rhesus monkeys in which the A-ACT for cardiopulmonary bypass varied between 2.5 and 10 times normal. The appearance of fibrin monomer was measured by a special radioimmune technique before, during, and after bypass. This method of measuring fibrin monomer was developed by Kisker et al.[75] Unlike other tests for fibrin monomer, it is sensitive only to circulating soluble fibrin monomer as it is cleaved from fibrinogen and insensitive to fibrinogen, fibrin, fibrin monomer, and fibrin degradation product complexes. It is therefore a measure of active intravascular coagulation but not the byproducts of lysis. In animals where the A-ACT was always greater than 400 seconds, no abnormal fibrin monomer was detected. However, fibrin monomer became elevated whenever the A-ACT during bypass was less than 400 seconds. Additionally, the fibrinogen level, platelet count, and antithrombin III levels were significantly depressed in the fibrin monomer positive, as compared to the fibrin monomer negative animals, both during and following cardiopulmonary bypass, indicating that not only significant coagulation occurred during bypass when the A-ACT was less than 400 seconds but also consumption of coagulation factors (Fig. 9.6).

The oxygenator surface in the experimental perfusions, where the A-ACT was always greater than 400 seconds, contained little or no microscopic fibrin and platelet debris when examined by scanning electron microscopy. However, when the A-ACT was less than 400 seconds, abundant fibrin and platelet debris was observed (Fig. 9.7). The experimental findings in the fibrin monomer negative group were confirmed by assaying for fibrin monomer in six pediatric clinical perfusions. No abnormal fibrin monomer was detected when the A-ACT was greater than 400 seconds, and minimal or no debris was observed in the oxgenator[54] (Fig. 9.8).

It was concluded that "safe" anticoagulation occurred when the coagulation time was sufficiently prolonged to prevent the activation of the coagulation system, resulting in the appearance of fibrin monomer. Based on these experiments, using the A-ACT to monitor the coagulation time and a bubble oxy-

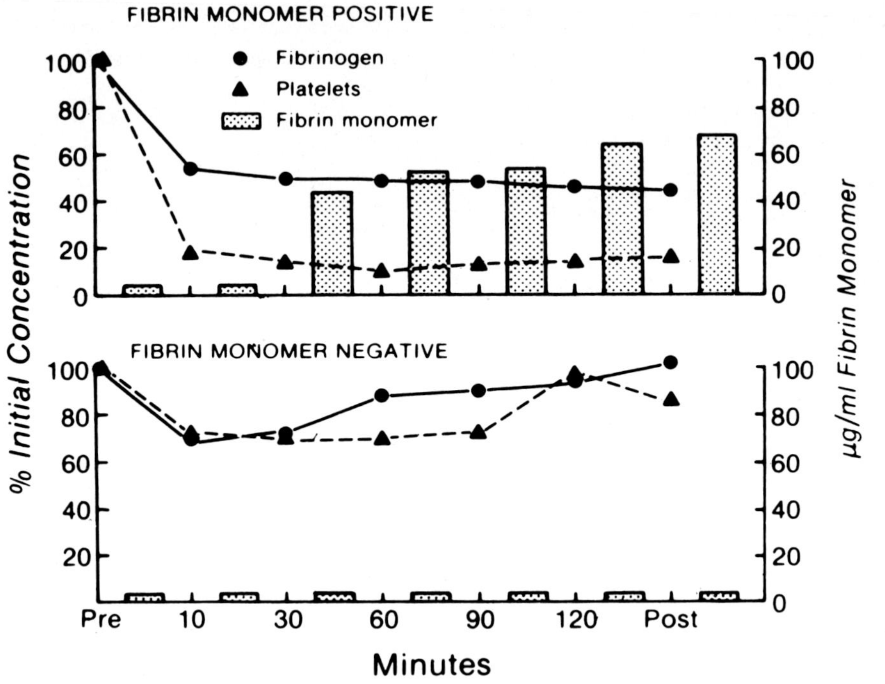

Figure 9.6. Fibrinogen and platelet counts, expressed as percentage of prebypass (control) concentration, are plotted against time on cardiopulmonary bypass for experiments in which fibrin monomer was positive (*top graph*) or negative (*bottom graph*). The mean percentage reduction in both fibrinogen and platelets was much greater in the fibrin monomer positive group and continued throughout CPB, suggesting continued consumption of these factors. The changes in the fibrin monomer negative group were much smaller and improved during cardiopulmonary bypass (CPB)[54]

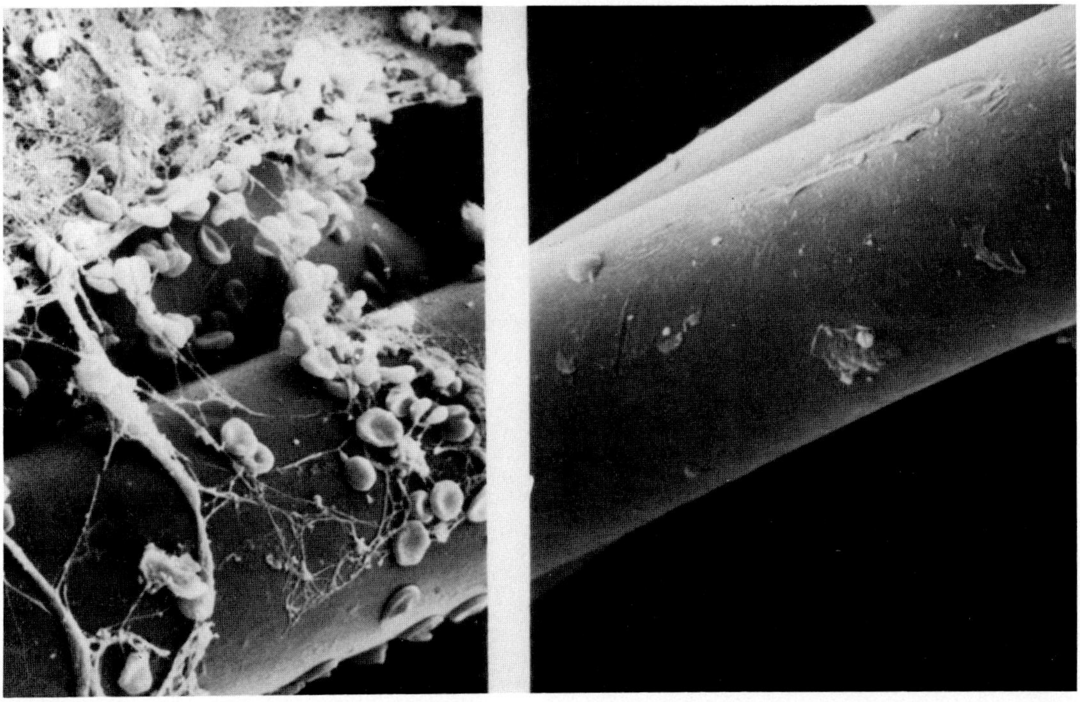

Figure 9.7. Scanning electron micrographs of oxygenator filter mesh. *Panel* on *left* is from a fibrin monomer positive experiment (ACT, 400 seconds), showing abundant fibrin, platelet debris, and cells. *Panel* on *right* is from a fibrin monomer negative experiment (ACT > 700 seconds), showing only a few platelets on the surface. (Original magnification × 1000.)[54]

genator for perfusion at 30°C, the lowest acceptable prolongation of the coagulation time is thought to be 400 seconds, or 4 times normal. It is probably preferable, however, for the A-ACT to be between 450 and 500 seconds when bypass is commenced. This is consistent with the middle ACT range of 480 seconds, which Bull et al.[61] considered to be optimal.

Active coagulation when blood interfaces with the perfusion apparatus may have two major deleterious effects. First, factor consumption may result in inadequate substrate for clot formation following bypass. Second, since the strongest stimulus for fibrinolysis is the activation of Factor 12 by surface contact, the fibrinolytic mechanisms should be fairly active at the conclusion of an inadequately anticoagulated perfusion. Significant amounts of fibrin degradation products may also be liberated into the circulation from the oxygenator reservoir, causing an anticoagulant effect independent of heparin effect following a perfusion in which anticoagulation has been suboptimal. If coagulation has become severely deranged by factor consumption, fibrinolysis, and circulating fibrin degradation products during an inadequately anticoagulated perfusion, the ACT will be prolonged in excess of heparin effect, resulting in an erroneously high protamine dose calculation by this method.

Adequate anticoagulation sufficient to prevent the activation of the coagulation system should prevent perfusion-related fibrinolysis and significant coagulation factor depletion.[63] The mechanics of cardiopulmonary bypass itself, however, may result in the release of plasminogen activators into the circulation independent of coagulation-dependent mechanisms. Excessive liberation of thromboplastic substances into the circulation can occur with improperly adjusted roller pump heads or extensive and continuous use of cardiotomy suction, resulting in hemolysis and red cell fragmentation. These same situ-

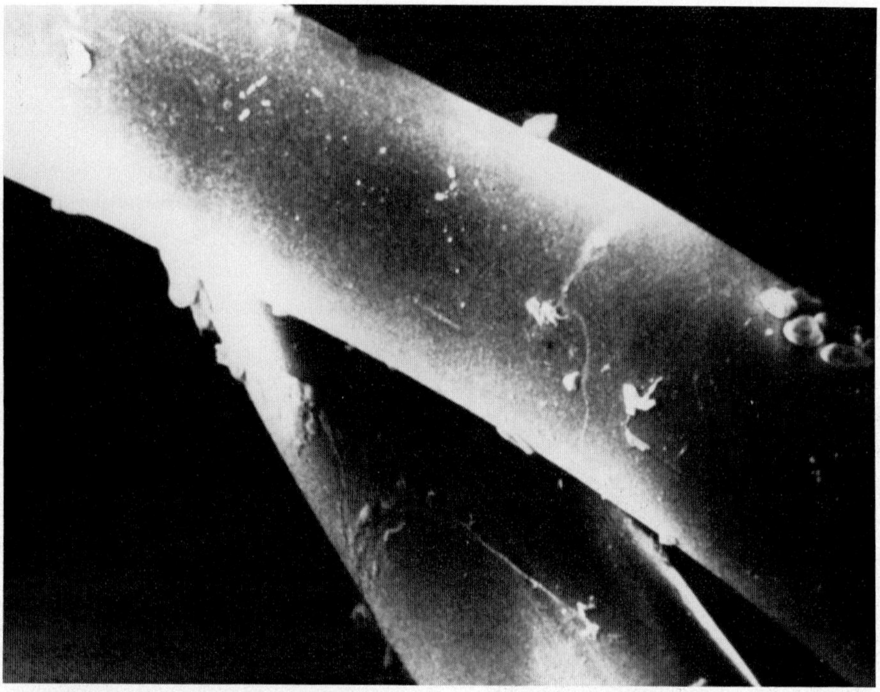

Figure 9.8. Scanning electron micrograph from oxygenator filter of a clinical case in which whole-blood activated clotting time was maintained above 450 seconds. Little debris is present, and fibrin monomer remained negative, suggesting that this bypass was free of appreciable coagulation. (Original magnification, × 1000).[54]

ations, of course, can occur during inadequately anticoagulated perfusions prone to coagulation-induced fibrinolysis, setting the stage for severe postperfusion coagulation problems[70] (Fig. 9.3).

MANAGEMENT OF POSTOPERATIVE COAGULATION PROBLEMS

The diagnosis of surgical bleeding is made when there is excessive bleeding in the face of a normal coagulaton profile. Although many patients will have an abnormal coagulation profile in the early postoperative period, treatment is indicated only when there is an associated bleeding diathesis. Although an abnormal profile does not exclude surgical bleeding, treatment should be undertaken to correct the abnormalities in the coagulation profile.

A PT, PTT, platelet count, fibrinogen level, and hemogram are usually obtained for most patients returning from the operating room. A thrombin time and other tests of lysis may also be obtained routinely. Mild to moderate elevations of the PT, PTT, and thrombin time are very common. The platelet count is usually somewhat depressed when compared to the prebypass platelet count, but even if normal, platelet function may not be normal. As previously indicated, the tests for fibrin degradation products provide indirect evidence for fibrinolysis and frequently are elevated after cardiopulmonary bypass in patients without bleeding problems. The euglobin lysis time, although not as time consuming as the fibrin plate method, is generally considered to be of little or no value in the diagnosis of significant fibrinolysis in the postperfusion patient.[74, 77, 78] Unfortunately, the differential diagnosis of bleeding when abnormalities of these commonly used coagulation tests exist is not specific and includes quantitative and qualitative platelet dysfunction, inadequate coagulation factors, circulating anticoagu-

CAUSE OF BLEEDING	PT >19 sec	PTT >45 sec	FIBRINOGEN <225 mg/100 ml	TFT ≤1:32	TREATMENT
FIBRINOLYSIS	NO	NO	NO	YES	AMICAR
HYPERFIBRINOLYSIS	YES/NO	YES	YES	YES	AMICAR; CRYOPRECIPITATE; FFP
HEPARIN	YES/NO	YES	NO	HEPARIN EFFECT	PROTAMINE
SURGICAL	NO	NO	NO	NO	REEXPLORATION

Figure 9.9. Recommended treatment in presence of significant bleeding. The Tri-F-Titer (*TFT*) should be interpreted in light of *PT* and *PTT* and fibrinogen level. Appropriate medical treatment is recommended if a positive Tri-f-Titer is associated with significant bleeding.

lants, and fibrinolysis and/or fibrinogenolysis. In order to treat all of these possible defects, additional protamne sulfate, fresh frozen plasma, fresh platelets, and ϵ-aminocaproic acid should be administered, even though the coagulopathy may have a relatively specific cause.

Tri-F Titer

In order to circumvent the lack of specificity associated with most of the standard laboratory tests used in the perioperative period, the Tri-F Titer was developed by Lambert et al.,[26] which when combined with a PT, PTT, and bleeding time, provides a rapid bedside method to distinguish between the various possible coagulation defects (Fig. 9.9). While the Tri-F Titer is being performed, a bleeding time can be done. The bleeding time is the only method for determining *in vivo* platelet function. A normal bleeding time irrespective of the absolute number of platelets is an indication that platelet function is normal. An abnormal bleeding time, however, indicates that a qualitative or quantitative platelet defect exists and is an indication for fresh platelet infusions. A normal bleeding time should take less than 15 minutes, which is about the time required to perform the Tri-F titer.

The Tri-F titer is a modification of the thrombin time, protamine corrected thrombin time, and protamine sulfate test for soluble fibrin monomer previously discussed. The Tri-F titer provides semiquantitative information about the presence or absence of heparin, fibrin degradation products, clinically significant fibrin(ogen)olysis, and the fibrinogen level. The Tri-F titer is performed by adding protamine sulfate to the first tube of the first row and protamine sulfate and amicar to the remaining tubes of that row. Amicar is added to each of the tubes in the second row and normal saline to each tube in the third row. The same amount of purified thrombin is then added to each of the 24 tubes. The purpose of amicar is to inhibit fibronogenolysis. The purpose of protamine sulfate is to neutralize heparin and inhibit the anticoagulant effect of fibrin degradation product. The patient's plasma (0.3 ml) is added to the first tube of each row, and eight serial doubling dilutions are carried out. The test is performed at 37°C and can be accurately interpreted within 10 minutes, although the sensitivity is increased slightly at 30 minutes (Fig. 9.10).

The first row containing protamine sulfate and ϵ-aminocaproic acid is used to estimate the fibrinogen level. The higher the dilution in which clots form, the higher the fibrinogen level. A titer between 128 and 256 is equivalent to a fibrinogen level of greater than 300 mg% when the fibrinogen level is determined by the standard method for quantitating fibrinogen described by Ratnoff. A titer of between 32 and 64 is equivalent to a fibrinogen level greater than 200 mg%.

The presence of significant fibrin degradation products can be estimated by comparing the titer in row 1 with that in row 2. Row 2 contain only ϵ-aminocaproic acid, and

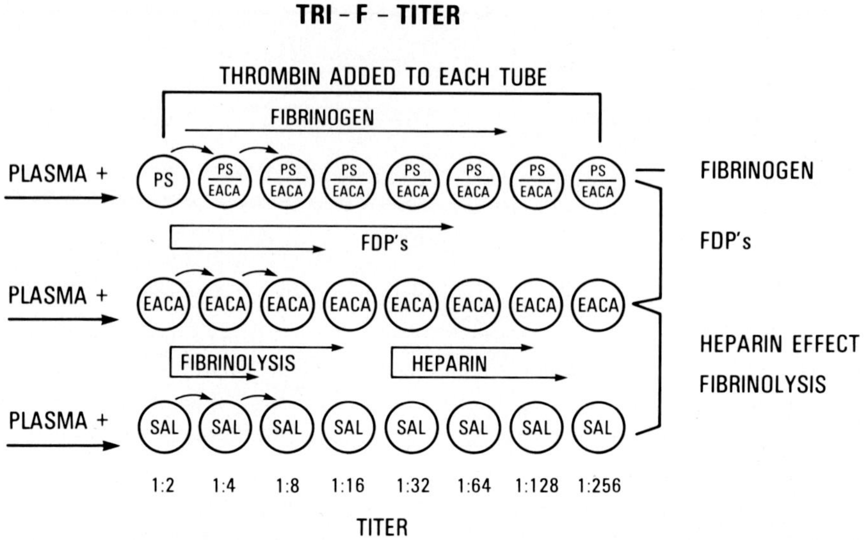

Figure 9.10. Layout of tubes in Tri-F-titer test. (PS, protamine sulfate; *EACA*, ε-aminocaproic acid; *SAL*, saline; *FDP*, fibrin degradation products.[12]

therefore plasminogen activation and plasmin activity are inhibited but not the anticoagulant effect of fibrin degradation products. A titer 1–2 tubes less in row 2, compared to row 1, indicates that significant circulating fibrin degradation products are present. As with other tests for measuring fibrin degradation products, a positive Tri-F titer for fibrin degradation products is indirect evidence for intravascular fibrinolysis but does not correlate with bleeding in the postoperative period.[12]

Evidence for heparin effect and fibrin(ogen)olysis is determined by comparing row 2 and 3. Since each tube contains the same amount of thrombin, heparin effect on thrombin will be less while the thrombin effect on fibrinogen will be greater with increasing dilutions. Therefore, in the presence of circulating heparin, no clot will form in the lower dilutions to the left, but will form at higher dilutions to the right as the heparin to thrombin ratio decreases.

Evidence of significant fibrin(ogen)olysis can be inferred by comparing the highest titer at which clotting occurs in row 2 containing ε-aminocaproic acid and row 3 containing only saline. The higher the titer, the less fibrin(ogen)olysis is occurring. The greater the difference between rows 2 and 3, the greater the level of fibrin(ogen)olysis. When significant fibrin(ogen)olysis occurs, the titer at which clot forms will be greater in row 2, compared to row 3. The significance of fibrin(ogen)olysis can best be interpreted in the context of the fibrinogen level, either directly measured or derived from the first row of the Tri-F titer, the PT, and the PTT. If the PT is greater than 19 seconds, the PTT greater than 45 seconds, the fibrinogen level less than 225 mg%, and the Tri-F titer is positive for fibrin(ogen)olysis in the presence of significant postoperative bleeding, then treatment should include aggressive factor replacement and ε-aminocaproic acid infusions.

Using the Tri-F titer to evaluate the coagulation status of the 20% of 750 open heart surgery patients who demonstrated excessive bleeding in the postoperative period, Lambert[79] attributed the bleeding to fibrin(ogen)olysis or hyperfibrin(ogen)olysis in most cases. In only 1% of the patients having excessive bleeding postoperatively were surgical bleeding or circulating heparin associated with the bleeding diathesis.

In summary, the basic properties of the coagulation system and its response to cardiopulmonary bypass have been outlined. The importance of adequate anticoagulation during cardiopulmonary bypass for the maintenance of coagulation homeostasis at the conclusion of bypass cannot be overstated. In the absence of adequate anticoagulation during cardiopulmonary bypass, fibrinolysis and/or fibrinogenolysis probably represent the most common causes of failure of hemostasis. Treatment of coagulation defects, however, should be directed at the specific causes as they occur.

References

1. von Kaulla KN, Swan H: Clotting deviations during cardiac bypass: Fibrinolysis and circulating anticoagulant. J Thorac Surg 36:519, 1958.
2. Crafoord C, Norberg B, Senning Å: Clinical studies in extracorporeal circulation with a heart-lung machine. Acta Chir Scand 112:220, 1957.
3. Nilsson IM, Swedberg J: Coagulation studies in cardiac surgery with extracorporeal circulation using a bubble-oxygenator. Acta Chir Scand 117:47, 1959.
4. Davie EW, Ratnoff OD: Waterfall sequence of intrinsic blood clotting. Science 145:1310, 1964.
5. Prentice CRM, Ratnoff OD: Genetic disorders of blood coagulation. Semin Hematol 4:93, 1967.
6. Ratnoff OD: Studies on the proteolytic enzyme in human plasma. IX. Fibrinogen and fibrin as substrate for the proteolytic enzyme of plasma. J Clin Invest 32:473, 1953.
7. Sherry S: Fibrinolysis. Ann Rev Med 19:247, 1968.
8. Risberg B: Surgery and fibrinolysis. J Surg Res 26: 698, 1979.
9. Porter GH III: Fibronolysis: An unusual cause of bleeding. Med Clin North Am 51:1061, 1967.
10. Bick RL: Alterations of hemostasis associated with cardiopulmonary bypass: Pathophysiology, prevention, diagnosis and management. Semin Thromb Hemostas 3:59, 1976.
11. Griffin JD, Ellman L: Epsilon-aminocaproic acid (EACA). Semin Thromb Haemostas 5:27, 1978.
12. Lambert CJ, Marengo-Rowe AJ, Levenson J, Alivizatos P, Geisler GF, Adam M, Mitchel BF Jr, Thiele JP: The Tri-F titer. A rapid test for estimation of plasma fibronogen and detection of fibrinolysis, fibrin(ogen) split products and heparin. Ann Thorac Surg 18:357, 1974.
13. Bachmann F, McKenna R, Cole ER, Najafi H: The hemostatic mechanism after open-heart surgery. I. Studies on plasma coagulation factors and fibrinolysis in 512 patients after extracorporeal circulation. J. Thorac Cardiovasc Surg 70:76, 1975.
14. Kladetzky RG, Popov-Cenı́c S, Büttner W, Müller N, Egli H: Studies of fibrinolytic and coagulation factors during open heart surgery. I. Fibrinolytic problems during open heart surgery with ECC. Thromb Res 7:579, 1975.
15. Müller NS, Popov-Cenı́c S, Büttner W, Kladetzky RG, Egli H: Studies of fibrinolytic and coagulation factors during open heart surgery. II. Postoperative bleeding tendency and changes in the coagulation system. Thromb Res 7:589, 1975.
16. Blombäck M, Norén I, Senning Å: Coagulation disturbances during extracorporeal circulaton and postoperative period. Acta Chir Scand 127:433, 1964.
17. Kevy SV, Glickman RM, Bernhard WF, Diamond LK, Gross RE: The control of the hemorrhagic defect in open heart surgery. Surg Gynecol Obstet 123:313, 1966.
18. Tice DA, Worth MH Jr: Recognition and treatment of postoperative bleeding associated with open-heart surgery. Ann NY Acad Sci 146:745, 1968.
19. Gralnick HR, Fischer RD: The hemostatic response to open-heart operations. J Thorac Cardiovasc Surg 61:909, 1971.
20. Tsuji HK, Redington JV, Kay JH, Groesswald RK: The study of fibrinolytic and coagulation factors during open-heart surgery. Ann NY Acad Sci 146: 763, 1968.
21. Dieter RA Jr, Neville WE, Pifarre R, Jasuja, M: Preoperative coagulation profiles and posthemodilution cardiopulmonary bypass hemorrhage. Am J Surg 121:689, 1971.
22. Gomes MMR, McGoon DC: Bleeding patterns after open-heart surgery. J Thorac Cardiovasc Surg 60:87, 1970.
23. Kalter RD, Saul CM, Wetstein L, Soriano C, Reiss RF: Cardiopulmonary bypass. Associated hemostatic abnormalities. J Thorac Cardiovasc Surg 77:427, 1979.
24. Dybkjaer E, Berg E, Kissmeyer-Nielsen F: Coagulation studies in extracorporeal circulaton. Acta Chir Scand 128:350, 1964.
25. Bentall HH, Allwork SP: Fibrinolysis and bleeding in open-heart surgery. Lancet 1:4, 1968.
26. Bick RL, Schmalhorst WR, Arbegast NR: Alterations of hemostasis associated with cardiopulmonary bypass. Thromb Res 8:285, 1976.
27. Mammen EF: Natural proteinase inhibitors in extracorporeal circulation. Ann NY Acad Sci 146:754, 1968.
28. Porter JM, Silver D: Alterations in fibrinolysis and coagulation associated with cardiopulmonary bypass. J Thorac Cardiovasc Surg 56:869, 1968.
29. Signori EE, Penner JA, Kahn DR: Coagulation defects and bleeding in open-heart surgery. Ann Thorac Surg 8:521, 1969.
30. Lee RI, White PD: A clinical study of the coagulation time of blood. Am J Med 145:495, 1913.
31. Wintrobe MM: *Clinical Hematology*. Philadelphia, Lea & Febiger, 1967.
32. Goodman TL, Todd ME, Goldsmith EI: Laboratory observations and clinical implications of monitoring the effect of heparin by bioassay. Surg Gynecol Obstet 142:673, 1976.
33. Colman RW, Oxley L, Giannusa P: Statistical comparison of the automated activated partial thromboplastin time and the clotting time in the regulation of heparin therapy. Am J Clin Pathol 53:904, 1970.
34. Schriever HG, Epstein SE, Mintz MD: Statistical correlation and heparin sensitivity of activated partial thromboplastin time, whole blood coagulation time and automated coagulation time. Am J Clin Pathol 60:323, 1973.
35. Hattersley PG: Activated coagulation time of whole blood. JAMA 196:436, 1966.
36. Bull BS, Korpman RA, Huse WM, Briggs BD: Heparin therapy during extracorporeal circulation. I. Problems inherent in existing heparin protocols. J Thorac Cardiovasc Surg 69:674, 1975.

37. Baele G, De broe M, De Weerdt GA, Ringoir S, Barbier F: Limitations of the activated partial thromboplastin time for determination of plasma heparin concentration and half-life in human subjects. Thromb Diath Haemorrh 27:107, 1972.
38. Biggs R: Intrinsic prothrombin activation. In: *Human Blood Coagulation Haemostasis and Thrombosis*. Oxford, Alden & Mobray, 1972.
39. Proctor RR, Rapaport SI: The partial thromboplastin time with Kaolin. A simple screening test for first stage plasma clotting factor deficiencies. Am J Clin Pathol 36:212, 1961.
40. Quick AJ: The prothrombin in hemophilia and in obstructive jaundice. J Biol Chem 109:LXXIII, 1935.
41. Esnouf MP: Extrinsic activation of prothrombin. In *Human Blood Coagulation, Haemostasis and Thrombosis*, edited by R. Biggs. 1922, p. 55. Oxford, Scientific Publications.
42. Biggs R, Douglass AS: The thromboplastin generation test. J Clin Pathol 6:23, 1953.
43. Hougie C: *Fundamentals of Blood Coagulation in Clinical Medicine.* New York, McGraw-Hill, 1963.
44. Call FL, Schroeder ET, Parker FB Jr, Davey FR: Fibrin-fibrinogen degradation products in cardiovascular surgery. Arch Surg 107:834, 1973.
45. Leavelle De, Bowie EJW, Mertens BF, McDuffie FC, Owen CA Jr: Assay of fibrinolytic split products: Comparison of staphylococcal clumping and hemagglutination-inhibition tests. J Lab Clin Med 77:993, 1971.
46. Smith RT, Ts'ao C: Fibrin degradation products in the postoperative period. Evaluation of a new latex agglutination method. Am J Clin Pathol 60:644, 1973.
47. Merskey C, Kleiner GJ, Johnson AJ: Quantitative estimation of split products of fibrinogen in human serum: Relation to diagnosis and treatment. Blood 28:1, 1966.
48. Astrup T, Müller S: The fibrin plate method for estimating fibrinolytic activity. Arch Biochem 40:34, 1952.
49. Gans H, Krivit W: Problems in hemostasis during open-heart surgery. III. Epsilon amino caproic acid as an inhibitor of plasminogen activator activity. Ann Surg 155:268, 1962.
50. Gurewich V, Hutchinson E: Detection of intravascular coagulation by serial dilution protamine sulfate test. Ann Intern Med 75:895, 1971.
51. Rosenberg RD: Heparin action. Circulation 603, 1974.
52. Gervin AS: Complications of heparin therapy. Surg Gynecol Obstet 140:789, 1975.
53. Bick RL, Kovacs I, Fekette LF: A new two-stage functional assay for antithrombin-III (heparin cofactor): Clinical and laboratory evaluation. Thromb Res 8:745, 1976.
54. Young JA, Kisker CT, Doty DB: Adequate anticoagulation during cardiopulmonary bypass determined by activated clotting time and the appearance of fibrin monomer. Ann Thorac Surg 26:231, 1978.
55. Bick RL, Bick MD, Fekete LF: Antithrombin III Patterns in disseminated intravascular coagulation. Am J Clin Pathol 73:577, 1980.
56. Abbott WM, Warnock DF, Austen WG: The relationship of heparin source to the incidence of delayed hemorrhage. J Surg Res 22:593, 1977.
57. McMahon FG, Jain AK, Ryan JR, Lefton TE: Anticoagulant potency of mucosal and lung heparin. Clin Pharmacol Ther 17:79, 1975.
58. Lowary LR, Smith FA, Coyne E, Dunham NW: Comparative neutralization of lung- and mucosal-derived heparin by protamine sulfate using *in vitro* and *in vivo* methods. J Pharm Sci 60:638, 1971.
59. Senning Å: Plasma-heparin concentration in extracorporeal circulation. Acta Chir Scand 117:555, 1959.
60. Monkhouse FC, MacMillan RL, Brown KWG: The relation between heparin blood levels and blood coagulation times. J Lab Clin Med 42:92, 1953.
61. Bull BS, Huse WM, Braver FS, Korpman RA. Heparin therapy during extracorporeal circulaton. II. The use of a dose-response curve to individualize heparin and protamine dosage. J. Thorac Cardiovasc Surg 69:685, 1975.
62. Ellison N, Beatty CP, Blake DR, Wurzel HA, MacVaugh H III: Heparin rebound: Studies in patients and volunteers. J Thorac Cardiovasc Surg 67: 723, 1974.
63. O'Shea MJ, Flute PT, Pannell GM: Laboratory control of heparin therapy. J Clin Pathol 24:542, 1971.
64. Griffin JD, Ellman L: Epsilon-AminoCaproic Acid (EACA). Semin Thromb Hemostas 5:27, 1978.
65. Ellison N, Ominsky AJ, Wollman H: Is protamine a clinically important anticoagulant? A negative answer. Anesthesiology 35(6):621, 1971.
66. Gans H, Subramanian V, John S, Casteneda AR, Lillehei CW: Theoretical and practical (clinical) considerations concerning proteolytic enzymes and their inhibitors with particular reference to changes in the plasminogen-plasmin system observed during assisted circulation in man. Ann NY Acad Sci. 146: 721, 1968.
67. Wright TA, Dante J, Mustard WT: Postoperative bleeding after extracorporeal circulation. Law J Surg 2:142, 1959.
68. Gans H, Castaneda AR: Problems in hemostasis during open heart surgery. VII. Changes in fibrinogen concentration during and after cardiopulmonary bypass with particular reference to the effect of heparin neutralization on fibrinogen. Ann Surg 165: 551, 1967.
69. Douglas AS, McNicol GP, Bain WH, Mackey WA: The haemostatic defect following extracorporeal circulation. Br J Surg 53:455, 1966.
70. Mattox RL, Guinn GA, Rubio PA, Beall AC Jr: Use of the activated coagulation time in intraoperative heparin reversal for cardiopulmonary operations. Ann Thoracic Surg 19:634, 1975.
71. Michelson EL, Torosian M, Morganroth J, MacVaugh H III: Early recognition of surgically correctable causes of excessive mediastinal bleeding after coronary artery bypass graft surgery. Am J Surg 139: 313, 1980.
72. McClure PD, Izsak J: The use of epsilon aminocaproic acid to reduce bleeding during cardiac bypass in children with congenital heart disease. Anesthesiology 40(6):604, 1974.
73. Roth JA, Cukingman RA, Scott CR: Use of activated coagulation time to monitor heparin during cardiac surgery. Ann Thoracic Surg 28:69, 1979.
74. Graeff H, Beller FK: Fibrinolytic activity in whole blood, dilute blood, and euglobulin clot lysis time - tests. In: *Thrombosis and Bleeding Disorders: The-*

ory and Methods, edited by NU Bang, FR Beller, E Deutsch, and EF Mammen. New York, Academic Press, 1970, p 328.
75. Kisker CT, Plummer G, Taylor B, Rush R: A method for measurement of fibrin monomer with the use of an immune precipitate of fibrinogen. J Lab Clin Med 89:653, 1977.
76. Verska JJ: Control of heparinization by activated clotting time during bypass with improved postoperative hemostasis. Ann Thoracic Surg 24:170, 1977.
77. Menon, IS: A study of the possible correlation of euglobulin lysis time and dilute blood clot lysis time in the demonstration of fibrinolytic activity. Lab Pract 17:334, 1968.
78. Katz J, Lurie A, Becker D, Metz J: The euglobulin lysis time test: An ineffectual monitor of the therpeutic inhibition of fibrinolysis. J Clin Pathol 23:529, 1970.
79. Lambert C: Personal communication, 1980.

CHAPTER 10

PLATELET PHYSIOLOGY DURING CARDIOPULMONARY BYPASS

L. HENRY EDMUNDS, JR., M.D.
V. PAUL ADDONIZIO, JR., M.D.

Cardiopulmonary bypass exposes blood to synthetic solid surfaces, atmospheric and anesthetic gases, and nonendothelial cell-lined tissues. Not surprisingly, this exposure injures various blood constituents and stimulates reactions from both formed and nonformed blood elements. Modern bypass systems have reduced the injury to blood constituents for short-term cardiopulmonary bypass to tolerable limits. In most instances the body can remove injured blood elements and replace those that are lost sufficiently rapidly and adequately to ensure that the multiple functions of the blood will continue.

In addition to other blood elements platelets are profoundly affected by cardiopulmonary bypass. During bypass, platelets react with both solid and gaseous surfaces, adhere to solid surfaces, form aggregates, and release a variety of vasoactive substances into the circulation. Bypass reduces the number of circulating platelets and stimulates the mobilization of new platelets. However, the most important consequence is that bypass interferes with platelet function. As a result of platelet dysfunction, postoperative bleeding times are prolonged, wound closure is delayed, and postoperative blood losses are increased.

This chapter will review the pathologic physiology of platelets during cardiopulmonary bypass. Necessarily, a synopsis of platelet structure and reactivity will be presented followed by a brief review of the interaction of plasma proteins and synthetic surfaces. Then the reactions of platelets exposed to synthetic surfaces and bypass systems *in vitro* will precede a summary of platelet reactivity *in vivo* during cardiopulmonary bypass with both membrane and bubble oxygenator systems.

THE PLATELET

Platelets are cell fragments ultimately derived from megakaryocytes and lacking a nucleus.[1] In the circulation platelets are discus-shaped structures averaging 1.5 μm in diameter and 0.5 to 1 μm in thickness.[2] Platelets are active participants in blood coagulation, but also have a separate hemostatic function.[1] In the coagulation cascade, platelets release various proteins and lipoproteins that activate or react with other coagulation factors. At sites of vascular injury, platelets secure hemostasis by forming platelet plugs and eventually fibrin-platelet meshes.

The ultrastructure of platelets is complex, but some understanding is necessary to follow the pathologic physiology of platelets during cardiopulmonary bypass. The most external surface of the platelet, called the glycocalyx, is rich in glycoproteins and may contain receptors for various agents that stimulate platelets.[3] Some of the external glycoproteins are important in the development of platelet aggregation and adhesiveness.[4] A trilaminar membrane is beneath the glycocalyx, and a submembrane area containing specialized filaments is beneath the trilaminar membrane. These structures are contiguous with a system of multiple channels—the open cannicular system—that penetrates into the interior of the platelet[3] (Fig. 10.1). The open cannicular system greatly expands the surface area of the platelet and permits egress of platelet secretory products and access of plasma constituents to reach the interior of the platelet.

The matrix of the platelet cytoplasm is called the sol-gel zone.[3] Microtubules and microfilaments are present within the sol-gel zone, as well as platelet organelles and a second separate, descrete membrane system called the dense tubular system. The microtubules and microfilaments within the sol-gel zone are involved in maintaining the platelet discoid shape and in producing platelet shape change, pseudopod formation, and internal contraction and secretion.[3] The microtubules and microfilaments contain actin and myosin in a ratio of 100:1 and are activated by an increase in cytoplasmic calcium ion.[3]

A circumferential band of microtubules present just beneath the third lamina of the peripheral zone plays an important role during the release reaction.[3] When adequately stimulated, microfilaments contract to draw circumferential microtubules around randomly dispersed platelet organelles. This internal contraction produces a compact mass of platelet organelles surrounded by microtubules and a mesh of microfilaments in the interior of the platelets. If release occurs, the contents of the secretory granules are discharged into the open cannicular system and plasma.

Platelets contain a heterogenous group of organelles dispersed throughout the cytoplasm or sol-gel zone. Mitochondria, electron dense bodies, and several different types of granules are present.[3] Alpha granules contain platelet factor 4, low affinity platelet factor 4, β-thromboglobulin,[5] fibrinogen, and possi-

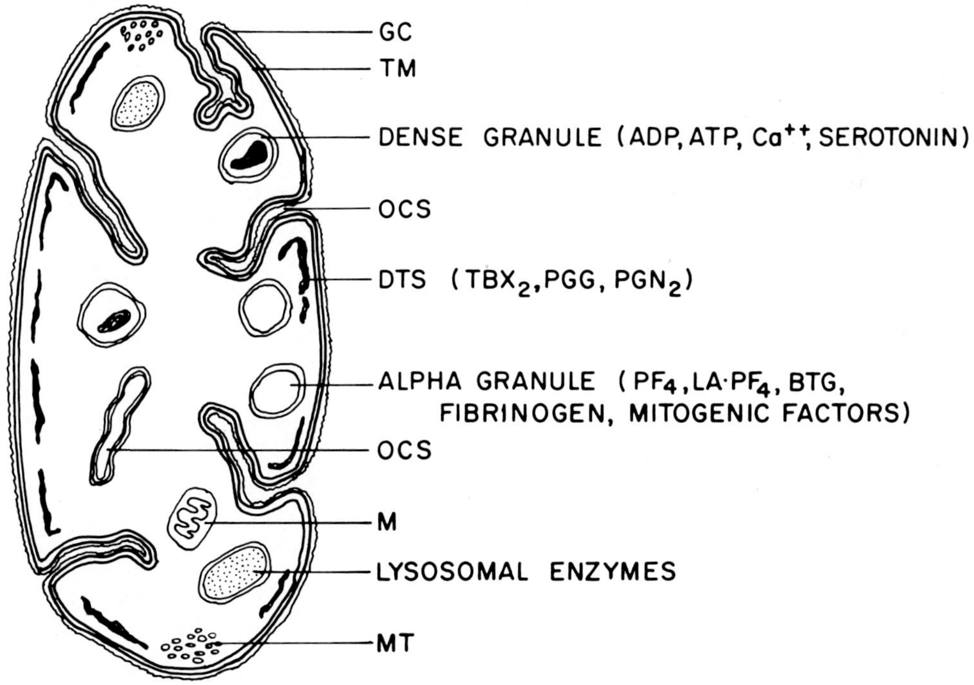

Figure 10.1. Diagram of some subcellular platelet structures. *BTG*, beta-thromboglobulin; *GC*, glycocalyx; *TM*, trilaminar membrane; *OCS*, open cannular system; *DTS*, dense tubular system; *TBX_2*, thromboxane A_2; *M*, mitochondria; *MT*, circumferential microtubules.

bly a mitogenic factor.[6] Some small granules contain catalase,[7] and others contain lysosomal enzymes: acid phosphatase, *n*-acetyl glucosaminidase and β-glucuronidase.[5,8] Electron dense bodies contain stores of adenine nucleotides (independent of those involved in platelet metabolism), calcium,[9] and serotonin.[10]

The dense tubular system is distinct from the open cannicular system and is the site of the platelet calcium pump and repository of calcium ions in the unactivated platelet.[3] Stimulation causes release of calcium into the platelet cytoplasm and contraction of microtubules and microfilaments to produce shape change, pseudopods, and internal contraction and secretion. This activity coincides with a decrease in cytoplasmic C-AMP.[11] The dense tubular system is also the site of platelet cyclooxygenase which converts platelet arachidonic acid derived from membrane phospholipids into prostaglandin endoperoxides (PGG_2, PGH_2),[12] stable prostaglandins (PGE_2, PGD_2, and PGF_2), and thromboxane A_2.

PLATELET FUNCTION

Platelets can adhere to nonendothelial cell surfaces and to each other (aggregation) and release secretory products into the circulation. A variety of chemical stimuli, also called aggregating agents, can stimulate platelets. Adenosine diphosphate (ADP), epinephrine, thrombin, collagen, vasopressin, serotonin, arachidonic acid, and thromboxane A_2 are examples of naturally occurring aggregating agents.[13] A variety of pharmacologic aggregating agents such as ionophore A-23187, ristocetin, and phorbol myristate acetate are also known.

Aggregating agents stimulating platelet membrane receptors cause release of calcium stored in the dense tubular system into the platelet cytoplasm or sol-gel zone. The increased calcium concentration causes contraction of microtubules and microfilaments and also synthesis of prostaglandin endoperoxides and thromboxane A_2. The extent of the platelet reaction depends upon the type and magnitude of the stimulus.[13] Different aggregating agents may cause different degrees of platelet activation.[13]

Platelet activation occurs in four stages, as observed when ADP is added to platelet-rich plasma[14] (Fig. 10.2). After a very brief delay (first stage), *in vitro* platelets change from discoid structures into spiny spheres with extended pseudopods (shape change) (Fig. 10.2). Shortly thereafter, first wave aggregation (third stage) occurs as the spiny platelets collide and adhere to each other. This process, as measured turbometrically in an aggregometer, requires the presence of ionized calcium and fibrinogen as cofactors and is reversible.[13] However, as first wave aggregation proceeds, increasing amounts of ADP, serotonin, platelet factor 4, and other secreted chemicals are detectable in the suspending medium.[15]

With higher concentrations of ADP or different aggregating agents, such as collagen or thrombin, second wave aggregation or the release reaction occurs (Fig. 10.2). This process results from internal contraction of microtubules and microfilaments within the platelet. In addition, platelets synthesize and secrete thromboxane A_2,[13,16] which is both a powerful platelet activator and the most potent vasoconstrictor known.[17] Synthesis of thromboxane A_2 requires oxygen which is taken up from the surrounding medium during second wave aggregation at an accelerated rate.[13] The release reaction depletes platelets

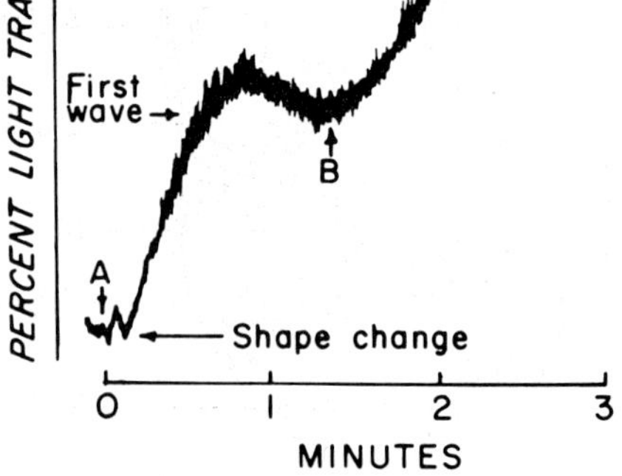

Figure 10.2. Aggregation of platelets in response to ADP. *Arrows* indicate addition of 50 μM ADP. *BTG*, beta-thromboglobulin.

of granule contents and is irreversible.[14] Since many of the released and secreted chemicals are potent platelet activators, release creates a local chain reaction by stimulating additional nearby platelets to aggregate and release.[13]

Many compounds inhibit platelet activation by increasing the concentration of cyclic AMP within the platelet. The concentration of cyclic AMP affects the platelet calcium pump and also cyclooxygenase activity.[18] Drugs which increase cyclic AMP (e.g., prostacyclin (PGI_2), PGE_1, dipyridamole, theophylline) primarily inhibit platelet aggregation. Aspirin and other drugs which inhibit cyclooxygenase prevent second wave aggregation (release).

Platelet activation can also occur in response to physical stimuli.[11,19] The magnitude of the platelet response is proportional to the intensity of the stimulus.[19] Once activated by a physical stimulus, activation occurs in identical sequence, as with chemical aggregating agents.

SURFACE ADSORPTION OF PLASMA PROTEINS

When blood contacts a solid, nonendothelial cell surface, plasma proteins are immediately adsorbed onto the synthetic surface. Within 5 seconds the protein layer is 50 Å thick and reaches 125 Å by 1 minute.[20] Plasma proteins are adsorbed from plasma selectively and competitively and not in proportion to their bulk concentrations.[21] Fibrinogen is most rapidly adsorbed and in greater amounts than either γ-globulin or albumin.[20,22] Albumin is least well adsorbed. Other proteins, including coagulation proteins and lipoproteins, are adsorbed, but the predominant protein is fibrinogen.[20] The final concentration of the adsorbed proteins varies somewhat with the composition of the surface material.

Adsorbed proteins, particularly fibrinogen and globulin, undergo conformational changes and changes in reactivity, but retain their alpha helical or random chain structures.[20,22] Some adsorbed proteins lose their ability to react with antigens, other proteins, and formed blood elements.[22] The degree of conformational change varies and may be more pronounced at the synthetic surface than at the fluid blood interface.[23] Conformational changes in proteins, together with adsorption of lipids, fatty acids, and lipoproteins, may lead to "passivation" of the surface and may decrease the affinity of the surface for circulating platelets and leukocytes.[24,25]

The "passivation" process involves a change in adsorbed fibrinogen. Within 20–30 seconds, depending upon the surface, adsorbed fibrinogen is "converted" by normal plasma containing high molecular weight kininogen to a molecule which does not react with antihuman fibrinogen.[22] There is evidence that conversion involves replacement of adsorbed fibrinogen with high molecular weight kininogen.[27] Platelets adhere in great numbers to adsorbed, unconverted fibrinogen,[28] but do not adhere or adhere very sparsely to surfaces in contact with plasma from afibrinogenic patients,[22] serum (which lacks fibrinogen), or albumin solutions.[29]

Coagulation factors are also adsorbed onto solid surfaces, but most of the measured decreases observed during cardiopulmonary bypass are due to dilution.[30,31] Salzman et al.[29] observed that Factors IX, XI, and XII decrease in plasma when surface contact is made. Harker et al.[31] found that Factor V decreases more during bypass than can be accounted for by dilution and that Factor VIII is rapidly mobilized during bypass so that its concentration remains within the normal range. With adequate heparin, fibrin formation and fibrinolysis usually do not occur during bypass,[31] but occasionally small amounts of fibrin breakdown products can be detected.[32] Except in rare instances, bypass does not reduce soluble coagulation factors sufficiently to cause abnormal bleeding postoperatively.[30,31,33]

The most important interaction between coagulation proteins and solid surfaces is the activation of Factor XII (Hageman factor).[34] There is little evidence that other coagulation proteins are directly activated by contact with nonendothelial cell solid surfaces, except for Factor XII and platelets. Within 30 seconds of contact, surfaces induce a conformational change in the 80,000 molecular weight protein.[35] This activation of Factor XII is facilitated by high molecular weight kininogen and by kallikrein. Kallikrein itself is formed from circulating prekallikrein by activated Factor XII. Plasmin also enhances activation of Factor XII. Activated Factor XII converts Factor XI to its active form, Factor XI[36], which in turn activates Factor IX. Kallikrein causes formation of bradykinin from high molecular weight kininogen and also converts plasminogen to plasmin. During renal dialysis, kallikrein esterase activity increases in venous blood, indicating activation of Factor XII by the extracorporeal circuit.[37] Heparin does not interfere with surface activation of Factor XII.[38]

PLATELET-SURFACE REACTIONS IN VITRO

Synthetic solid surfaces activate the coagulation system which eventually leads to thrombus formation. When coagulation is prevented by heparin, citrate, or other anticoagulants, Factor XII is activated, but the cascade is stopped. Platelets, however, react with all solid surfaces, except those lined with endothelial cells which secrete the powerful platelet inhibitor prostacyclin (PGI_2).[39] Heparin, citrate, and other anticoagulants do not inhibit platelet activation.

Physical and chemical properties of the surface affect both initiation of coagulation and platelet activation and adherence. The term thromboresistance refers to the ability of a synthetic surface to resist thrombus formation or activation of both the coagulation cascade and platelets. As noted above, adsorption of plasma proteins precedes platelet adherence and activation. Chemical and physical properties of various synthetic surfaces affect the sequential and competitive adsorption of plasma proteins[40]; consequently, these properties affect initiation of coagulation and platelet adherence. Properties such as surface texture (smoothness), free energy, electrocharge, and wettability are thought to affect the surface[41]; however, none of these properties or combinations of these properties has consistently predicted thromboresistance. The surface chemistry of various polymers differs, and each polymer presents different reactive groups and combinations to interact with circulating plasma proteins.[40,42] Although some relatively thromboresistant materials are known (segmented polyurethane, polyether urethane, pyrolytic carbon, polyalkylsulfones, copolymers of polyether urethane and polydimethyl siloxane, etc.), the configurations, types and combinations of surface radicals that result in thromboresistance are not well defined. Thromboresistance remains empirically determined by *in vivo* testing.

Anticoagulants may affect adsorption of plasma proteins and subsequent adhesion of platelets.[25,58] Thrombus does not form, but platelets nevertheless adhere, depending upon protein adsorption, which in turn is primarily determined by the physical, and more especially, chemical properties of the synthetic surface.[42] Using citrated blood, Merrill et al.[42] have studied some of the chemical properties of surfaces which affect platelet adhesion. Although the authors indicate the data are preliminary, surfaces which bind hydrogen ion or have ionic or aromatic groups seem more likely to attract platelets.[42]

Within 30 seconds of blood contact, platelets adhere to synthetic solid surfaces. Fibrinogen clearly enhances platelet adhesion to surfaces, and in fact, may be a necessary cofactor, as it is for platelet aggregation. Fibrinogen is gradually "converted" and subsequently demonstrates decreased affinity for platelets.[26] Gamma globulin preferentially binds white cells,[43] although it may also bind a few platelets.[44] Platelet adhesion is not affected by inhibition of coagulation sequences or absence of Factors VIII, IX, or XII.[45]

Adsorbed albumin does not bind platelets or white cells and, in fact, precoating surfaces with albumin or platelet-free plasma greatly reduces platelet adhesion.[9,46] The effect lasts several hours[46] until eventual desorption of albumin and adsorption of fibrinogen and γ-globulin result in platelet adhesion. The mechanism for this albumin effect is thought to be related to the absence of carbohydrate receptors on albumin molecules. Fibrinogen and γ-globulin are glycoproteins and have carbohydrate receptors which may form complexes with similar receptors on platelets.[21] The reaction may involve glycosyl transferase.[40]

At blood-air interfaces, platelets probably adhere to a plasma protein film that contains unconverted fibrinogen.[22] Platelets adhere to this film in large numbers; thus the destruction of platelets occurs at air-blood interfaces.[22] Blood-gas interfaces have long been known to denature plasma proteins.[47]

Platelet reactions to synthetic surfaces have been studied in a variety of *in vitro* test systems.[11,25,26,48] When blood is passed through columns of tightly packed beads, platelets adhere to the beads and are activated.[11] Initially, individual platelets adhere to the surface. Platelets coalesce, forming an irregular monolayer (Fig. 10.3), and eventually raised masses as more platelets are recruited. In the bulk phase, platelet aggregates form.[49,50] Activated platelets release granule contents. With some solids, many platelets adhere and few release; with others few adhere and many release and form aggregates.

As a result of a variety of *in vitro* tests, other factors beside surface characteristics and adsorbed plasma proteins have been found to affect platelet adhesion, aggregation, and release. The presence of red cells enhances platelet adhesion to synthetic surfaces.[51] The ratio of blood volume to surface area affects platelet loss with low ratios being detrimental.[52] High flow rates increase platelet adhesion.[48] Turbulence increases platelet aggregation and release.[49,53] Shear stress does not induce platelet adhesion,[53] but shear stress can cause membrane damage.[54] Release of soluble aggregating agents, particularly ADP from red cells, can activate platelets.[55]

Study of platelets in *in vitro* extracorporeal perfusion systems has provided further information regarding platelet-surface interactions.[24,56] These systems, utilizing human blood and actual components of cardiopulmonary bypass systems, have advantages over *in vivo* studies in that animals cannot add or remove platelets and released materials from the test system.[24] When heparinized human blood is recirculated at 37°C in an extracorporeal perfusion system containing a silicone rubber venous reservoir, spiral coil membrane oxygenator, and roller pump, platelet count decreases to approximately 20% of control values within 2 minutes of blood surface contact[24] (Fig. 10.4). Over the next 6 hours, platelet count progressively increases to 50% of control values. Scanning electron micrographs show individual and groups of platelets attached to synthetic surfaces. Platelets remaining in the recirculated blood lose their ability to aggregate in response to ADP and epinephrine within 2 minutes of the start of recirculation.[24] Furthermore, low affinity platelet factor 4 (LA-PF_4), which is stored in dense granules, is progressively released. The amount of stored LA-PF_4 in platelets decreases.[24] Thromboxane B_2, the stable end product of thromboxane A_2, appears and progressively increases.[57] Unlike LA-PF_4, which appears immediately after blood contact, thromboxane B_2 does not appear for at least 2 minutes and then increases rapidly during the first hour of recirculation.[57] Lastly, acid phosphatase, a lysomal enzyme, is released in progressively increasing amounts during the first 2 hours of recirculation.[58]

Several physical and hemodynamic variables affect platelet-surface interaction during *in vitro* recirculation of human blood at 37°C. The ratio of blood volume to surface area (1 ml to 19 cm^2 in above studies) affects the magnitude of platelet alterations.[24,48,52] When the ratio of blood volume to surface area is reduced, the decrease in platelet count, loss of platelet function to soluble aggregating agents, and release of LA-PF_4 are attenuated.[24] Other studies have shown that high flow rates increase platelet adhesion[48,59] and that geometry of flow within the system also affects platelet adhesion.[48,59]

Available data indicate that not all platelets are similarly activated during *in vitro* recirculation in membrane oxygenator systems. When blood volume to surface area ratio is high, some platelets adhere to the synthetic surfaces and a few release (second wave aggregation), but the majority are not activated. When the blood volume-surface area ratio is low, more platelets adhere to solid surfaces and more are activated to release granule contents and acid phosphatase and to synthesize thromboxane A_2. To a significant degree, the magnitude of the platelet response is directly proportional to the blood volume-surface area ratio.

The platelet response to *in vitro* recirculation in membrane oxygenator systems can be attenuated in several ways. Precoating the circuit with albumin[60] (Fig. 10.5), and addition of PGE_1[61] or prostacyclin (PGI_2)[60] (Fig.

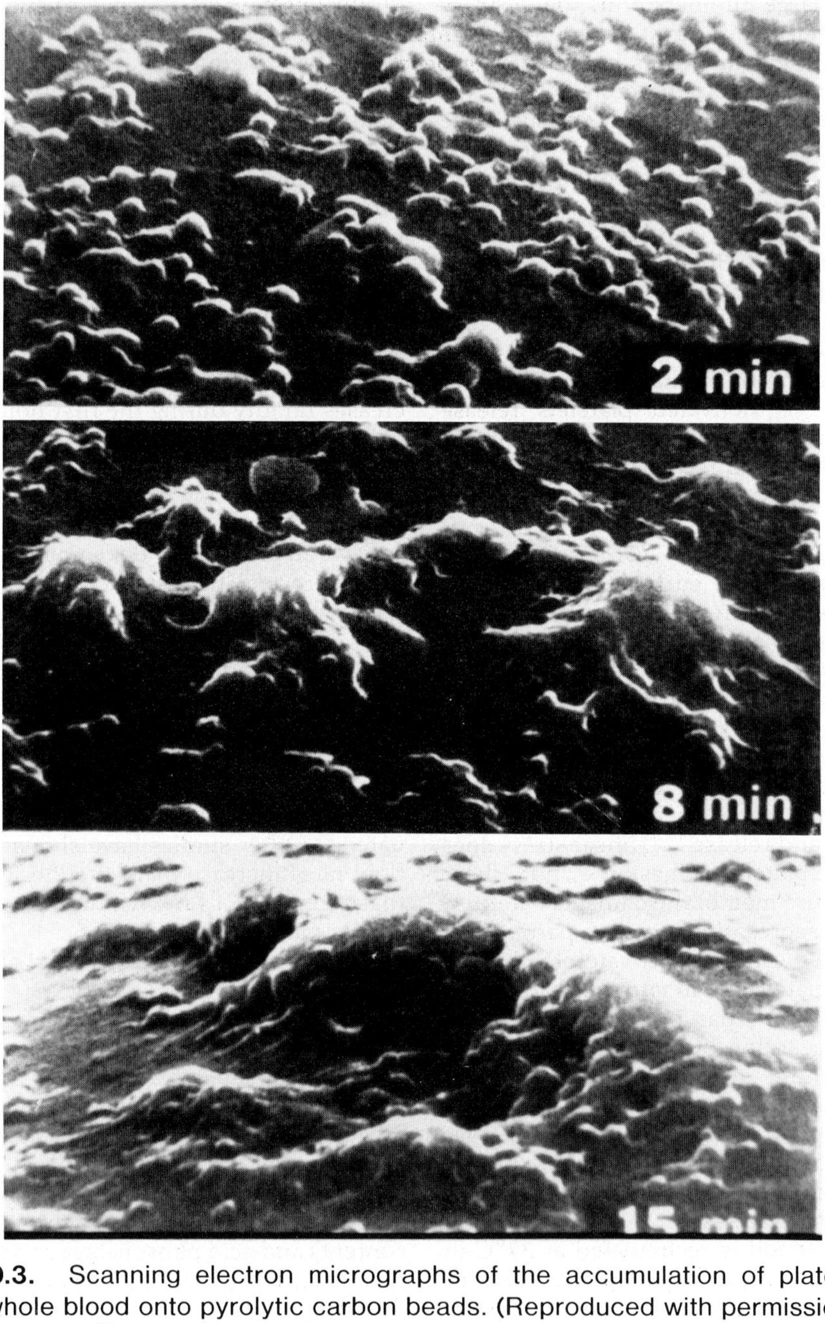

Figure 10.3. Scanning electron micrographs of the accumulation of platelets from citrated whole blood onto pyrolytic carbon beads. (Reproduced with permission from E. W. Salzman et al.[11])

10.6) prevents platelet adhesion and release of LA-PF_4. Precoating with albumin also attenuates platelet responses to ADP and epinephrine. Platelet aggregation is inhibited in the presence of PGE_1 and PGI_2; therefore, platelets cannot respond to soluble aggregating agents. However, since PGI_2 is rapidly metabolized in plasma, platelet function returns after several minutes of recirculation. These fully functional platelets, however, do

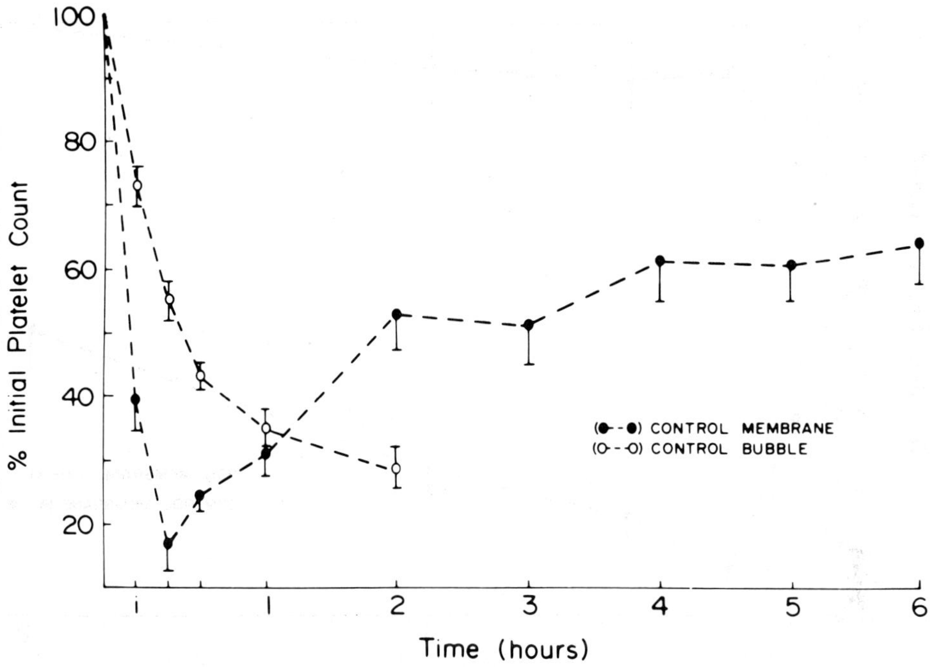

Figure 10.4. Change in circulating platelet count during recirculation of heparinized human blood in membrane and bubble oxygenator circuits.[24,62]

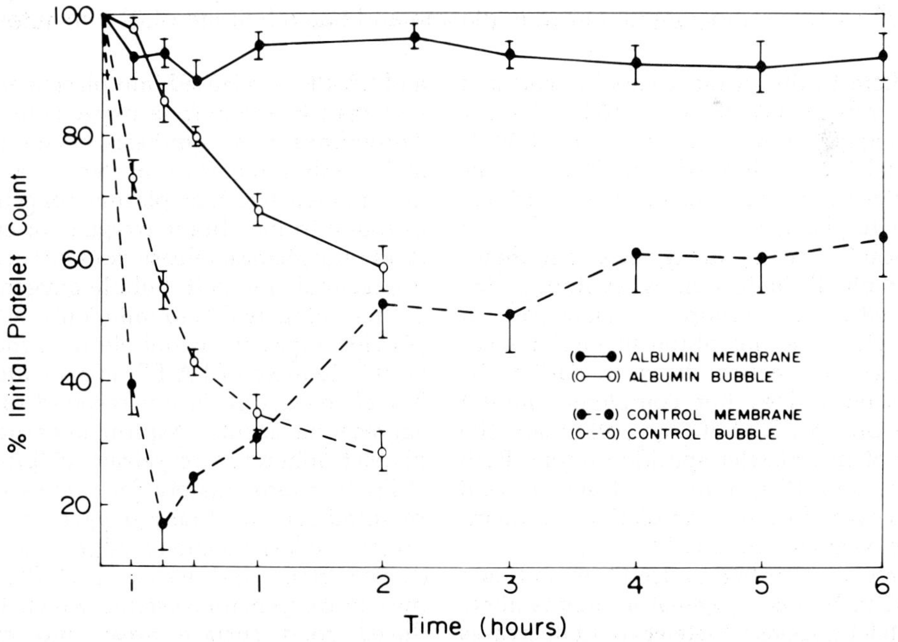

Figure 10.5. Circulating platelet counts during recirculation of heparinized human blood in membrane and bubble oxygenator circuits with and without prior exposure of the circuit to 5% albumin.[60,62]

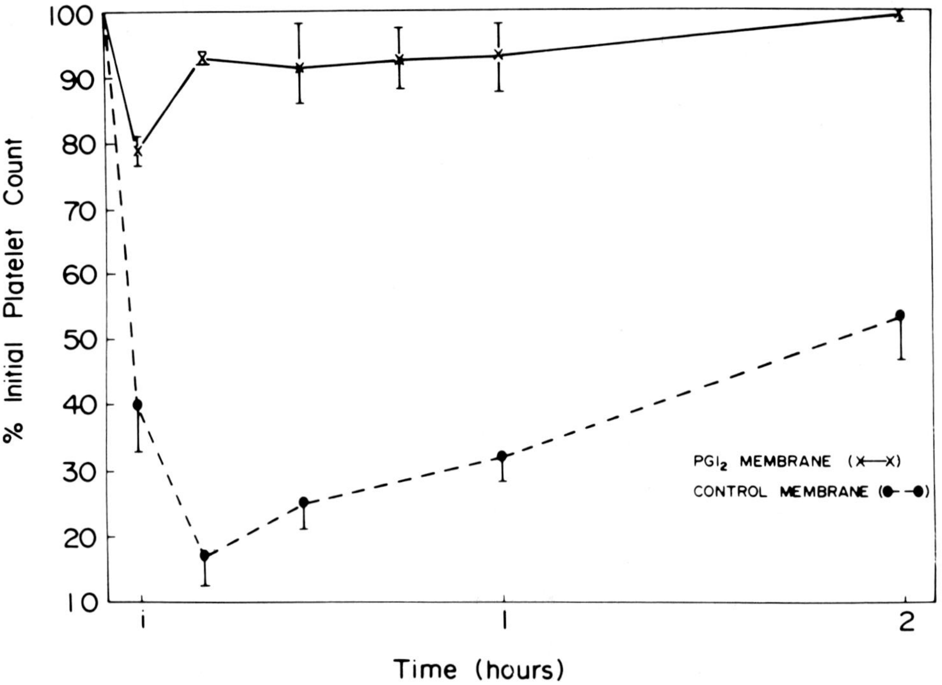

Figure 10.6. Effect of a single bolus of prostacyclin (PI_2) on the circulating platelet count during recirculation of heparinized human blood in a membrane oxygenator circuit.[60] PGI_2 is rapidly metabolized in plasma and has a half-life of 3–5 minutes.

not adhere to the extracorporeal circuit and do not release LA-PF_4 (Fig. 10.7), thereby indicating that prior exposure to blood while the platelets are inhibited with PGI_2 permits the surface to become "passivated" and less reactive to platelets.[60]

Aspirin inhibits cyclooxygenase and therefore inhibits thromboxane A_2 synthesis during *in vitro* extracorporeal circulation.[57] *In vitro* aspirin does not inhibit shape change or first wave aggregation. In recirculation circuits, aspirin does not completely inhibit release of LA-PF_4, but does attenuate the release of this platelet-specific protein. Both albumin and PGI_2 inhibit release of acid phosphatase during recirculation in membrane oxygenator circuits.[58]

Recirculation of heparinized human blood at 37°C in bubble oxygenator circuits alters the platelet response. Platelet count decreases progressively during the period of recirculation and not precipitously within the first 2–5 minutes of recirculation.[62] Bulk platelets do not respond to soluble aggregating agents, and LA-PF_4 is released into plasma at a lower rate than in membrane oxygenator circuits. Thromboxane A_2 synthesis begins immediately within the start of recirculation, but does not reach as high plasmic concentrations as found in membrane oxygenator circuits.[63] Acid phosphatase release does not occur during recirculation with bubble oxygenators.[58]

Precoating with albumin only attenuates platelet adhesion in bubble oxygenator circuits.[60] Release of LA-PF_4 is also attenuated, but platelets still do not respond to soluble aggregating agents. Aspirin does not affect platelet adherence or release of LA-PF_4.[57,63] PGE_1 in approximately four times the dose required for membrane oxygenator systems greatly reduces platelet adherence to synthetic surfaces and release of LA-PF_4.[62] Thus, bubble oxygenator systems which have reduced solid surface areas and extensive blood-gas interfaces appear to cause a different pattern of platelet activation and response than membrane systems. Bubble oxygenators systems may cause a direct injury to platelet

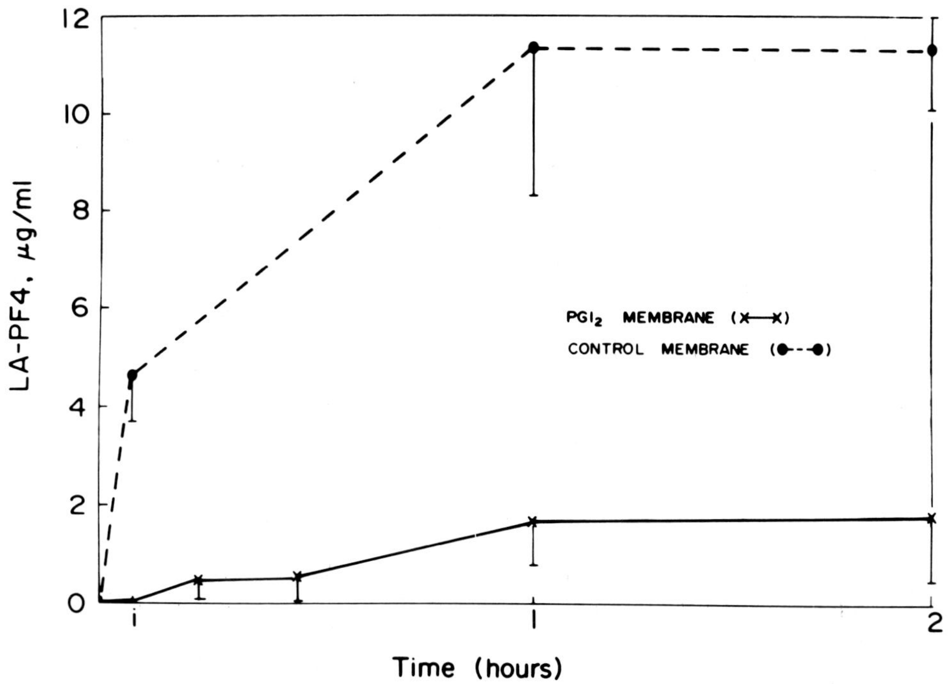

Figure 10.7. Plasma LA-PF_4 concentrations during recirculation of heparinized human blood in membrane oxygenator circuits.[60]

membranes at the blood-gas interface, but simultaneously reduce the magnitude of platelet-solid surface interaction. Membrane oxygenator systems, devoid of blood-gas interfaces, seem to offer more potential than bubble oxygenator systems for pharmacologic preservation of platelets since direct physical injury to platelets and platelet membranes appears to be less.

PLATELET REACTIONS DURING *IN VIVO* CARDIOPULMONARY BYPASS

Early studies showed that platelet counts decrease markedly within the first few minutes of clinical cardiopulmonary bypass.[64,65] Salzman[66] later observed that during bypass the ability of platelets to adhere to glass spheres was reduced.[66] Recently, investigators have shown renewed interest in the pathologic physiology of platelets during clinical cardiopulmonary bypass.

During clinical perfusions with membrane oxygenator bypass systems, actual platelet counts decrease significantly during and after the period of bypass.[67,68] Dilution accounts for most of the decrease in actual platelet counts; however, when corrections for dilution are made, corrected platelet counts are also significantly reduced during clinical bypass. Platelet aggregates are formed and can be counted in the arterial perfusion line.[69] Platelet aggregation to ADP is reduced during and 1 hour after bypass, and plasma concentrations of LA-PF_4 are significantly increased. No change in platelet LA-PF_4 or adenine nucleotides (ATP, ADP), or their ratio occurs. As a result of bypass, postoperative bleeding times are significantly prolonged.

Changes in platelets during cardiopulmonary bypass with bubble oxygenator systems have been more extensively studied.[31,32,67,68,70] Although actual platelet counts decrease significantly during bypass, counts corrected for dilution do not decrease, but either stay the same or increase slightly.[31,68,70] Smaller, older platelets appear in the circulation, suggesting selective removal of larger, younger platelets.[71] Platelet aggregates are formed.[69] These vary widely in size and number, but experimental evidence suggests that these disaggregate in the distal capillary circulation.[72] Although experimental evidence in dogs suggests platelets may be temporarily sequestered in the liver and spleen during bypass,[73] this does not appear to occur in humans.

Platelet aggregation to ADP and collagen decrease significantly during bypass with bubble oxygenators and remain reduced for a variable period after bypass.[31,68,70] During bypass, plasma concentrations of LA-PF_4, PF_4, and B-thromboglobulin[31,68], and thromboxane B_2[32] increase. Although one study showed a significant decrease in platelet adenine nucleotides,[74] another failed to confirm this change.[31] As with membrane oxygenator systems, postoperative bleeding times are prolonged.[31,68,70]

During clinical cardiopulmonary bypass, the cardiotomy suction return system is utilized to aspirate blood from the operative field. This blood, which has been in contact with pericardium and epicardium and exposed to air, is filtered and held in a reservoir before it is returned to the bypass circuit. Cardiotomy sucker systems are a major cause of hemolysis during cardiopulmonary bypass,[75,76] but few studies of the effect of cardiotomy sucker systems on platelets have been made. Contact with tissues and air activates platelets,[77]; filtration removes platelet aggregates, but may also induce aggregate formation.[69] The volume of blood aspirated by the cardiotomy suction system and the percentage of total perfusate aspirated correlate directly with decreases in actual platelet count during cardiopulmonary bypass.[78]

Attempts to preserve platelets by precoating membrane or bubble oxygenator systems with albumin have failed. No significant preservation of platelets or reduction in bleeding times have been observed.[79] Administration of dipyridamole reduces losses of platelets during clinical bypass, but platelets remain inhibited by the drug after bypass stops.[80] In monkeys, infusion of PGE_1 results in temporary inhibition of platelets during cardiopulmonary bypass with either membrane or bubble oxygenator systems.[81] Following bypass, bleeding times are only slightly increased over preoperative controls[62,80] (Fig. 10.8). However, when PGE_1 is infused in humans, profound hypotension prevents infusion of sufficient drug to inactivate platelets.[79] Recently, PGI_2 has been infused during bypass in humans. Although profound hypotension occurred in some patients (mean blood reached 20 torr), no ill effects were observed. In these patients, postoperative blood losses were reduced.

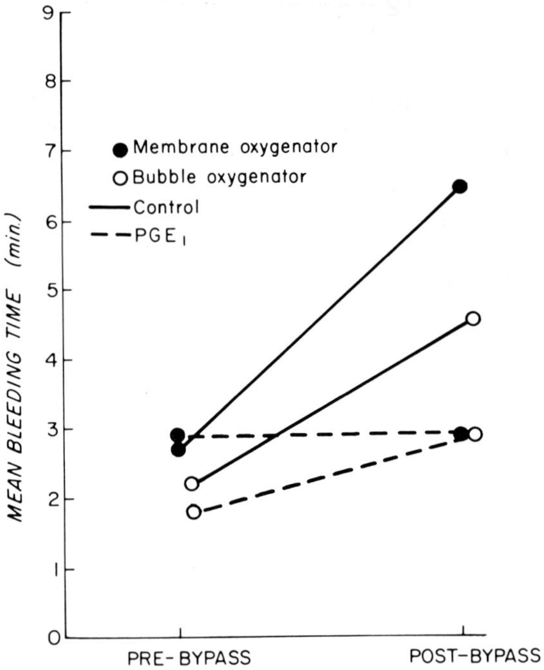

Figure 10.8. Effect of an effusion of PGE_1 during 1 hour of cardiopulmonary bypass in rhesus monkeys. With PGE_1, postoperative bleeding times did not differ significantly from preoperative measurements.

The pathogenesis of platelet changes during cardiopulmonary bypass is not clear. Clearly, some platelets are activated, some platelets adhere to synthetic surfaces, others form circulating aggregates, and others release granule contents. Remaining platelets are temporarily less responsive to soluble aggregating agents, which is reflected in the observed prolongation of postoperative bleeding times. It is possible that the number of platelets that adhere to synthetic surfaces, form circulating aggregates, or release are wholly or partially replaced by new platelets entering the circulation. When platelet counts are corrected for dilution, one must conclude that a minority of platelets are activated and that the majority (including new platelets) circulate, but with reduced function.

Currently, three hypotheses have been advanced to explain the reduced function of circulating platelets during and immediately after bypass.[68] Surface contact with the extracorporeal system may alter platelet membrane receptors so that platelets are refractory to activating physical and chemical stimuli. Alternatively, all platelets may partially release stored granule contents and lose function as a result of this depletion. Thirdly, platelets may be inhibited by a circulating inhibitor, possibly released by activating platelets since this inhibitor is not effective if initial platelet activation is prevented.

The reduced platelet function caused by bypass is temporary, since Harker observed that bleeding times return toward normal within 2–4 hours after bypass.[31] This return of function may indicate recovery of circulating inhibited platelets or the appearance of a substantial number of new platelets. Although bleeding times are only temporarily prolonged, this consequence of platelet dysfunction occurs at the time the surgeon is attempting to close the chest.

References

1. Wintrobe MM: *Clinical Hematology*, Ed. 7. Philadelphia, Lea & Febiger, 1974.
2. Hovig T: The ultrastructure of blood platelets in normal and abnormal states. Sci Haematol 1:3–64, 1968.
3. White JG, Gerrard JM: Platelet function and its disorders: Anatomy and structural organization of the platelet. In *Textbook of Haemostasis & Thrombosis*, Chap. 21, edited by RW Colman, J Hirsh, V Marder, and EW Salzman. Philadelphia, Lippincott, in press, 1981.
4. Nurden AT and Caen JP: Membrane glycoproteins and human platelet function. Br J Haematol 38:155, 1978.
5. Niewiarowski S: Proteins secreted by the platelet. Thromb Haemostas 38:924, 1977.
6. Paul D, Niewiarowski S, Varma KG, Rucinski B, Rucker S, Lange E: Human platelet basic protein associated with antiheparin and mitogenic activities: Purification and partial characterization. Proc Natl Acad Sci USA 77:5914, 1980.
7. Bretòn-Gorius J, Guichard J: Two different types of granules in megakaryocytes and platelets as revealed by the diaminobenzidine method. J Microsc Biol Cell: 23, 197, 1975.
8. Bentfeld ME and Bainton DF: Cytochemical localization of lysosomal enzymes in rat megakaryocytes and platelets. J Clin Invest 56:1635, 1975.
9. Martin JH, Carson FL, Race GJ: Calcium-containing platelet granules. J Cell Biol 60:775, 1974.
10. DaPrada M, Pletcher A, Tanzer JP, Knuchel H: Subcellular localization of 5-hydroxytryptamine in blood platelets. Nature 56:1315, 1967.
11. Salzman EW, Lindon J, Brier D, Merrill EW: Surface-induced platelet adhesion, aggregation and release. Ann NY Acad Sci 283:114, 1977.
12. Bills TK, Silver MJ: Phosphatidylcholine is the primary source of arachidonic acid utilized by platelet prostaglandin synthetase. Fed Proc 34:790, 1975.
13. Marcus AJ: Platelet function and its disorders: Platelet aggregation. In *Textbook of Haemostasis & Thrombosis*, Chapter 23, edited by RW Colman, J Hirsh, V Marder, and EW Salzman. Philadelphia, Lippincott Co., in press, 1982.
14. Weiss HJ: Platelet physiology and abnormalities of platelet function. N Engl J Med 293:531, 580, 1975.
15. Packham MA, Guccione MA, Greenberg JP, Kinlough-Rathbone RL, Mustard JF: Release of ^{14}C-serotonin during initial platelet changes induced by thrombin, collagen or A23187. Blood 50:915, 1977.
16. Gorman RR: Modulation of human platelet function by prostacyclin and thromboxane A_2. Fed Proc 38: 83, 1979.
17. Hamberg M, Svensson J, Samuelsson B: Thromboxanes: A new group of biologically active compounds derived from prostaglandin endoperoxides. Proc Natl Acad Sci USA 72:2994, 1975.
18. Steer M, Salzman EW: Intracellular respiratory processes in platelets. In *Textbook of Haemostasis & Thrombosis*, Chapter 31, edited by RW Colman, J Hirsh, V Marder, and EW Salzman. Philadelphia, Lippincott, in press 1982.
19. Salzman EW, Lindon JN, Rodvien R: Cyclic AMP in human blood platelets: Relation to platelet prostaglandin synthesis induced by centrifugation or surface contact. J Cyclic Nucleotide Res 2:25, 1976.
20. Baier RE, Dutton RC: Initial events in interactions of blood with a foreign surface. J Biomed Mater Res 3: 191, 1969.
21. Lee RG, Kim SW: Adsorption of proteins onto hydrophobic polymer surfaces: Adsorption isotherms and kinetics. J Biomed Mater Res 8:251, 1974.
22. Vroman L, Adams AL, Klings M, Fischer G: Fibrinogen, globulin, albumin, and plasma at interfaces. Adv Chemistry 145:255, 1975.
23. Kochwa S, Litwak RS, Rosenfield RE, Leonard EF: Blood elements at foreign surfaces: A biochemical appraoch to the study of the adsorption of plasma proteins. Ann NY Acad Sci 283:37, 1977.
24. Hennessey VL Jr, Hicks RE, Niewiarowski S, Edmunds LH Jr, Colman RW: Function of human platelets during extracorporeal circulation. Am J Physiol 232:H622, 1977.
25. Lindon J, Rosenberg R, Merrill E, Salzman E: Interaction of human platelets with heparinized agarose gel. J Lab Clin Med 91:47, 1978.
26. Vroman L, Adams AL: Findings with the recording ellipsometer suggesting rapid exchange of specific plasma proteins at liquid/solid interfaces. Surface Science 16:438, 1969.
27. Vroman L, Adams AL, Fischer, GC, Munoz PC: Interaction of high molecular weight kininogen, Factor XII and fibrinogen in plasma at interfaces. Blood 55:156, 1980.

28. Zucker MD, Vroman L: Platelet adhesion induced by fibrinogen adsorbed onto glass. Proc Soc Exp Biol Med 131:318, 1969.
29. Salzman EW, Merrill EW, Binder A, Wolfe CFW, Ashford TPA, Austin WG: Protein-platelet interaction on heparinized surfaces. J Biomed Mater Res 3: 69, 1969.
30. Bachman F, McKenna R, Cole ER, Najafi H: The hemostatic extracorporeal mechanism after open heart surgery. I. Studies on plasma coagulation factors and fibrinolysis in 512 patients after extracorporeal circulation. J Thorac Cardiovasc Surg 70:76, 1975.
31. Harker LA, Malpass TW, Branson HE, Hessel EA II, Slichter SJ: Mechanism of abnormal bleeding in patients undergoing cardiopulmonary bypass: Acquired transient platelet dysfunction association with selective α-granule release. Blood 56:824, 1980.
32. Davies GC, Sobel M, Salzman EW: Elevated plasma fibrinopeptide A and thromboxane B_2 levels during cardiopulmonary bypass. Circulation 61:808, 1980.
33. Woods JE, Kirklin JW, Owen CA Jr, Thompson JH Jr, Taswell HF: Effect of bypass surgery on coagulation-sensitive clotting factors. Mayo Clinic Proc 42:724, 1967.
34. Meier HL, Scott CF, Mandle R Jr, Webster ME, Pierce JV, Colman RW, Kaplan AP: Requirements for contact activation of human Hageman factor. Ann NY Acad Sci 28:93, 1977.
35. Margolis J: The interrelationship of coagulation of plasma and release of peptides. Ann NY Sci 104:133, 1963.
36. Ratnoff OD: Studies on the product of the reaction between activated Hageman factor (Factor XII) and plasma thromboplastin antecedent (Factor XI). J Lab Clin Med 80:704, 1972.
37. Wardle EN, Piercy DA: Studies of contact activation of blood in hemodialysis. J Clin Pathol 25:1045, 1972.
38. Rosenberg RD: Heparin action. Circulation 49:603, 1974.
39. Moncada S, Higgs EA, Vane JR: Human arterial and venous tissues generate prostacyclin (prostaglandin X), a potent inhibitor of platelet aggregation. Lancet 1:18, 1977.
40. Kim SW, Wisniewski S, Lee ES, Winn ML: Role of proteins and fatty acid adsorption at the blood-polymer interface. J Biomed Mater Res Symp 8:23, 1977.
41. Baier RE: The organization of blood components near interfaces. Ann NY Acad Sci 283:17, 1977.
42. Merrill EW, Salzman EW, DaCosta SA, Brier-Russell D, Wolfe, LC, Dincer A, Wu JJ, Pape P, Lindon JN: Molecular factors in blood polymer interactions: Hydrophobic, hydrophilic, and hydrogen bonding. (work in progress).
43. Vroman L, Adams AL, Klings M, Fischer GC, Munoy PC, Solensky RP: Reactions of formed elements of blood with plasma proteins at interfaces. Ann NY Acad Sci 283:65, 1977.
44. Mason RG, Shermer RW, Zucker WH: Effects of certain purified plasma proteins on the compatibility of glass with blood. Am J Pathol 73:183, 1973.
45. Mason RG, Shermer RW, and Rodman NF: Reactions of blood with nonbiologic surfaces. Ultrastructural and clotting studies with normal and coagulation factor deficient bloods. Am J Path 69:271, 1972.
46. Packham MA, Evans G, Glynn MF, Mustard JF: The effect of plasma proteins on the interaction of platelets with glass surfaces. J Lab Clin Med 73:686, 1969.
47. Lee WH Jr, Hairston P: Structural effects on blood proteins at the gas-blood interface. Fed Proc 30:1615, 1971.
48. Friedman LI, Liem H, Grabowski EF, Leonard EF, McCord CW: Inconsequentiality of surface properties for initial platelet adhesion. Trans Amer Soc Artif Intern Organs 16:63, 1970.
49. Yu SK, Goldsmith HL: Behavior of model particles and blood cells at spherical obstructions in tube flow. Microvasc Res 6:5, 1973.
50. Morton WA, Parmentier EM, Petschek HE: Study of aggregate formation in regions of separated blood flow. Thromb Diath Haemorrh 34:840, 1975.
51. Brash JL, Brophy JM, Feuerstein IA: Adhesion of platelets to artificial surfaces: Effect of red cells. J Biomed Mater Res 10:429, 1976.
52. Olsson P, Lagergren H, Larsson R, Rådegran K: Prevention of platelet adhesion and aggregation by a glutardialdehyde-stabilized heparin surface. Thromb Haemostas 37:274, 1977.
53. Goldsmith HL, Marlow JC, Yu SK: The effect of oscillatory flow on the release reaction and aggregation of human platelets. Microvasc Res 11:335, 1976.
54. Bernstein EF, Marzec U, Clayman MD, Swanson S, Johnston GG: Platelet function following surface injury and shear stress: Adhesion, aggregation, release, Factor 3 activity. Ann NY Acad Sci 283:138, 1977.
55. Mustard JF, Packham MA: Factors influencing platelet function, adhesion, release and aggregation. Pharmacol Rev 22:97, 1970.
56. Tamari Y, Aledort L, Puszkin E, Degnan TJ, Wagner N, Kaplitt, MJ, Pierce EC II: Functional changes in platelets during extracorporeal circulation. Ann Thorac Surg 19:639, 1975.
57. Addonizio VP Jr, Smith JB, Guiod LR, Strauss JF III, Colman RW, Edmunds LH Jr: Thromboxane synthesis and platelet protein release during simulated extracorporeal circulation. Blood 54:371, 1979.
58. Addonizio VP Jr, Chang LK, Strauss JR III, Colman RW, Edmunds LH Jr: Release of lysosomal hydrolases during extracorporeal circulation, Submitted for publication to Journal of Thoracic and Cardiovascular Surgery, 1980.
59. Addonizio VP Jr, Colman RW, Edmunds LH Jr: The effect of blood flow rate and circuit surface area on platelet loss during extracorporeal circulation. Trans Am Soc Artif Intern Organs 24:650, 1978.
60. Addonizio VP Jr, Macarak EJ, Nicolaou KC, Edmunds LH Jr, Colman RW: Effects of prostacyclin and albumin on platelet loss during *in vitro* stimulation of extracorporeal circulation. Blood 53:1033, 1979.
61. Addonizio VP Jr, Macarak EJ, Colman RW, Niewiarowski S, Edmunds LH Jr: Preservation of human platelets with prostaglandin E_1 during *in vitro* stimulation of cardiopulmonary bypass. Circ Res 44:350, 1979.
62. Addonizio VP Jr, Strauss JF III, Colman RW, Ed-

munds LH Jr: Effects of prostaglandin E_1 on platelet loss during *in vivo* and *in vitro* extracorporeal circulation with a bubble oxygenator. J Thorac Cardiovasc Surg 77:119, 1979.

63. Addonizio VP Jr, Smith JB, Strauss JF III, Colman RW, Edmunds LH Jr: Thromboxane synthesis and platelet secretion during cardiopulmonary bypass with bubble oxygenator. J Thorac Cardiovasc Surg 79:91, 1980.
64. Kendall AG, Lowenstein L: Alterations in blood coagulation and hemostasis during extracorporeal circulation. Can Med Assoc J 87:786, 859, 1962.
65. Kay EB, Zimmerman HA, Berne RM, Hirose Y, Jones RD, Cross FS: Certain clinical aspects of the use of a pump oxygenator. JAMA 162:639, 1956.
66. Salzman EW: Measurement of platelet adhesiveness. J Lab Clin Med 62:724, 1963.
67. Clark RE, Beauchamp RA, Magrath RA, Brooks JD, Ferguson TB, Weldon CS: Comparison of bubble and membrane oxygenators. J Thorac Cardiovasc Surg 78:655, 1979.
68. Edmunds LH Jr, Ellison N, Colman RW, Niewiarowski S, Rao AK, Addonizio VP Jr, Stephenson LW, Edie RN: Platelet function during open heart surgery: Comparison of membrane and bubble oxygenators, submitted for publication to J Thorac Cardiovasc Surg, 1981.
69. Dutton RC, Edmunds LH Jr, Hutchinson JC, Roe BB: Platelet aggregate emboli produced in patients during cardiopulmonary bypass with membrane and bubble oxygenators and blood filters. J Thorac Cardiovasc Surg 67:258, 1974.
70. McKenna R, Bachman F, Whitaker B, Gilson JR, Weinberg M Jr: The hemostatic mechanism after open heart surgery. J Thorac Cardiovasc Surg 70: 298, 1975.
71. Laufer N, Merin G, Grover NB, Pessachowicz B, Borman JB: The influence of cardiopulmonary bypass on the size of human platelets. J Thorac Cardiovasc Surg 70:727, 1975.
72. Hicks RE, Dutton RC, Ries CA, Price DC, Edmunds LH Jr: Production and fate of particulate emboli during veno-venous perfusion. Surg Forum 24:250, 1973.
73. deLaval ME, Hill JD, Mielke CH et al. Blood platelets and extracorporeal circulation. J Thorac Cardiovasc Surg 69:144, 1975.
74. Beurling-Harbury C, Galvan CA: Acquired decrease in platelet secretory ADP associated with increased postoperative bleeding in post-cardiopulmonary bypass patients and in patients with severe valvular heart disease. Blood 52:13, 1978.
75. Morris KN, Kinross FM, Stirling GR: Hemolysis of blood in the pericardium: The major source of plasma hemoglobin during total body perfusion. J Thorac Cardiovasc Surg 49:250, 1965.
76. Osborn JJ, Cohn K, Hait M, Russi M, Sald A, Harkins G, Gerbode F: Hemolysis during perfusion. Sources and means of reduction. J Thorac Cardiovasc Surg 43:459, 1962.
77. Dutton RC and Edmunds LH Jr: Formation of platelet aggregate emboli in a prototype hollow fiber membrane oxygenator. J Biomed Mater Res 8:163, 1974.
78. Edmunds LH Jr, Saxena NC, Hillyer P, Wilson TJ: Relationship between platelet count and cardiotomy suction return. Ann Thor Surg 25:306, 1978.
79. Ellison N, Addonizio VP, Niewiarowski S, MacVaugh H III, Harken AH, Colman RW, Edmunds LH Jr: Platelet protection during cardiopulmonary bypass with albumin prime and prostaglandin E_1 infusion. Anesthesiology 53:S168, 1980.
80. Nuutinen LS, Mononen P: Dipyridamole and thrombocyte count in open-heart surgery. J Thorac Cardiovasc Surg 70, 707, 1975.
81. Addonizio VP Jr, Strauss JF III, Macarak EJ, Colman RW, Edmunds LH Jr: Preservation of platelet number and function with prostaglandin E_1 during total cardiopulmonary bypass in rhesus monkeys. Surgery 83:619, 1978.

CHAPTER 11

BLOOD CONSERVATION DURING CARDIOPULMONARY BYPASS

LELAND B. HOUSMAN, M.D.

In the last 10 years, there has been almost an exponential increase in the number of open heart surgical procedures carried out in the United States.[1,2] Most of this increase is attributable to coronary artery bypass operations. Whereas less than 25,000 such procedures were performed in 1973, by 1977 an estimated 70,000 patients underwent coronary artery bypass surgery,[3] and the numbers will surely have exceeded an annual rate of greater than 100,000 per year by the end of 1980.

In 1971 and again in 1978, surveys indicated that the number of units of bank blood utilized per case averaged 8.5. Recent studies have shown, however, that most routine open heart procedures can be carried out safely without the use of autologous banked blood in fully 70–90% of all cases.[2,4–6] As we look into the future, an overall reduction in blood usage is becoming mandatory, because if the current trend in number of cases performed continues its upward spiral, a burden will be placed upon blood banks which they may be unable to meet.

In this chapter, the various techniques of blood conservation currently in use will be reviewed, current research endeavors analyzed, and future directions in blood conservation during open heart surgery discussed.

HISTORICAL REVIEW

During the early days of cardiac surgery, the heart-lung machine was most often primed with whole blood or blood products.[7,8] As the number of cases increased together with the inevitable demand on blood banks, and the complications of blood transfusions became manifest,[9,10] various studies were undertaken in the research laboratory[11,12] and at the clinical level[13,14] investigating the feasibility and practicality of performing open heart surgery with reduced amounts of blood (Fig. 11.1). In certain clinical situations, the religious preference of patients severely curtails or eliminates the opportunity for blood transfusion. The successful management of these individual cases without transfusion proved conclusively that open heart surgery could indeed be performed without the use of blood.[15]

Another major impact on blood usage in cardiac surgery was the rapid improvement in existing extracorporeal circuits and the application of newer material technology to the clinical setting.[16] Early extracorporeal circuits made use of pumps or discs that resulted in high levels of hemolysis and increased red cell damage. Transfusion became necessary to prevent severe, clinically significant anemia. As the newer pump-oxygenators were developed with particular attention to these problems, the hemolysis and protein denaturation seen with the early generation oxygenators was markedly reduced.[17]

The two major types of oxygenators currently in use clinically are the bubble oxygenator and the membrane oxygenator. The bubble oxygenator affords clinically accept-

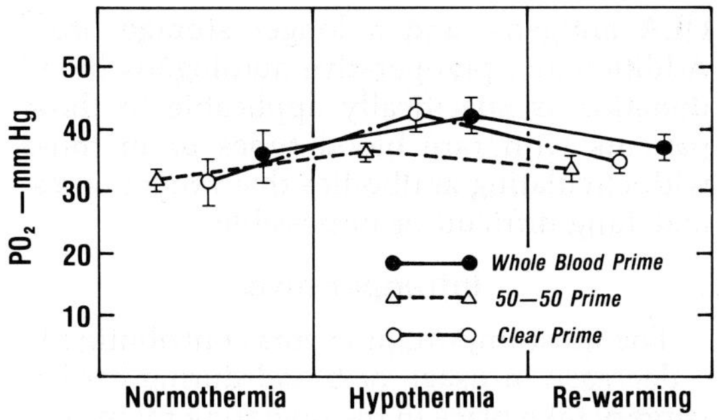

Figure 11.1. Mean mixed venous pO_2 values > 25–28 mm Hg were achieved in animals and verify that adequate tissue perfusion had taken place regardless of the type of priming solution used in the heart-lung machine.

able low levels of hemolysis, especially when the duration of cardiopulmonary bypass is kept below 2½ hours. When perfusion time exceeds 3 hours, the membrane oxygenator, which has no direct blood-gas interface, is clearly superior and would seem to be the oxygenator of choice whenever longer periods of perfusion are necessary.[12,18]

Since cardiac surgeons now have oxygenators available which do not have an associated high obligatory destruction of red blood cells the amount of blood needed for individual operations and postoperative care has been greatly reduced.

Hemodilution

It had been erroneously assumed that normal or near-normal hemoglobin levels had to be maintained during and after cardiopulmonary bypass. It was thought that with lower levels, the oxyhemoglobin dissociation curve would be altered in such fashion that oxygen in adequate amounts would be unable to be delivered to the body tissues which would culminate in extensive, progressive, and theoretically fatal acidosis.

As stated previously, studies carried out in the laboratory showed hemodilution to be not only feasible, but quite practical and highly advantageous in terms of improved tissue perfusion.[11] This led to the routine incorporation of hemodilution in cardiac surgical operations requiring extracorporeal circulation. Today, the ability to prime the heart-lung machine with nonhemic solutions and the acceptance of low hemoglobin levels while on bypass has obviously resulted in a dramatic decrease in blood utilization during open heart surgery.

Despite the use of these current generation oxygenators and hemodilution, the average number of units of banked blood utilized per case remains unacceptably high. As we shall see, a multitude of other techniques are available and currently in use in certain centers which can significantly reduce blood usage associated with cardiac surgery. Indeed, it has now become quite practical to perform cardiac surgery routinely without the use of autologous banked blood.

TECHNIQUES OF BLOOD CONSERVATION

Preoperative

To minimize blood transfusion, one must maximize blood conservation. These efforts must begin in the preoperative period. One aspect most commonly overlooked is the nutritional status of the cardiac surgery patient.

In many instances, patients are clinically malnourished or undernourished. This is most often seen in advanced valvular heart disease in adults, but no subset of the patient population is immune.[19] Furthermore, these nutritional deficits are often clinically undetectable (muscle wasting in a mildly obese patient) and frequently quite subtle. Careful measurements by clinical nutritionists have made it possible to accurately quantitate the nitrogen and caloric deficits as well as specific needs of patients.[20] It is often advantageous to defer surgery in severely depleted patients until their nutritional status has been improved. This delay has resulted in significant decreases in both mortality and morbidity. In particular, a well nourished patient is much easier to wean from mechanical ventilation than one suffering from cardiac cachexia and overall muscle weakness.

Specific nutritional deficiencies directly affect the hematopoietic system. Among these are iron and the various vitamins such as B_6 and B_{12} which are necessary for effective hematopoiesis. The simple preoperative correction of an iron deficiency anemia can raise depressed hemoglobin levels to normal values and thereby reduce the need for blood during surgery and in the postoperative period. Similarly, adequate tissue stores of specific vitamins and minerals essential for red blood cell manufacture ensure rapid repletion of blood components in the postoperative period. As will be shown later, this rebuilding of normal hemoglobin levels is much more rapid than previously appreciated and has contributed significantly to the overall reduction in transfusion requirements in patients having undergone cardiac surgery.

Although oral hyperalimentation is always preferable when possible and is associated with almost no complications, maximal utilization of this method is not always available. Limiting features in cardiac surgical patients include fluid restriction, lack of patient compliance, and inability, because of extreme weakness, of the patient to ingest the tremendous amounts of foodstuffs required to correct their nutritional deficiencies. Intravenous hyperalimentation has proven to be quite satisfactory and can be used to supplement oral intake or serve as the sole nutritional source.[21] Obviously, a combination of oral and intravenous hyperalimentation is the most rapid and effective means of correcting nutritional deficiencies in any individual patient.

Finally, the preoperative storage of the patients' own blood has had a major impact on blood conservation. In those patients undergoing elective procedures, autologous blood can be drawn off prior to admission and transfused at appropriate times during future hospitalization.[22] If this collection takes place 20–30 days preoperatively, the patient often enters the hospital with near normal hemoglobin values.

Certain groups of patients have elevated central blood volumes and are ideal candidates for preoperative autologous blood collection. The most common example are those patients with valvular heart disease and congestive heart failure and patients with intracardiac shunts, cyanosis, and markedly elevated hemoglobin values (tetralogy of Fallot). Some centers store whole units of donor blood, whereas others advocate frozen red blood cells whenever repeated donation is carried out prior to an elective surgical procedure. Advantages of frozen cells include higher levels of 2,3-diphosphoglycerate, a lower incidence of both serum hepatitis and HLA antigens, and a longer storage life.[23] Additionally, preoperative autologous blood donation is specifically applicable to those patients with rare blood types or in those with circulating antibodies that render cross-matching difficult or impossible.

Intraoperative

The most important events contributing to a decrease in usage of blood during cardiac surgery take place in the operating room. The first of these are the prebypass withdrawal of autologous blood.

Many studies have shown that the immediate prebypass removal of one or two units of the patients' own blood and subsequent reinfusion following bypass has significantly reduced the requirements for blood bank transfusion.[24,25] This has certainly been consistent with our own experience and is used routinely, regardless of the hematocrit at the time of induction of anesthesia. If the hematocrit value is likely to drop below 15–18 vol% during bypass, red blood cells are added at the appropriate time, but we feel it is imperative to withdraw autologous blood in all patients even if banked blood must be given simultaneously to maintain hemoglobin levels high enough to deliver oxygen to the tissues. This level of hemoglobin is much lower than generally realized, and as long as the hemoglobin is 5 gm or greater, no significant adverse effects on the oxyhemoglobin dissociation curve are noted.[11]

There are many ways to withdraw the autologous blood prior to bypass. The simplest seems to be the slow, gradual removal through a large-bore central venous pressure (CVP) catheter. The removal is usually begun following endotracheal intubation. This allows the anesthesiologist more time for simultaneous replenishment of the intravascular volume which is necessary for maintenance of a satisfactory cardiac output.

Other methods of withdrawal include removal through the arterial monitoring line or from the arterial or venous cannula. The latter is usually accomplished through an attached side arm and is done following cannulation. Often times this more rapid withdrawal may result in clinical instability and increased hemolysis. Furthermore, since heparinization is carried out prior to cannulation this heparinized blood that is withdrawn may alter the patient's coagulation status during or after surgery.

Additional advantages of autologous blood removal include the immediate postoperative availability of fresh blood with nontraumatized platelets and abundant coagulation factors. This has significantly reduced postoperative bleeding in several reported series.[26,27]

One of the more important intraoperative maneuvers in blood conservation is that of surgical technique. Meticulous attention to hemostasis during all phases of the operation can prevent large amounts of blood loss. The liberal use of electrocautery, especially when opening the chest, has proven extremely rewarding in this regard. In coronary artery bypass procedures, the leg wound is a major potential source of blood loss. Again, meticulous hemostasis during harvesting of the saphenous vein and careful approximation of the various wound layers with elimination of all dead space will greatly reduce needless blood loss (Fig. 11.2).

The next major innovation is the use of autotransfusion techniques. Utilizing various types of machines, these "cell-savers" (Haemonetics Cell Saver II; Haemonetics Corp., Braintree, Mass.) employ a form of regional anticoagulation by introducing heparin into the suction tubing at its tip. This allows all discard suction material to be anticoagulated, collected, centrifuged, washed, and returned to the patient as red blood cells. In this fashion, blood that ordinarily would be discarded can be saved. We have been able to salvage an average of one unit of packed cells per elective case, and addition of these autotransfusion techniques has raised the percentage of cases performed without the use of blood from 85%[26] to 94% (Figs. 11.3 and 11.4). Others have had a similar experience.[28]

BLOOD LOSS PER PATIENT

	Group I	Group II
In Surgery Chest Tubes	1630cc 870cc	280cc 530cc
Total (mean)	2500cc	810cc

Figure 11.2. Meticulous attention to surgical technique has resulted in a significant decrease in surgical blood loss. Group I, Early series with free utilization of blood. Group II, Current series using maximal blood conservation techniques.

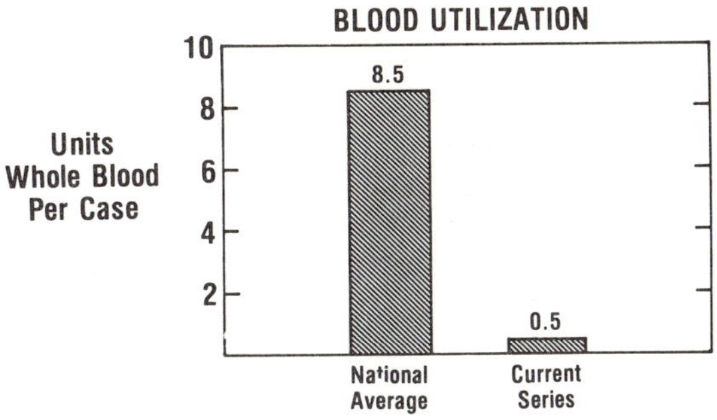

Figure 11.3. Significant reductions in blood utilization can be obtained when conservation techniques are routinely employed.

UNITS OF WHOLE BLOOD USED PER PATIENT

	Group I	Group II
Surgery S.I.C.U. Floor	4.87 3.70 0	.20 .29 0
Total (mean)	8.57	.49

Figure 11.4. Numerical breakdown of blood usage with respect to location. Group I, Early series with free utilization of blood. Group II, Current series using maximal blood conservation technique.

Autotransfusion is associated with potential but definite problems. These include technical difficulties with the equipment, citrate intoxication, coagulopathy, sepsis, air embolism, and anticoagulation with resultant bleeding.[29] Overall, however, the use of autotranfusion techniques intraoperatively and even in the postoperative period for the retrieval of shed mediastinal blood seems to far outweigh the risks and small incidence of complications.[30] We now use autotransfusion on all cases, whether elective or emergent.

Another integral part of blood conservation is the reinfusion of all red cells that remain in the oxygenator at the conclusion of bypass.[31] Various maneuvers can be employed to facilitate transfusion of the remaining fluid volume in the oxygenator. Vasodilatation with intravenous nitroglycerine or nitroprusside allows reinfusion of oxygenator blood in varying amounts after the termination of bypass and removal of the venous cannulae. In those patients in whom filling pressures are high and cannot be lowered for one reason or another, the oxygenator blood can simply be transferred to the autotransfusion equipment, the cells spun down, washed, and given back to the patient at the appropriate time postoperatively.

Finally, the careful monitoring and administration of both heparin and protamine therapy can significantly reduce blood loss. The use of the activated clotting time can avoid either the administration of too much or too little heparin or protamine. Thus, there can be a reduction in postoperative blood loss secondary to prolonged clotting times on an iatrogenic basis.[32]

The combination of autologous blood removal and later infusion, meticulous attention to intraoperative hemostasis, collection and salvage of wound and shed mediastinal blood, close monitoring of the anticoagulation status, and the knowledge that extreme hemodilution can be utilized safely has proven to be a most effective method of blood conservation during the performance of cardiac surgery and has significantly lowered blood usage.[26]

Postoperative

The techniques of blood conservation must continue into the postoperative period. As has been mentioned, shed mediastinal blood can be processed and autotransfused into the patient. This is especially useful in patients with excessive bleeding, such as dissecting aneurysms or re-do operations.[33]

As soon as the patient is extubated and able to take medications by mouth, oral ferrous sulfate is begun. This usually commences on the first postoperative day in the intensive care unit, and the starting dosage in adults is 300 mg three times a day with meals. When given in this fashion, many of the side effects, such as nausea, are avoided.

As long as the patient is hemodynamically stable and there is no impairment in the delivery of oxygen to the tissues, transfusion can be avoided unless the hematocrit drops below 20–24 vol%, regardless of the patient's age. Although arterial pO_2 and cardiac output can help assess the adequacy of tissue oxygenation, there is no question that the single best measurement for this purpose is the mixed venous oxygen saturation.[11,26] If the temperature-corrected mixed venous saturation remains normal, which in our experience has been equal to or greater than 75%, the simultaneous pO_2 and cardiac output or indices are satisfactory for the patients' need at that particular time.

Another important application of mixed venous saturation values was found during and following open heart surgery.[34] Despite hematocrit values less than 30 vol%, blood or plasma need not be utilized for volume replacement. Instead, Ringer's lactate has proven quite satisfactory for volume replacement before, during, and after cardiac surgery. The monitoring of arterial pO_2, mixed venous oxygen saturation, and left atrial pressure enables one to intelligently make decisions concerning volume replacement. The use of Ringer's lactate, which is inexpensive, readily available, and virtually without side effects (i.e., hepatitis) has led to a significant decrease in blood usage, especially in the postoperative period. Whereas patients previously received fresh frozen plasma or blood for volume replacement, we now administer only two units of fresh frozen plasma immediately following protamine administration in the operating room. These two units supply abundant amounts of the coagulation factors necessary following bypass, and we now use Ringer's lactate exclusively for volume replacement at all times during hospitalization, unless blood is specifically indicated in cases where hematocrit values are less than 20–24 vol% or there is an impairment in oxygen delivery to the tissues which is correctable by increasing the red cell mass of the patient.

Despite having hematocrit values in the mid-20s when entering the intensive care unit, following the profound diuresis seen in the first few hours after bypass the hematocrit is generally 28–35 vol% by the 1st post-

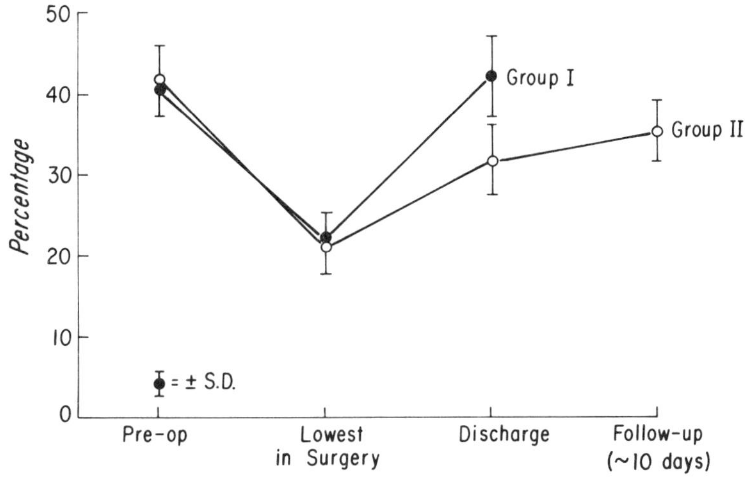

Figure 11.5. Whether patients are (Group I) or are not (Group II) routinely transfused, normal Hct values are seen in the majority of patients 10–12 days following discharge.

operative day. There continues to be a slow increase in these values so that the majority of patients have hematocrits of 32–38 vol% at the time of discharge from the hospital. On oral iron supplementation alone, which is continued on an outpatient basis, hematocrit values are restored to normal in over 85% of all patients at the time of their 1st postoperative office visit, which is usually 10 to 14 days following discharge (Fig. 11.5). The application of the aforementioned techniques has made it possible to avoid blood transfusion in over 90% of all patients undergoing open heart surgery.[34]

ADVANTAGES OF BLOOD CONSERVATION

The marked increase in the volume of cardiac surgery being performed in the United States has created tremendous supply difficulties for blood banks that are trying to meet these demands. In many communities, it has often become necessary to cancel elective surgical procedures because the demand for blood and blood products exceeds the supplies available. Simple mathematics dictates that a 50% reduction in blood usage would result in a doubling of the number of potential open heart cases that could be performed. Therefore, the voluntary efforts at blood conservation should be employed by all teams performing open heart surgery because, if the numbers of procedures continue to increase at the predicted and expected rate, these very measures may become mandatory as the amounts of banked blood continue to dwindle according to the laws of supply and demand.

Another benefit of blood conservation by cardiac surgeons is that it makes massive amounts of banked blood available for other patient populations where avoidance of blood transfusion may not be a viable alternative. Such instances include massive gastrointestinal bleeding, hematologic disorders, and trauma. As long as cardiac surgeons continue to have the option of blood conservation, albeit at a slight increase in effort and time, it should be exercised to the utmost.

If and when blood is needed, component therapy should always be utilized. Again, the reasons for this are a reflection of supply and demand. When a patient needs an increase in red cell mass, that patient should receive packed red blood cells. Whole blood is unnecessary and the remaining components, such as fresh plasma, platelets, white blood cells, and specific coagulation factors can be fractionated and selectively transfused to patients in whom they are needed. The use of component therapy is an important concept and further maximizes the usage and supply of banked blood.[35,36]

Furthermore, since the incidence of complications associated with transfusion, such as hemolytic reactions and infections (syphilis, malaria, hepatitis, bacterial), are directly proportional to the incidence of exposure, if blood is not used, the complications can be avoided.[37] If a patient receives one unit of blood instead of two, his chances of contracting hepatitis are reduced by 50%. Therefore, although absolute avoidance of transfusion is not always possible, conservation and reduction in usage is always a sound clinical principle and should be employed whenever possible.

In addition to a reduction in the morbidity and rare mortality associated with blood transfusions there are certain physiologic advantages in using fluids other than blood in patients undergoing cardiac surgery. It has been shown that priming the heart-lung machine with clear fluids and employing hemodilution results in better tissue perfusion, higher mixed venous oxygen saturation, and less acidosis than when whole blood is used in the oxygenator prime.[11] Additionally, postoperative pulmonary, renal, and hemotologic function is generally better when hemodilution is used.[4,38]

The lower the body temperature, the safer hemodilution becomes. Therefore, the lower the perfusion temperature during bypass, the lower the simultaneous hemoglobin level can be and still provide adequate tissue oxygenation. This inverse relationship between hemoglobin levels and body temperature has led us to cool all patients to at least 25°C. Furthermore, this greater degree of cooling enhances myocardial preservation when cold potassium cardioplegic arrest is used for this purpose.

Summary

In conclusion, the pronounced increase in the number of open heart procedures performed annually in the United States has imposed great difficulties on community and commercial blood banks throughout the country. There are many ways cardiac surgeons can dramatically reduce the amount of blood utilized during the performance of open heart surgery. The most important of these include maximizing preoperative hemoglobin levels, withdrawal and storage of autologous blood at varying times preoperatively where possible, and the reinfusion of this autologous blood at the conclusion of bypass.

Additionally, modifications in surgical technique to include meticulous control of hemostasis, the use of hemodilution and autotransfusion techniques has greatly enhanced blood conservation during cardiac surgery. The avoidance of transfusion unless specifically indicated by an impairment in the ability of the body to provide adequate tissue oxygenation has further contributed to a reduction in blood usage in these patients. Volume replacement can be satisfactorily accomplished with the use of crystalloid solutions eliminating the need to give blood for this purpose alone. The appreciation of these concepts and incorporation of the aforementioned techniques have made it possible to greatly reduce the amounts of blood used in these patients and indeed, it should be possible to routinely perform open heart surgery without the use of blood. In the few instances where transfusion is necessary, specific component therapy should always be employed. The realization that low levels of circulating hemoglobin postoperatively are not detrimental, and that with oral iron supplementation and time alone, the overwhelming majority of patients undergoing open heart surgery will require no blood has made it possible to routinely perform open heart surgery in over 90% of all cases without the use of blood transfusion.

References

1. Roche JK, Stengle JM: Open-heart surgery and the demand for blood. JAMA 225:1516, 1973.
2. Schaff HV, Hauer JM, Brawley RK: Autotransfusion in cardiac surgical patients after operation. Surgery 84:713, 1978.
3. Braunwald E: Coronary-artery surgery at the crossroads. N Engl J Med 297:661, 1977.
4. Zubiate P, Kay JH, Mendez AM, Krohn BG, Hochman R, Dunne EF: Coronary artery surgery: A new technique with use of little blood, if any. J Thorac Cardiovasc Surg 68(2):263, 1974.
5. Cooley DA, Bloodwell RD, Beall AC Jr, Hallman GL: Cardiac valve replacement without blood transfusion. Am J Surg 112:743, 1966.
6. Tector AJ, Gabriel RP, Mateicka WE, Oparah SS,

Flemm RJ, Lepley D Jr: Reduction of blood usage in open heart surgery. Chest 70(4):454, 1976.
7. Gomes MMR, McGoon DC: Bleeding patterns after open-heart surgery. J Thorac Cardiovasc Surg 60:87, 1970.
8. Hardesty RL, Bayer WL, Bahnson HT: A technique for the use of autologous fresh blood during open heart surgery. J Thorac Cardiovasc Surg 56:683, 1968.
9. Knodell RG, Conrad ME, Dienstag JL, Bell CJ: Etiological spectrum of post-transfusion hepatitis. Gastroenterology 69:1278, 1975.
10. National transfusion hepatitis study: Risk of post-transfusion hepatitis in the United States. A prospective cooperative study. JAMA 220(5):692, 1972.
11. Housman LB, Turina M, Braunwald NS: Use of hemodilution during total cardiopulmonary bypass in neonates: Experimental evaluation employing a miniaturized heart-lung machine. Surgery 72(3):460, 1972.
12. Housman LB, Braunwald NS: Experimental evaluation of the Travenol and Landé-Edwards membrane oxygenators for use in neonate perfusions. Ann Thorac Surg 14(2):150, 1972.
13. Cohn LH, Angell WW, Shumway NE: Body fluid shifts after cardiopulmonary bypass. I. Effects of congestive heart failure and hemodilution. J Thorac Cardiovasc Surg 62:423, 1971.
14. Dieter RA Jr, Neville WE, Pifarré R: Serum electrolyte changes after cardiopulmonary bypass with Ringer's lactate solution used for hemodilution. J Thorac Cardiovasc Surg 59:168, 1970.
15. Sandiford FM, Chiariello L, Hallman GL, Cooley DA: Aorto coronary bypass in Jehovah's witnesses: Report of 36 patients. J Thorac Cardiovasc Surg 68(1):1, 1974.
16. Cooley DA, Beall AC Jr, Grondin P: Open-heart operations with disposable oxygenators, 5% dextroxe prime and normothermia. Surgery 52:713, 1962.
17. Pierce EC II, Corrigan JJ, Kent BB, Cate CL, Johnson RL, Dreves AE: Comparative trauma to blood in the disc oxygenator and membrane lung. Trans Am Soc Artif Intern Organs 15:33, 1969.
18. Landé AJ, Edwards L, Bloch JH, Carlson RG, Subramanian VA, Ascheim RS, Scheidt S, Fillmore S, Killip T, Lillehei CW: Clinical experience with emergency use of prolonged cardiopulmonary bypass with a membrane pump-oxygenator. Ann Thorac Surg 10:409, 1970.
19. Dudrick SJ, Long JM, Steiger E, Rhoads JE: Intravenous hyperalimentation. Med Clin North Am 54: 577, 1970.
20. Dudrick SJ, Wilmore DW, Vars HM, Rhoads JE: Long-term total parenteral nutrition with growth, development and a positive nitrogen balance. Surgery 64:134, 1968.
21. Dudrick SJ, Wilmore DW, Vars HM, Rhoads JE: Can intravenous feeding as the sole means of nutrition support growth in the child and restore weight loss in an adult? An affirmative answer. Ann Surg 169:974, 1969.
22. Kaplan JA, Cannarella C, Jones EL, Kutner MH, Hatcher CR Jr, Dunbar RW: Autologous blood transfusion during cardiac surgery. A re-evaluation of these methods. J Thorac Cardiovasc Surg 74(1):4, 1977.
23. Umlas J, Sakhuja R: The effects on blood coagulation of the exclusive use of transfusions of frozen red cells during and after cardiopulmonary bypass. J Thorac Cardiovasc Surg 70(3):519, 1975.
24. Cohen LH, Fosberg AM, Anderson WP, Collins JJ Jr: The effects of phlebotomy, hemodilution and autologous transfusion on systemic oxygenation and whole blood utilization in open heart surgery. Chest 68(3):283, 1975.
25. Hallowell P, Bland JHL, Chir B, Buckley MJ, Lowenstein E: Transfusion of fresh autologous blood in open-heart surgery: A method for reducing blood bank blood requirements. J Thorac Cardiovasc Surg 64(6):941, 1972.
26. Housman LB, Litchford B, Mazur JH: The routine performance of open-heart surgery without blood. J Extra-Corporeal Technol 11:163, 1979.
27. Wagstaffe JG, Clarke AD, Jackson PW: Reduction of blood loss by restoration of platelet levels using fresh autologous blood after cardiopulmonary bypass. Thorax 27:410, 1972.
28. Cosgrove DM, Thurer RL, Lytle BW, Gill CG, Peter M, Loop FD: Blood conservation during myocardial revascularization. Ann Thorac Surg 28(2):184, 1979.
29. Mattox KL: Comparison of techniques of autotransfusion. Surgery 84(5):700, 1978.
30. Brawley RK, Hauer JM: Autotransfusion seminar. Surgery 84(5):693, 1978.
31. Yeh T Jr, Shelton L, Yeh TJ: Blood loss and bank blood requirements in coronary bypass surgery. Ann Thorac Surg 26(1):11, 1978.
32. Berg E, Stenbjerg S, Albrechtsen OK: Monitoring heparin and protamine therapy during cardiopulmonary bypass by activated clotting time. J Extra-Corporeal Technol 11(6):229, 1979.
33. Schaff HV, Hauer JM, Bell WR, Gardner TJ, Donahoo JS, Gott VL, Brawley RK: Autotransfusion of shed mediastinal blood after cardiac surgery: A prospective study. J Thorac Cardiovasc Surg 75(4):632, 1978.
34. Housman LB, Virgilio R, Kinyon G, Zamost B: The use of crystalloid vs. colloid in the management of patients undergoing coronary artery bypass surgery. Presented at the 7th World Congress of Anesthesiologists, Hamburg, Germany, Sept. 14–21, 1980.
35. Hummer GJ: Advances in blood component therapy. Anesthesiology 34:309, 1971.
36. Valeri CR: Blood components in the treatment of acute blood loss: Use of freeze-preserved red cells, platelets and plasma proteins. Anesth Analg (Cleve) 54(1):1, 1975.
37. Kay AB: Some complications associated with the administration of blood and blood products. Clin Haematol 5(1):165, 1976.
38. Laks H, Standeven J, Blair O, Hahn J, Jellinek M, Willman VL: The effects of cardiopulmonary bypass with crystalloid and colloid hemodilution on myocardial extravascular water. J Thorac Cardiovasc Surg 73(1):129, 1977.

CHAPTER 12

CARDIOPULMONARY BYPASS WITH HEMOGLOBINOPATHIES AND RED CELL ABNORMALITIES

DIANE J. SANSONETTI, M.D.

Patients who have genetically determined alterations in the structure of the protein components of hemoglobin, the red cell membrane, or red cell metabolism may require special considerations during cardiopulmonary bypass. These alterations produce dysfunction through a variety of mechanisms. The impairment may be clinically detectable or may become apparent only under stress of cardiopulmonary bypass. Hemoglobinopathies and red cell abnormalities merit special consideration related to management of cardiopulmonary bypass.

PATHOPHYSIOLOGY OF HEMOGLOBIN

Normal human hemogloblin molecules are tetramers (polymers composed of four molecules) formed by the reversible association of two pairs of polypeptide chains. The chains are designated as alpha and non-alpha (e.g., beta, sigma), and each possess a reversibly bound heme group. The structural genetic loci for alpha chains segregate independently from the loci for non-alpha chains.

Hemoglobin A is conventionally the sum of HbA_1 and HbA_3 fractions. It comprises about 96–97% of the total normal adult hemoglobin and consists of two α and two β polypeptide chains. Hemoglobin A_2 constitutes 2–3% of the total hemoglobin and is composed of two alpha and two sigma chains. Increased amounts of HbA_2 are found in individuals with β-thalassemia and megaloblastic anemia.[1]

Abnormal Hemoglobins

Fetal hemoglobin (HbF) with two alpha and two sigma chains contributes less than 1% to the normal adult hemoglobin pool. Hemoglobin F is increased to a variable extent in thalassemia, sickle cell anemia, and other genetic disorders.[1]

Hemoglobin abnormalities alter red cell function by changing the properties of the membrane and the cell's metabolism. The red cell membrane is responsible for the cell's biconcave disc shape. This shape is the result of dynamic factors operating within, inside, and outside the membrane. The biconcavity affords a greater surface area per cell volume and is a feature of the mature erythrocyte, but not the reticulocyte.[2] The membrane shape can be changed by an altered configuration of the hemoglobin molecules which it envelopes. Mechanical trauma to the membrane structure may also change the cell shape. This property is known as the cell's mechanical fragility. The ionic composition of the red cell and its environment affects mechanical fragility. Red blood cell abnormalities may alter the cell's ability to maintain membrane integrity in an environment of ionic gradients. A large inequality exists between the concentration of sodium and potassium in the red cell and plasma. Transmembrane migration of these ions involves several mechanisms, including passive diffusion and energy-dependent transport.[2] Osmotic lysis of the erythrocyte occurs when the plasma is hypotonic, whereas hypertonic plasma causes cell shrinkage or crenation.

Oxygen diffuses passively through the erythrocyte membrane and moves to the cell's interior by both passive and hemoglobin-facilitated oxygen diffusion.[2] The oxygen dissociation curve of hemoglobin represents the percentage of hemoglobin saturated with oxygen at a specific partial pressure of oxygen. It is sigmoid-shaped, such that minor changes in the low range of PO_2 bring about the association or dissociation of large amounts of oxygen from hemoglobin. In the higher range of oxygen tension, proportionately larger changes are necessary to exact further oxygen saturation. The shape of the oxygen dissociation curve results from an altered affinity of hemoglobin once the oxygen binds to the first heme group. Although the mechanism of the heme-heme interaction is unknown, it has been observed that one oxygenated heme group confers increased affinity to oxygen binding on the other heme groups in the molecule.[2]

The major factors altering the properties of the oxygen dissociation curve include pH, temperature, and the concentration of 2-3 diphosphoglycerate. At standard conditions, the oxygen pressure at which 50% of hemoglobin is saturated with oxygen is expressed as the P_{50} value.

Sickle Cell Disease

Sickle cell syndromes are found among Africans, Greeks, Italians, Saudis, Israeli Arabs, and Southern Indians. About 8% of American blacks carry the trait and 0.2% exhibit the anemic form of the disease.[2] The presence and severity of the disease are determined by hemoglobin electrophoresis. However, the genotype cannot always be inferred from the phenotype. Determination of heterozygosity or homozygosity requires clinical and biochemical data supplemented by genetic observations.

The molecular bases of sickling relate to the deoxygenation of sickle hemoglobin (HbS). Bonds form which result in individual hemoglobin molecules linking together in long chains which increase the viscosity of the solution. The sickled erythrocyte is basically bundles of hemoglobin chains covered by a distorted cell membrane. The membrane deformity is ordinarily reversible upon reoxygenation; however, repeated sickling permanently damages the membrane, and the abnormal shape persists. Sickled cells are rigid, mechanically friable, are phagocytized more readily, and have a shortened life span.[3] The cellular basis of sickling depends on hemoglobin composition, cell age, membrane integrity, and the rate of oxygen dissociation.

Deoxygenated, rigid, sickled cells may obstruct blood flow in small vessels. The resulting stasis engenders local hypoxia and acidosis which promotes further deoxygenation and sickling of cells. Distribution of vessels and rate of blood flow affect the severity of the local phenomenon. An additional factor includes endothelial disruption secondary to anoxia of the microvasculature, which causes collagen to be released into the circulation, activating the intrinsic coagulation system. Exposed subendothelial surfaces favor platelet adhesion and aggregation. However, "hypercoagulability" is not the primary etiological event in the thrombotic problem of sickling.[4]

In vitro studies show that under physiologic conditions homozygotic HbS red cells initiate sickling at oxygen saturations below 85% and are completely sickled at 38%. Heterozygotic HbS cells initiate sickling at 40% oxygen saturation.[1] In sickle cell disease, the oxygen dissociation curve is shifted to the right, representing a lower affinity of hemoglobin for oxygen. Any shift to the right or higher P_{50} value is detrimental in sickle cell disease because it facilitates sickling by increasing the proportion of reduced hemoglobin.

Hypothermia causes increased viscosity and oxygen saturation (left shift in the oxygen dissociation curve) in both normal and sickle cell blood. In sickle cell disease, however, the increased oxygen saturation is offset by the direct effect of hypothermia on blood viscosity, which is disadvantageous.

Operative Management

Patients with HbS require special considerations during cardiopulmonary bypass to avoid the factors which may initiate the cycle of sickling. In the anemic form of the disease, low hemoglobin levels may provide inadequate oxygen-carrying capacity. These patients should be transfused preoperatively to a hemoglobin level of 15 gm/100 ml. In heterozygotic and nonanemic homozygotic patients, preoperative partial exchange transfusions have been advocated to reduce the level of HbS. The HbA cells do not develop the sickling phenomenon, and dilution of the concentration of potentially sickled cells serves as a protective factor. In nonanemic patients, the exchange may be accomplished by using HbA blood in the oxygenator prime. Plasma hemoglobin concentrations can be obtained at the initiation of cardiopulmonary bypass and throughout the immediate postoperative period. The normal range of plasma hemoglobin is less than 5 mg/100 ml. Yacoub et al.[5] showed that plasma hemoglobin peaked at 41 mg% at the conclusion of bypass and returned to normal range within 8 hours in an adult sickle cell trait patient who underwent mitral valve replacement and who demonstrated no clinical hemolytic problems.

Hypoxia in the preoperative period should be avoided by frequent arterial blood gases. Increased inspired oxygen concentrations, especially at times of anesthetic induction and extubation, may prevent sickling. Inhaled gas mixtures should contain at least 50% oxygen.

Acidosis shifts the oxygen dissociation curve to the right and favors sickling. Acidosis should be treated by sodium bicarbonate.

In patients with HbS, local or systemic hypoperfusion may be produced by several factors, including hypothermia and underhydration. Poor positioning on the operating table or use of tourniquets may also produce regions of poor perfusion.

Localized sickling in the myocardium can be produced by low oxygen tension while the aorta is cross-clamped. Washout of HbS cells from the myocardium with warm HbA blood or crystalloid solution may precede the infusion of cold cardioplegic solutions.

Should sickling occur intraoperatively, the increased mechanical fragility of the cells and the corpuscular trauma of extracorporeal circulation may cause an increased hemolysis. Some sickling is reversible by reoxygenation. HbA blood should be transfused. Tissue infarction secondary to sickle cell thrombi may not be avoidable. One report documents multisystem infarctions from sickle cell thrombi in a patient with unsuspected sickle cell trait who underwent aortic valve replacement. In this instance, the cycle of sickling was initiated intraoperatively or in the immediate postoperative period; the process was not recognized until the patient failed to fully regain consciousness. Sickling was demonstrated only at postmortem examination.[6] Many reports have been published of successful cardiac surgery using cardiopulmonary bypass in patients with sickle cell trait disease.[7–9]

OTHER ABNORMALITIES

Thalassemia

Thalassemia minor patients have increased amounts of HbA_2. The erythrocytes have decreased osmotic fragility and normal mechanical fragility in comparison to the normal red cell. Therefore, blood trauma from cardiopulmonary bypass or valve prosthesis should not be a problem. These patients can exhibit anemia, which is treatable by transfusion but no other special precautions are necessary.[10]

Spherocytosis

Erythrocytes in hereditary spherocytosis are both mechanically and osmotically more fragile than normal red cells. The red cells have shortened half-life that can be returned to normal by splenectomy despite the cellular defects remaining unchanged. Special treatment of these patients should include splenectomy prior to cardiopulmonary bypass and use of valve prostheses. Cardiopulmonary bypass in patients with spherocytosis has not resulted in increased hemolysis.[11]

Elliptocytosis

The defect in hereditary elliptocytosis is unknown, and studies of cell fragility are incomplete. A small proportion of patients have hemolysis and anemia for which splenectomy is the preferred treatment.

Glucose-6-Phosphate Dehydrogenase Deficiency

The trait for a glucose-6-phosphate dehydrogenase deficiency (G-6-PD) is present in nearly 3 million Americans and affects 10% of the black male population.[10] The enzyme is part of the pentose phosphate pathway, a source of energy for the red cell. Erythrocytes deficient in G-6-PD undergo a variable degree of hemolysis in response to different stimuli, including infection, diabetic acidosis, and hemolytic drugs. Over 40 drugs have been shown to induce hemolysis in G-6-PD patients, not on an immune basis. Drugs commonly used in cardiac surgery which should be avoided are chloramphenicol, sulfonamides, sulfasoxazole, aspirin, acetophetidin, vitamin K, and quinidine. Even in the absence of induced hemolysis, G-6-PD cells have 20% shortened life span.[2] Their mechanical fragility is normal, and the osmotic fragility is slightly decreased. Therefore, prosthetic valves and cardiopulmonary bypass should not cause special problems. A successful repair of tetralogy of Fallot in a girl with both sickle cell anemia and G-6-PD deficiency has been reported.[12]

References

1. Bunn HF, Forget BG, Ranney HM: *Human Hemoglobins*. Philadelphia, W. B. Saunders, 1977.
2. Harris JW, Kellermeyer RW: *The Red Cell*. Cambridge, Harvard University Press, 1970.
3. Flye MW, Silver D: The role of surgery in sickle cell disease. Surg Gynecol Obstet 137:115, 1973.
4. Rickles FR, O'Leary DS: Role of coagulation system in pathophysiology of sickle cell disease. Arch Intern Med 133:635, 1974.
5. Yacoub MH, Baron J, Et-Etr A, Kittle CF: Aortic homograft replacement of the mitral valve in sickle cell trait. J Thorac Cardiovasc Surg 59:568, 1970.
6. Leachman RD, Miller WT, Atias IM: Sickle cell trait complicated by sickle cell thrombi after open-heart surgery. Am Heart J 74:268, 1967.
7. Heiner M, Teasdale SJ, David T, Scott AA, Glynn MFX: Aorto-coronary bypass in a patient with sickle cell trait. Can Anaesth Soc J 26:428, 1979.
8. Harris LC, Haggard ME, Travis LB: The coexistence of sickle cell disease and congenital heart disease: A report of three cases, with repair under cardiopulmonary by-pass in two. Pediatrics 33:562, 1964.
9. Craenen J, Kilman J, Hosier DM, Weinberger M: Mitral valve replacement in a child with sickle cell anemia. J Thorac Cardiovasc Surg 63:797, 1972.
10. deLeval MR, Taswell HF, Bowie EJW, Danielson GK: Open heart surgery in patients with inherited hemoglobinopathies, red cell dyscrasias and coagulopathies. Arch Surg 109:618, 1974.
11. Moyes DG, Rogers MA, Coleman AJ: Cardiopulmonary bypass in hereditary spherocytosis: A case report. Thorax 26:131, 1971.
12. Szentpetery S, Robertson L, Lower RR: Complete repair of tetralogy associated with sickle cell anemia and G-6-PD deficiency. J Thorac Cardiovasc Surg 72:276, 1976.

CHAPTER 13

THE IMMUNE RESPONSE TO CARDIOPULMONARY BYPASS

JOE R. UTLEY, M.D.

Infection fortunately has become a rare event following cardiac surgery requiring cardiopulmonary bypass; however, an understanding of the factors which alter the patient's susceptibility to infection and the effect of cardiopulmonary bypass on them is important to enhance the cardiac surgeon's ability to prevent infection. Depressed function of virtually all components of the immune system have been described following cardiopulmonary bypass. Many of the effects are due to the dilution, cellular destruction, and particle production by the heart-lung machine, while others are due to the anesthetic agents, trauma, and blood transfusion. Alteration of the immune mechanism has been implicated in postcardiac surgery syndromes and effects. The postpericardiotomy syndrome is related to the development of autoimmune antiheart antibodies often with antiviral antibodies as well.

REVIEW OF NORMAL IMMUNE MECHANISM

The physiology of immunity includes local factors which protect tissues exposed to endogenous or exogenous microorganisms from invasive infections. Such specialized mechanisms protect the pharynx, trachea, bronchi, lungs, gastrointestinal tract, skin, eye, bladder, and vagina from invasive infection. Alteration of local immunity has not been studied in relation to cardiopulmonary bypass, but invasion of microorganism at these locally protected sites may be the source of infection following cardiac surgery.

The systemic immune response includes cellular and humoral factors. Circulating and tissue leucocytes and fixed macrophages compose the cellular components to immunity. Humoral immunity depends principally on immunogloblulins and complement.[1-3]

Cellular Immunity

Phagocytosis, the process whereby cells ingest particles, is the most important event in cellular immunity. Cells capable of phagocytosis include polymorphonuclear leukocytes, circulating monocytes, and macrophages. All tissues contain wandering macrophages. Fixed macrophages include the Kupffer cells of the liver, the alveolar macrophages of the lung, the primordial macrophages of spleen, lymph nodes, bone marrow and adrenal gland, and the glial cells of the brain. Circulating neutrophils and macrophages wander across capillary membranes and through tissue toward regions of microbes, foreign material, or injury in response to a chemical gradient, called chemotaxis. Most chemotactic factors require the interaction of the microbes with the host for their production. While some do not require host interaction, the classic process begins with the microbial antigen-host antibody interaction. The antigen-antibody complex then activates the cascade of complement. Complement includes a system of 15 serum proteins which generate many chemotactic substances.[1-3]

The ingestion and destruction of microbes is facilitated by opsonization, a process of coating microbes with serum-immune proteins. Antibody and complement are the best characterized opsonins. Only IgG_2 and IgG_3 are opsonically active. One portion of the IgG molecule attaches to the microbe and the other portion to the neutrophil or macrophage, thus gluing the two together. A component of complement, C3, may increase the rate of ingestion of microbes without increasing the affinity of the microbe for the cell membrane.

The next steps of microbe killing are ingestion, cellular degradation, and enzymatic and chemical destruction of the microbe. The period after microbe ingestion is characterized by increased oxygen consumption and synthesis of hydrogen peroxide. Hydrogen peroxide production greatly speeds microbe death but may be altered by the presence of catalase, myeloperoxidase, halide ions, or low pH.[1-3]

The wandering and tissue macrophages perform a number of important functions in addition to ingestions of microorganisms. These include: secretion of biologically active materials, breaking down erythrocytes and processing iron for reuse, processing and presenting antigens to lymphocytes on the afferent limb of the immune response, killing neoplastic cells, and metabolizing ingested lipids. Circulating particulate matter such as bacteria, lipid emulsion, colloidal carbon, and protein aggregates are rapidly cleaved by the mixed macrophages. This function may be saturated by large amounts of circulating particulate matter producing reticuloendothelial "blockade." The liver accounts for 80–85% of the function of the reticuloendothelial system and the spleen constitutes 10%. The wandering and circulating macrophages are more easily isolated and collected and therefore are better understood than the fixed macrophages. They have a generation time of 19–25 hours and circulation time of 30–100 hours. They have no large reservoir in bone marrow.[1-3]

Disorders of phagocytic function may be classified into cellular and microbial factors related to microbe killing; ingestion, opsonization, and chemotaxis; altered neutrophil production, destruction, or concentration.[1-3]

An important part of cellular immunity are those lymphocytes capable of reaction with antigen specificity. There are two classes of lymphocytes. The T-cells differentiate under the influence of the thymus, and the B-cells differentiate under the influence of the bone marrow. In both humoral and cellular immune responses there is interaction between lymphocytes. Although B-cells are the precursors of antibody forming cells, they cannot produce antibody unless they interact with T-cells. Thus, T-cells are helper cells in antibody formation and the effector cells in cell-mediate responses. Even in these responses the T-cells may interact with each other so that one group of T-cells plays the role of effector while another plays the role of helper.

The incorporation of thymidine in response to mitogens (substances which induce mitosis) has become the standard technique for quantitating the response of lymphocytes. The mitotic proliferation of lymphocytes may be quantitated by the amount of labeled thymidine incorporated into their DNA. The mitogens most commonly used are phytohemagglutinin (PHA), concanavalin A (Con A), pokeweed mitogen (PWM), and bacterial lipopolysaccharide (LPS). Con A and PHA act as mitogens for T-cells but not B-cells. PWM and LPS act as B-cell mitogens but do not stimulate T-cells.[4]

Humoral Immunity

The most important components of humoral immunity are the immunoglobulins. These antibodies have a central role in allergic reactions, autoimmune responses, neutralization of toxins, and defense against infectious agents. Antibodies are produced by plasma cells which are the end product of antibody stimulation of B-lymphocytes of bone marrow origin. A complex interaction of macrophages, T-cells, and B-cells is required before antibody synthesis occurs. Immunoglobulins are made up of heavy chains and light chains. The five immunoglobulin classes, IgG, IgM, IgA, IgD, and IgE, are determined by the heavy chains. IgG, IgM, and IgA are most important in resistance to infection.

Antibodies play a variety of roles in defense against microbial infection. Antibodies neutralize toxins of bacteria-producing exotoxins. Viruses may be neutralized by antibodies. Antibodies and complement may lyse certain gram-negative bacteria; gram-positive bacteria are opsonized by antibody or complement rather than lysed. Antibodies may activate the inflammatory response and agglutinate bacteria to reduce the number of infectious units. They may also inhibit mobility and metabolic activity of extracellular organisms.

Complement is a system of 15 serum proteins that mediate the biologic function of antigen-antibody reaction. Eleven proteins make up the classic complement pathway, and four make up the alternate (properdin) complement pathway. Activation of complement has kinin-like activity, causing increased vascular permeability, tissue edema, and smooth muscle contraction. Certain components of complement function as opsonins. Complement activation results in lysis of erythrocytes, platelets, bacteria, viruses with lypoprotein envelopes, and lymphocytes. The complement system also interacts with the clotting system and kinin system through factor XII, Hageman factor.

Other soluble factors play a role in host defense, including alpha-2 surface binding glycoprotein, lysozyme, B-lysine, spermine, hematin, Tillet factor, Tuftsin, and interferon.

Evaluation of humoral immunity includes the qualitative and quantitative description of immunoglobulins, and the determination of levels of plasma cell and B-lymphocyte transformation. Immunoglobulin deficiency is complicated by infectious complications. Complement deficiencies are associated with infectious complications, and less frequent vascular changes including membranous glomerulonephritis, collagen vascular disorders, and Reynaud's phenomena. Deficiency of C_1 inhibitor has been associated with angioedema of skin, gastrointestinal tract, tongue, and larynx.[1-3]

EFFECT OF ANESTHESIA, OPERATION, AND TRAUMA ON IMMUNITY

Depression of many components of the immune system has been described at the time of operation. Conditions common in cardiac surgery patients which depress immune defense include very young or very old age and diabetes mellitus. Drugs and anesthetic agents which depress immunity include steroids and antibiotics, including tetracycline, chloramphenicol, clindamycin, oxytetracycline, streptomycin, gentamycin, kanamycin, and neomycin. B- and T-cell mitogenic capabilities are inhibited by halothane, cyclopropane, ether, and nitrous oxide. Pentobarbital produces a fall in leukocyte count. Both shock and fever have been shown to depress immune responsiveness. A study of healthy kidney donors has shown a global depression of the immune system. *In vitro* testing showed a depression of total blood lymphocyte counts, B-cell counts, T-cell counts, mitogen blastogenic response, and mixed leukocyte reactivity as both responder and stimulator. These returned to normal by the 5th postoperative day. *In vivo* delayed hypersensitivity response to recall antigen was still falling at the 5th day. Return of preoperative skin response was complete for streptokinase/streptodornase by 10–14 days but was incomplete in 2–3 weeks for mumps and *Candida* antigens. No changes in serum immunoglobulins were found.[5]

Depression of opsonic acitivty was found 24 hours after operation or trauma. Survivors had recovery of opsonic activity in 48–72 hours, while those who died had suppression of opsonic activity. The author characterized this opsonin as an alpha-2-globulin. This opsonin protein does not facilitate the phagocytosis of micro-organisms but acts as an opsonin for circulating microaggregates induced by disseminated intravascular coagulation that accompanied shock or low perfusion.[6]

CARDIOPULMONARY BYPASS

Effects on Humoral Immune Components

Hairston et al.[7] showed that the serum bacteriocidal capacity against *Escherichia coli* was diminished in 30 of 35 patients (Fig. 13.1). The serum bacteriocidal capacity against *Staphylococcus aureus* was decreased in 23 of 33 patients. These changes were

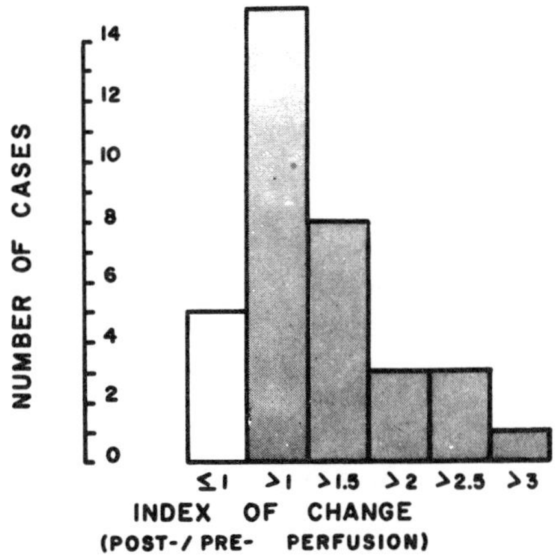

Figure 13.1. In the study the growth of *E. coli* (10^{-6} organisms) was compared in serum before and after cardiopulmonary bypass. The frequency and quantity of increased *E. coli* was greater in postperfusion serum. (Reproduced with permission from P. Hairston et al.[7] and Academic Press, Inc.)

rarely observed in surgical patients without cardiopulmonary bypass. These studies demonstrated diminished total complement (CH50) during perfusion with the depression greatest during rewarming. However, the depression of complement fraction (B1C globulin) was greatest postperfusion, not during rewarming. The pattern of depression of IgA, IgM, and IgC was similar to complement fraction. Surgical patients not having cardiopulmonary bypass showed no similar depression of any immune component.

Hemodilution causes a fall in concentration of serum proteins, both albumin and globulins. The decrease in protein concentration is proportional to the fall in hematocrit. Larmi et al.[8] found the concentration of albumin and globulin to continue to fall with cardiopulmonary bypass. He could not correlate the fall after hemodilution with any parameter of liver function. During 3 hours of perfusion serial studies of protein electrophoresis showed falling concentrations of alpha-2 and gamma-globulins, whereas the alpha-1- and beta-globulins tended to rise. Alpha-2-globulins tended to rise with hypothermia but not with normothermia. Higher globulin levels were correlated with BSP retention. Beta-globulin levels increased with a rise in venous pressure or a fall in arterial pressure or venous PO_2. He postulated that serum proteins were denatured and macroaggregated by the pump oxygenation then cleared by the reticuloendothelial system, producing the falling concentrations of protein and rising BSP retention. He also postulated that venous hypertension produced ischemic and congestive liver damage which led to decreased protein production.

Wallace et al.[9] studied glycoprotein concentration in surgical patients with and without cardiopulmonary bypass. Alpha-2-globulin was greater in the group with cardiopulmonary bypass. Alpha-2-macroglobulins were depressed postoperatively in the open heart group. The postoperative depression of IgG was more marked in the open heart group. IgM was markedly elevated in open heart patients on the 6th–8th postoperative day. They suggested the elevated IgM was due to production of an antibody against foreign protein produced or induced by cardiopulmonary bypass.

Direct denaturation of serum protein has been clearly demonstrated in the classical paper of Lee et al.[10] It has been repeatedly shown that contact of proteins with an air-fluid interface results in denaturation. Electrostatic surface forces cause globular proteins to be aligned with the polar groups toward the interface and the nonpolar groups away from the interface. These surface-polarizing forces result in the disruption of sulfhydryl and hydrogen bonds which stabilize the secondary and tertiary structure of the protein molecules. The consequent unfolding of the globular molecule exposes masked chemical groups and creates a randomly coiled, more asymmetric molecule. These changes in symmetry and chemical reactivity lead to formation of macromolecules which tend to flocculate. The denaturation of protein molecules concerned with lipid transport may lead to release of free lipid. Owens et al.[11] demonstrated fat emboli in capillaries after cardiopulmonary bypass, presumably due to changes in colloid solubility properties of lipids. Lee et al.[10] studied the effect of pump oxygenation on plasma and found that viscosity of plasma increased in a manner typical of denatured proteins.

He found slight increases in free sulfhydryl groups. Serum electrophoresis showed the appearance of an abnormal band in the beta-gamma region. Albumin fell with a corresponding rise in alpha-2-globulin, beta-globulin, and gamma-globulin. This effect increased with time. Lee concluded that this differential change in concentration is a direct effect of the pump oxygenation and not related to changes in capillary permeability. The study demonstrated the coating of sludged red cells caused by denatured protein.

Pruitt et al.[12] studied the effect of disc oxygenation on solutions of albumin and gamma-globulin. The disc oxygenator, which caused turbidity, produced precipitation of gamma-globulin solutions that was dependent on concentration. The gamma-globulin exposed to the oxygenator was highly reactive with complement when compared to control solutions. Such gamma-globulin may be antigenic and stimulate antibody production. These changes in gamma-globulin were reduced in the presence of plasma or albumin. Studies of solubility of albumin and gamma-globulin and the precipitates' fluorescence spectra in the presence of 1-anilino-naphthalene showed that a molecular species was produced when a mixture of albumin and gamma-globulin was exposed to the oxygenator rather than when either was exposed alone. The author proposed that the oxygenator denaturation is produced by an unfolding of the gamma-globulin molecule followed by interaction with albumin. These products of gamma-globulin-albumin mixture exposed to oxygenators tend to form more precipitates at low temperatures than in control solutions.[12]

The presence of albumin decreased the rate of denaturation of gamma-globulin (Fig. 13.2). Furthermore, molecular species containing both albumin and globulin components were produced when both were present in the oxygenator. Pruitt et al.[12] postulated that when unfolded gamma-globulin reacted with other globulin molecules a less soluble complex was formed than when the unfolded gamma-globulin reacted with albumin. He

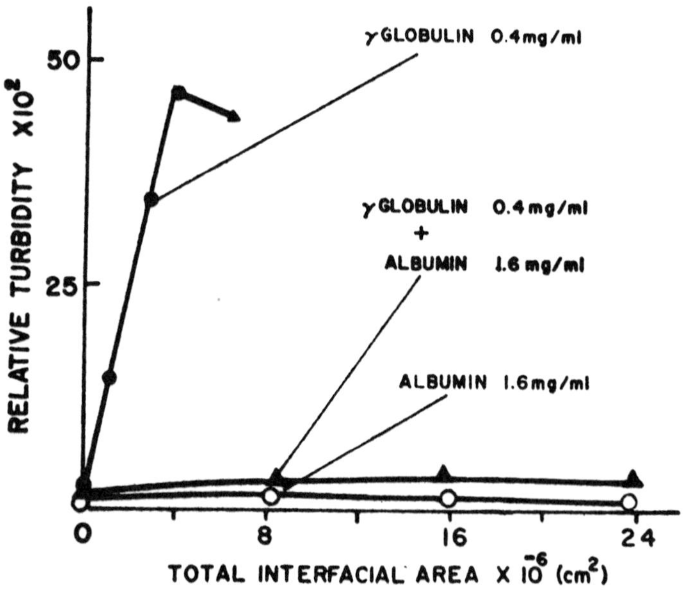

Figure 13.2. The denaturation of proteins was quantitated by the change in relative turbidity in this study. The solutions were exposed to various areas of foreign surfaces, the greatest for gamma-globulins alone and least for albumins. The denature of gamma-globulin was diminished in the presence of albumin. (Reproduced with permission from K. M. Pruitt et al.[12])

also postulated increased rate of precipitation of cryoprecipitable gamma-globulin complexes during hypothermic perfusion.

Pretty et al.[13] demonstrated anti-gamma-globulin antibodies commonly in patients undergoing open heart surgery but rarely demonstrated leukocyte and platelet antibodies.

Wright et al.[14] conducted experiments similar to those of Lee and confirmed the rise in viscosity. They also observed rise in optical density, sulfhydryl content, and an increased rate of mobility of the alpha-2-globulins in starch gel electrophoresis. The changes were greater with screen oxygenation than with membrane oxygenation. The studies show that chemical changes are a significant part of the alteration in immune protein function which occurs with cardiopulmonary bypass.[14] Studies of the effect of cardiopulmonary bypass on serum complement and immunoglobulins in patients showed a fall in IgG, IgA, and IgM but a much greater fall in complement with cardiopulmonary bypass. Denatured immunoglobulins are known to activate complement *in vitro*. The reduction in complement concentration could not be accounted for by hemodilution. The changes in complement are so rapid that increased complement utilization rather than decreased production would be a more likely cause. The authors believed the decreased complement was due to interaction with denatured immune globulins. They postulated this reaction to be a potential cause of diminished resistance to pneumococcal septicemia or cytomegalovirus infection. Complement activation may result in the increased formation of anaphylatoxins and kinins which alter capillary function. Other effects of complement activation include platelet aggregation and increased leukocyte and platelet adherence.[15,16]

A later study demonstrated the conversion of C_3 complement to C_3b following cardiopulmonary bypass. The studies demonstrated no difference in C_3 concentration in arterial and venous blood. The conversion was demonstrable only after cardiopulmonary bypass had been terminated and the pulmonary circulation restored. The mechanism for this complement activation is unknown. The effect of complement activation in this case may be enhanced phagocytotic and chemotactic migration of leukocytes. When complement levels are depleted host defenses are lost. Hairston and Pruitt have demonstrated diminished complement for more then 24 hours postoperatively. Pruitt showed that gamma-globulins exposed to the gas/liquid interface fixed complement at a greatly increased rate.

The effect of complement activation and granulocyte interaction has been demonstrated most strikingly in patients undergoing hemodialysis. These patients have complement activation by the dialysis membrane and develop white blood cell aggregation in the lungs. Repeated episodes with chronic dialysis may produce pulmonary fibrosis and calcinosis.[17]

EFFECTS ON CELLULAR COMPONENTS

The effect of cardiopulmonary bypass on cellular components of the immune system has been the subject of an increasing number of studies. Diminished white blood cell counts were recognized very early to be a consequence of cardiopulmonary bypass (Fig. 13.3).[18] Brinsfield et al.[19] did a more detailed study of the kinetics of white cells during cardiopulmonary bypass. He showed an immediate fall in leukocytes followed by later leukocytosis and appearance of immature leukocytes and nucleated red blood cells. The decrease in white cells was due to a fall in numbers of mature granulocytes and macronuclear cells. Animals perfused with disc or membrane oxygenators showed an increase in the relative numbers of myeloid elements in the bone marrow, while those perfused with bubble oxygenators showed a decrease in bone marrow myeloid elements. The bone marrow showed a stimulated response following cardiopulmonary bypass.[18]

Cardiopulmonary bypass produces significant changes in the myelopoietic and reticuloendothelial portions of the bone marrow. The erythropoietic series were only slightly affected. In the myelopoietic series there is increased mitosis immediately postoperatively. The number of stab cells and polymorphonuclear forms diminishes for 3 days but is increasing 1 week postoperatively. The cellular changes include vacuolization and

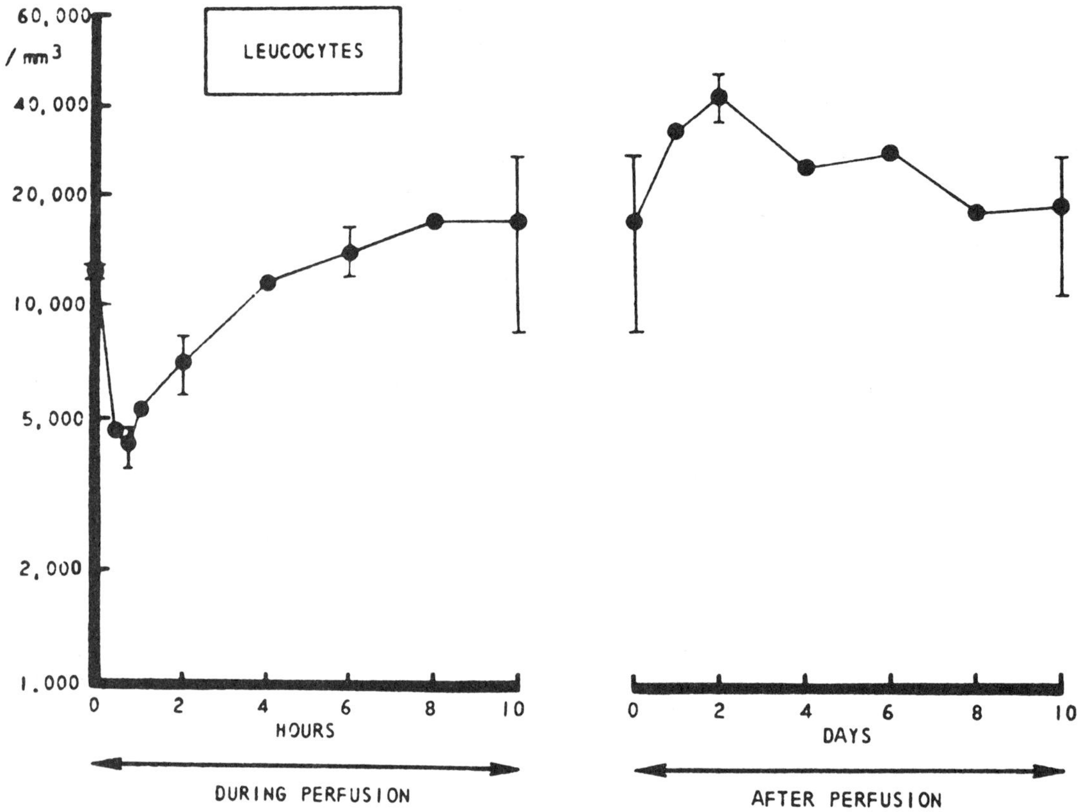

Figure 13.3. Leukocyte counts diminished immediately with the onset of cardiopulmonary bypass and then returned to increased levels. (Reproduced with permission from D. E. Brinsfield et al.[19])

nuclear lysis and pathologic granulation. There is a rapid decrease of bone marrow lymphoid cells while monocytes increase slightly.[20] Phagocytic function fell during operation and remained depressed for more than 15 days.[20]

Fall in white cell count has been observed with perfusion of blood through a pump oxygenator circuit. Kusserow showed that of the cells remaining, fewer demonstrated phagocytic activity, and those phagocytically active ingested fewer bacteria in a standard phagocytic test. Thus, not only destruction but also functional impairment of white cells is produced by the pump oxygenator. The study also demonstrated decreased oxygen utilization and decreased glucose utilization by white cells exposed to a pump oxygenator circuit (Fig. 13.4). The authors described a number of morphologic changes. Nuclear changes included distortion and confluence of lobes in granulocytes. Other nuclear changes included hyaloid transformation, homogenization, and vacuolization of nuclear substance and raggedness of nuclear contour. There was loss of cytoplasm, a raggedness of cytoplasmic contour, and a reduction in size of some cells. The absolute number of both polymorphonuclear and mononuclear cells diminished, but the decrease was greater in the mononuclear cells than in granulocytes.[21–23]

The leukocytosis in animals during cardiopulmonary bypass is due to the pump oxygenator and not due to surgical trauma. Animals were prepared in identical manner including cannulation, except that one group was not perfused. Only the animals perfused with the pump oxygenator developed the leukocytosis. Greater fall in white cell counts

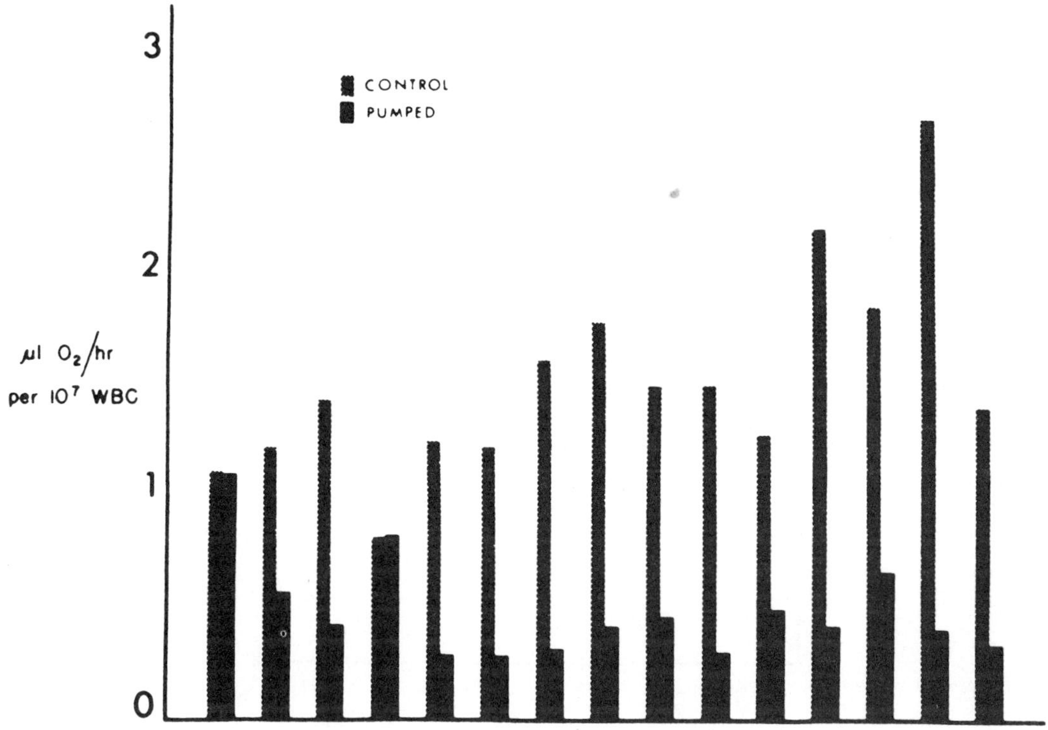

Figure 13.4. The oxygen utilization of leukocytes exposed to a pump oxygenator is diminished compared to control leukocytes. (Reproduced with permission from Transactions: American Society for Artificial Internal Organs, 15:40, 1969.)

was observed with bubble oxygenator than with the membrane oxygenator.[24]

Bubenik and Meakins[25] studied the random migration of neutrophils after cardiopulmonary bypass and found slight decreases. Studies of the migration of neutrophils in response to a chemotactic stimulation showed marked depression of neutrophil chemotaxis. The depressed chemotaxis remained low until 3 days postoperatively and did not return to normal until 7 days postoperatively (Fig. 13.5).

Phagocytic function and phagocytic intracellular oxidation has been shown to be reduced in a number of studies (Fig. 13.6). The quantitative nitroblue tetrazolium test (NBT) is a measure of a phagocyte's ability to produce hydrogen peroxide intracellularly, which is necessary for bacterial killing. Silva et al.[6] showed a decrease in NBT reduction during cardiopulmonary bypass with a rapid return to normal postoperatively. Of four patients studied, the bacteriocidal reaction to *E. coli* and *S. aureus* was diminished in two. The degree of bacteriocidal depression was greater for *E. coli* in one patient and greater for *S. aureus* in the other patient. The diminished bacteriocidal activity could not be correlated with the depression in NBT reduction. Taguchi et al.[26] have confirmed the decrease of NBT reduction in a group of patients undergoing hemodilution cardiopulmonary bypass. Palmbald[27] showed that bacteriocidal activity of polymorphonuclear leukocytes was decreased 2 days after cardiopulmonary bypass accompanied by the appearance of immature forms. He concluded that the increased bacteriocidal activity was due not to immature cells which normally have decreased bacteriocidal activity but to activation of the granulocytes in some way. This hypothesis is supported by the increase in NBT reduction and increased macrophage hemolytic activity demonstrated days following cardiopulmonary bypass.[27]

Other studies failed to show any depres-

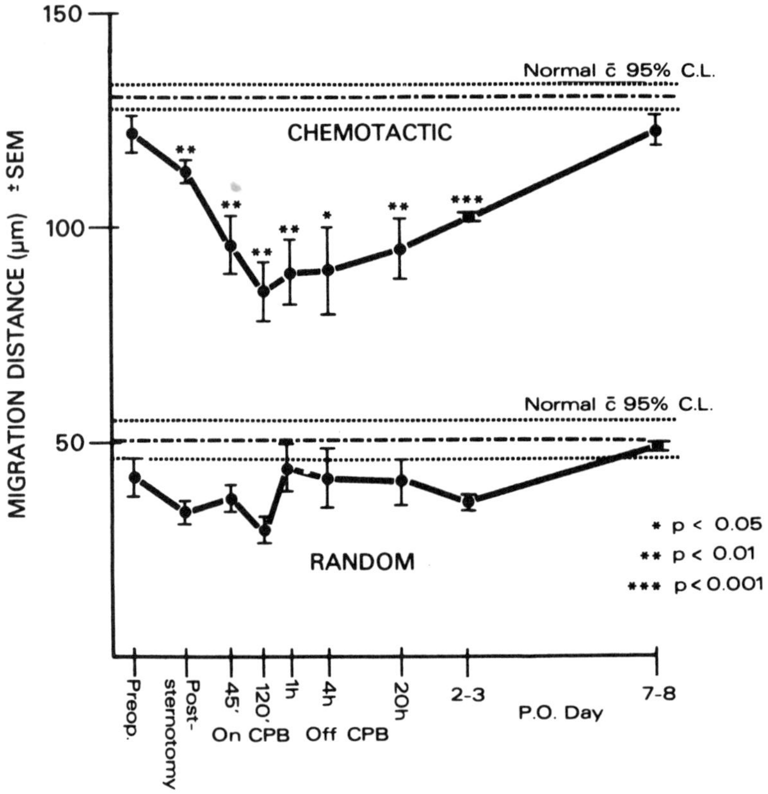

Figure 13.5. The migration of neutrophils in response to chemotactic stimulus is diminished by cardiopulmonary bypass and does not return to normal for 7 days. (Reproduced with permission from O. Bubenik and J. L. Meakins.[25])

sion of the ability of polymorphonuclear leukocytes to phagocytize or kill bacteria following cardiopulmonary bypass.[28]

NBT reduction has been used to monitor patients for potential infection after cardiac surgery. In children a positive NBT reduction after the 1st postoperative week was found to be predictive of endocarditis or pneumonia but not wound infection, nonbacterial febrile illnesses, or postpericardiotomy syndromes. There were many false positives in the 1st week postoperatively.[29] In another study of patients postoperatively it was suggested that a negative NBT Reduction Test was useful in ruling out bacterial infection but that a positive test was not diagnostic of infection.[30]

Studies of the lymphocyte response to cardiopulmonary bypass in patients undergoing value replacement showed that on the 2nd postoperative day the total lymphocyte count and the numbers in subclasses as characterized by E (T-cells), EA (fc receptor cells), and EAC (Bcells) were reduced. Rosette formation and the surface membrane immunoglobulin markers were diminished. These had returned to normal by the 7th postoperative day. Increases in the number of atypical lymphocytes characterized by morphology and autoradiography were observed up to 14 days postoperatively. The transformation responses of lymphocytes to phytohemagglutinin (PHA) and pokeweed mitogen (PWM) were diminished 2 days postoperatively but were at greater than preoperative levels 5 days postoperatively. The mixed lymphocyte culture (MLC) was decreased on the 2nd postoperative day and returned to normal by the 5th postoperative day. The stimulatory ability of lymphocytes in MLC and their response to purified tuberculoprotein was

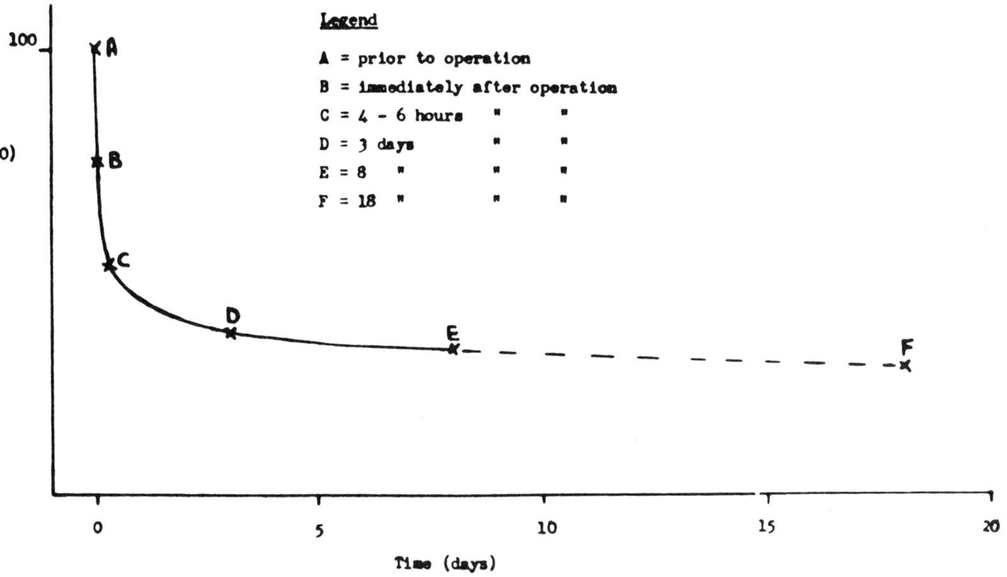

Figure 13.6. Effect of extracorporeal circulation on phagocytosis. The phagocytosis of leukocytes is diminished immediately after cardiopulmonary bypass and remained depressed for 20 days in this study. (Reproduced with permission from M. Lundstrom et al.[20])

diminished for up to 14 days postoperatively.[31]

There was no difference in response in patients perfused with bubble or membrane oxygenators or in patients who did or did not receive perenteral hyperalimentation. The authors found the fall in eosinophils and basophils to be similar to neutrophils. The decrease in monocytes was less postoperatively than polymorphonuclear cells. The increased atypical lymphocytes and the number of lymphocytes spontanously synthesizing DNA may be a response to transfusion products of tissue decomposition and certain infective factors. They are considered a polyclonal immune response to antigen stimulation.[31] Other studies confirmed the suppression of lymphocyte response to phytohemagglutinin (PHA) and concanavalin A during cardiac surgery (Fig. 13.7). Serial studies showed the change was not due to anesthesia or operation but mainly to cardiopulmonary bypass. The values were 1–5% of the preoperative values on the 1st postoperative day and did not return to normal until 2 to 3 months postoperatively. The sharpest changes were observed in patients undergoing coronary or valve surgery and lesser response in patients having atrial septal defect closure. The author postulates that decreased cellular immunity increases the cardiac surgical patient's susceptibility to viral, fungal, and certain bacterial infections.[32]

Other studies showed a decrease in transformation of lymphocytes in the presence of phytohemagglutinin, concanavalin A, and pokeweed mitogen. The abnormalities had returned only partially to normal at the 8th day and were associated with decrease in percent lymphocytes and increase in percent monocytes.[33] The depression of immunoglobulin-G levels after cardiac surgery was partially reversed by parenteral hyperalimentation.[34]

The ability of lymphocytes to incorporate tritiated thymidine is diminished following cardiac and noncardiac surgery. Incubation of the cells in normal plasma partially reversed this effect, while incubation in patients' plasma potentiated the effect. The depressed cellular immunity has been implicated in the development of postperfusion and postcardiotomy syndrome.[35]

An interesting corollary to the depression

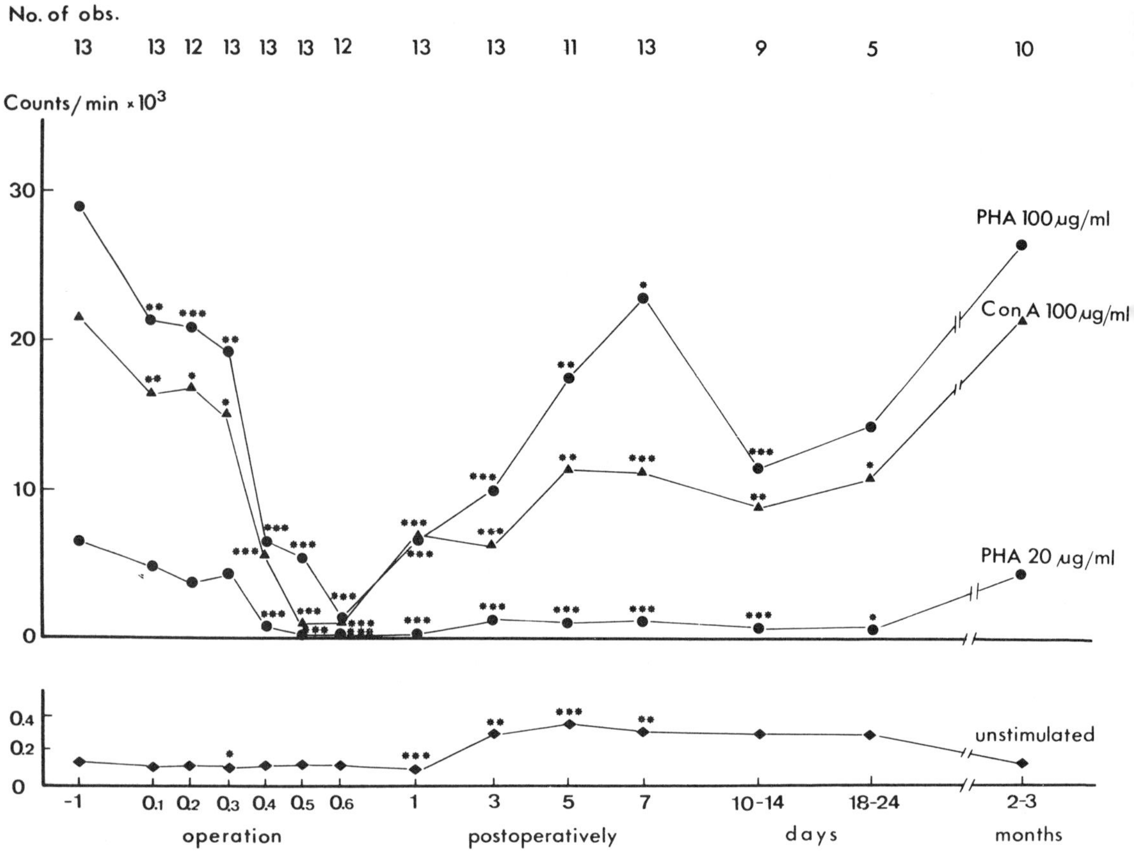

Figure 13.7. The mitogenic response of lymphocytes to PHA and Con-A is diminished by cardiopulmonary bypass and does not return to control values for several days. (Reproduced with permission from M. Salo.[32])

of immunity following cardiopulmonary bypass is the clearing of psoriasis following cardiopulmonary bypass. Psoriasis is known to be associated with increased chemotaxis of monocytes and polymorphonuclear leukocytes. Increased NBT reduction has been observed in the polymorphonuclear and monocytic leukocytes of psoriasis. Cardiopulmonary bypass suppresses these functions known to be enhanced in psoriasis.[36]

RETICULOENDOTHELIAL FUNCTION

Subramanian et al.[37] has performed a series of experiments demonstrating suppression of reticuloendothelial function following cardiopulmonary bypass. His first studies showed that blood that was recirculated in a pump oxygenator depressed the phagocytic function of the isolated perfused rat liver. This depression of phagocytic function was not accompanied by change of bile flow, blood flow, or weight of the perfused liver. The depressed phagocytosis of staphylococci was produced to a lesser extent by perfusion with plasma recirculated through the pump oxygenator. Thus, the effect was due mainly to the cellular elements exposed to the pump oxygenator. Plasma perfused through the pump oxygenator decreased phagocytosis of the large staphylococci more than of the small ^{198}Au particles.

The depressed phagocytosis was demonstrated by decreased clearance of ^{198}Au- and ^{59}Fe-labeled staphylococci (Fig. 13.8). The author concluded that the particles generated

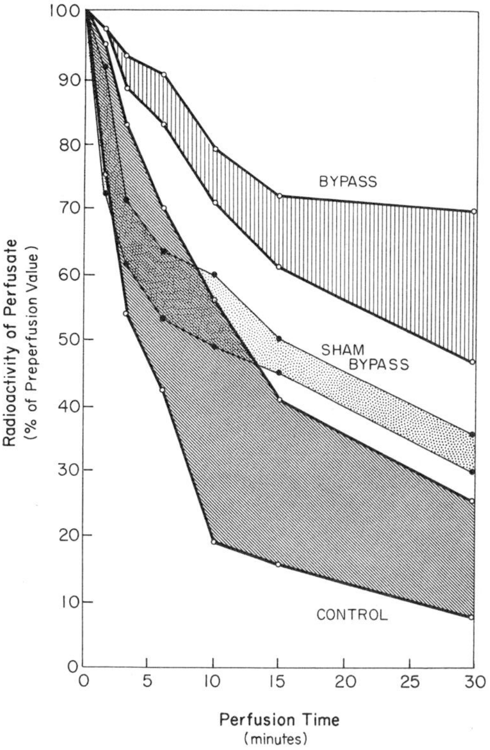

Figure 13.8. In this study the function of the reticuloendothelial system was studied by determining the role of clearance of colloidal radioactive gold (Au^{198}) (Reproduced with permission from V. Subramanian et al.[37] and C. V. Mosby Company.)

from both cellular breakdown and protein aggregation interfered with Kupffer cell function. The reticuloendothelial system is important in clearing circulating blood of bacteria, endotoxin, platelets, denatured proteins, chylomicrons, plasma hemoglobin, thrombin, fibrin, fibrin degradation products, thromboplastin, and plasminogen activator. In a second set of experiments this investigator demonstrated depression of phagocytic function in liver of rats who underwent cardiopulmonary bypass compared to animals not operated or subjected to sham bypass. Again there was no change in bile flow, blood flow, or liver weight.[38,39]

The most recent study showed that dogs subjected to cardiopulmonary bypass were unable to clear infused *Klebsiella aerogenes* compared to a group of sham-operated animals. Mortality was 16% in the cardiopulmonary bypass group and 0% in the sham-operated group.[40]

References

1. Howard RJ: Effect of burn injury, mechanical trauma, and operation on immune defenses. Surg Clin North Am 59(2):199, 1979.
2. Howard RJ: Host defense against infection-Part 1. Curr Probl Surg 17(5):267, 1980.
3. Howard RJ: Host defense against infection-Part 2. Curr Probl Surg 17(6):319, 1980.
4. Golub ES: *The Cellular Basis of the Immune Response: An Approach to Immunobiology.* Sunderland, Mass., Sinauer Associates, 1977.
5. Slade MS, Simmons RL, Yunis E, Greenberg LJ: Immunodepression after major surgery in normal patients. Surgery 78(3):363, 1975.
6. Silva J Jr, Hoeksema H, Fekety FR Jr: Transient defects in phagocytic functions during cardiopulmonary bypass. J Thorac Cardiovasc Surg 67(2):175, 1974.
7. Hairston P, Manos JP, Graber CD, Lee WH Jr: Depression of immunologic surveillance by pump-oxygenation perfusion. J Surg Res 9(10):587, 1969.
8. Larmi TKI, Kärkölä P: Plasma protein electrophoresis during a three-hour cardiopulmonary bypass in dogs. Scand J Thorac Cardiovasc Surg 8:152, 1974.
9. Wallace HW, Arai K, Blakemore WS: Comparison of postoperative glycoprotein responses in open-heart and nonopen-heart patients. J Appl Physiol 28(4):433, 1970.
10. Lee WH Jr, Krumhaar D, Fonkalsrud EW, Schjeide OA, Maloney JV Jr: Denaturation of plasma proteins as a cause of morbidity and death after intracardiac operations. Surgery 50(1):29, 1961.
11. Owens G, Adams JE, McElhannon FM, Youngblood RW: Experimental alterations of certain colloidal properties of blood during cardiopulmonary bypass. J Appl Physiol 14(6):947, 1959.
12. Pruitt KM, Stroud RM, Scott JW: Blood damage in the heart-lung machine. Proc Soc Exp Biol Med 137: 714, 1970.
13. Pretty HM, Fudenberg HH, Perkins HA, Gerbode F: Anti-γ globulin antibodies after open heart surgery. Blood 32(2):205, 1968.
14. Wright ES, Sarkozy E, Harpur ER, Dobell ARC, Murphy DR: Plasma protein denturation in extracorporeal circulation. J Thorac Cardiovasc Surg 44(4):550, 1962.
15. Parker DJ, Cantrell JW, Karp RB, Stroud RM, Digerness SB: Changes in serum complement and immunoglobulins following cardiopulmonary bypass. Surgery 71(6):824, 1972.
16. Parker DJ, Cook S, Turner-Warwick M: Serum complement studies during and following cardipulmonary bypass. In *Lung Metabolism*, edited by AF Junod and R de Haller. New York, Academic Press, 1975, p. 481.
17. Jacob HS: Granulocyte-complement interaction: A beneficial antimicrobial mechanism that can cause

disease. Arch Intern Med 138:461, 1978.
18. Brown IW Jr, Smith WW: Hemotologic problems associated with the use of extracorporeal circulation for cardiovascular surgery. Ann Intern Med 49:1035, 1958.
19. Brinsfield DE, Hopf MA, Geering RB, Galletti PM: Hematological changes in long-term perfusion. J Appl Physiol 17:531, 1962.
20. Lundstrom M, Olsson P, Unger P, Ekeström S: Effect of extracorporeal circulation on hematopoiesis and phagocytosis. J Cardiovasc Surg 4:664, 1963.
21. Kusserow B, Larrow R, Nichols J: Metabolic and morphological alterations in leukocytes following prolonged blood pumping. Trans Am Soc Artif Intern Organs 15:40, 1969.
22. Kusserow B, Larrow R, Nichols J: Perfusion- and surface-induced injury in leukocytes. Fed Proc 30(5): 1516, 1971.
23. Kusserow BK, Larrow R: Studies of leukocyte response to prolonged blood pumping-effects upon phagocytic capability and total white cell count. Trans Am Soc Artif Intern Organs 14:261, 1968.
24. Kvarstein B, Cappelen C Jr, Österud A: Blood platelets and leucocytes during cardiopulmonary bypass. Scand J Thorac Cardiovasc Surg 8:142, 1974.
25. Bubenik O, Meakins JL: Neutrophil chemotaxis in surgical patients: Effect of cardiopulmonary bypass. Surg Forum 27:267, 1976.
26. Taguchi K, Takamura K, Mochizuki T, Kishi D, Yokoyama T: Alteration of the phagocytic function in cardiopulmonary bypass. Hiroshima J Med Sci 25(1):7, 1976.
27. Palmbald J: Activation of the bacterial capacity of polymorphonuclear granulocytes after surgery, measured with a new in vitro assay. Scand J Haematol 23:10, 1979.
28. Kaplan EL, Castaneda AR, Ayoub EM, Quie PG: Effects of cardiopulmonary bypass on the phagocytic and bactericidal capacities of polymorphonuclear leukocytes. Circulation 37(2):158, 1968.
29. Lerer RJ, Treat K: Nitro blue tetrazolium dye reduction test in children after cardiac surgery. Am J Dis Child 127:846, 1974.
30. Freeman R, King B, Hambling MH: Infective complications of open-heart surgery and the monitoring of infections by the NBT test. Thorax 28:617, 1973.
31. Ryhanen P, Herva E, Hollmen A, Nuutinen L, Pihlajaniemi R, Saarela E: Changes in peripheral blood leukocyte counts, lymphocyte subpopulations, and in vitro transformation after heart valve replacement. J Thorac Cardiovasc Surg 77(2):1259, 1979.
32. Salo M: Effect of anaesthesia and open-heart surgery on lymphocyte responses to phytohaemagglutinin and Concanavalin A. Acta Anaesthesiol Scand 22: 471, 1978.
33. Schlaak M, Lehmann H, Zabel P, Bernhard A: Immunoglobulin levels and alterations of the lymphocyte function after extracorporal circulation and massive blood transfusion. Thoraxchir Vask Chir 23: 415, 1975.
34. Gierhake FW, Johannsen R, Meyer-Hoepfel W, Meyer-Hoepfel I, Herget HF, Stöcker R, Carlsson AB, L'Allemand H, Hehrlein FW: Immunologic aspects to the prevention of infection cardiac surgery. Thoraxchirurgie 23:417, 1975.
35. Park SK, Brody JI, Wallace HA, Blakemore WS: Immunosuppressive effect of surgery. Lancet 1:53, 1971.
36. Buselmeier TJ, Cantieri JS, Dahl MV, Nelson RS, Baumgaertner JC, Bentley CR, Goltz RW: Clearing of psoriasis after cardiac surgery requiring cardiopulmonary bypass oxygenation: A corollary to clearance after dialysis? Br J Dermatol 100:311, 1979.
37. Subramanian V, McLeod J, Gans H: Effect of extracorporeal circulation on reticuloendothelial function. I. Experimental evidence for impaired reticuloendothelial function following cardiopulmonary bypass in rats. Surgery 64(4):775, 1968.
38. Subramanian V, Lowman JT, Gans H: Effect of extracorporeal circulation on reticuloendothelial function: Impariment and its relationship to blood trauma. Arch Surg 97:330, 1968.
39. Subramanian V, Lande AJ, Gans H, Lowman JT, Lillehei CW: Depression of host-defense mechanism following extracorporeal circulation. Trans Am Soc Artif Intern Organs 15:165, 1969.
40. Subramanian VA, Gay WA Jr, Dineen PPA: Effect of cardiopulmonary bypass on in vivo clearance of live *Klebsiella* aerogens. Surg Forum 28:255, 1977.

CHAPTER 14

HYPOTHERMIA: LESSONS FROM COMPARATIVE PHYSIOLOGY*

FRED N. WHITE, Ph.D.

Cold-blooded animals (ectotherms) experience a wide range of body temperatures during diurnal and seasonal fluctuations in ambient thermal conditions. These alterations in thermal state are accompanied by shifting metabolic demands and alterations in blood gas transport and acid-base parameters. It is of interest from a comparative physiological and biochemical viewpoint to contrast the similarities and differences which characterize the regulatory strategies of warm-blooded (endothermic) vertebrates and ectotherms, especially in light of the subject of this monograph—the subjugation of mammalian tissues to hypothermia. We may ask, from such studies, whether the homeostatic responses of ectotherms offer a rationale for exploring new strategies by which the welfare of hypothermic mammalian tissues may be better guarded.

ALTERATIONS IN ACID-BASE HOMEOSTASIS AS A FUNCTION OF TEMPERATURE

It has become widely appreciated that a sample of blood held in a gas-tight syringe, i.e., at constant CO_2 content, exhibits a predictable ΔpH/°C equal to −0.014 when pH is measured in a closed electrode system at various temperatures.[1] Thus, if a sample of blood is taken at 22°C and measured in the blood gas laboratory, where pH electrodes are maintained at 37°C, the pH at 22°C may be approximated from the 37°C value: $pH_{22°C} = pH_{37°C} + (37 - 22)\ (0.014)$. A 37°C pH value of 7.16 may be translated as 7.37 at 22°C.

The temperature-dependent shift in pH of *in vitro* blood, held at constant CO_2 content, has been ascribed to the influence of imidazole of histidine. Imidazole, at appropriate concentrations, has been shown to convey to simple aqueous systems the ΔpH°C slope displayed by blood[2] (Fig. 14.1). Sufficient titratable imidazole groups (approximately 30 mmol/liter) exist in blood to account for the ΔpH/°C relationship described by Rosenthal.[1] Rahn[3] has pointed out that the arterialized blood of man represents a heterogeneity of pH's, depending on the temperature of the various tissues (Fig. 14.2). Thus, in the cold, blood perfusing the skin of man may fall from a core value of 37°C at pH 7.4 to 25°C and pH 7.6 in the periphery. Exercising skeletal muscle may rise to 41°C and pH_a equals 7.34. We should view arterial pH not as a sharply fixed value, but as a spectrum of values which depend upon the temperature of the various tissues with which the precapillary blood equilibrates. Once blood has completed its exchanges in the lungs, the $[H^+]_a$ is at the will of the thermal state of the tissues. This fact alone should raise concerns

* Supported in part, by NSF Grant PCM 80-05052.

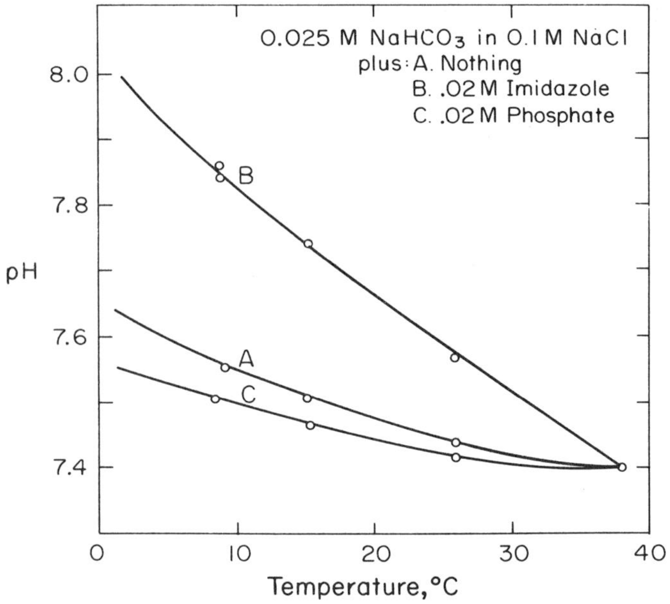

Figure 14.1. Change in pH with temperature of three simple aqueous solutions which were adjusted to have a pH of 7.4 at 38°C and then allowed to cool with no access to air. Note that ΔpH/°C for the imidazole system is approximately −0.014, similar to the behavior of *in vitro* arterial blood under similar conditions (Modified from R. B. Reeves.[2])

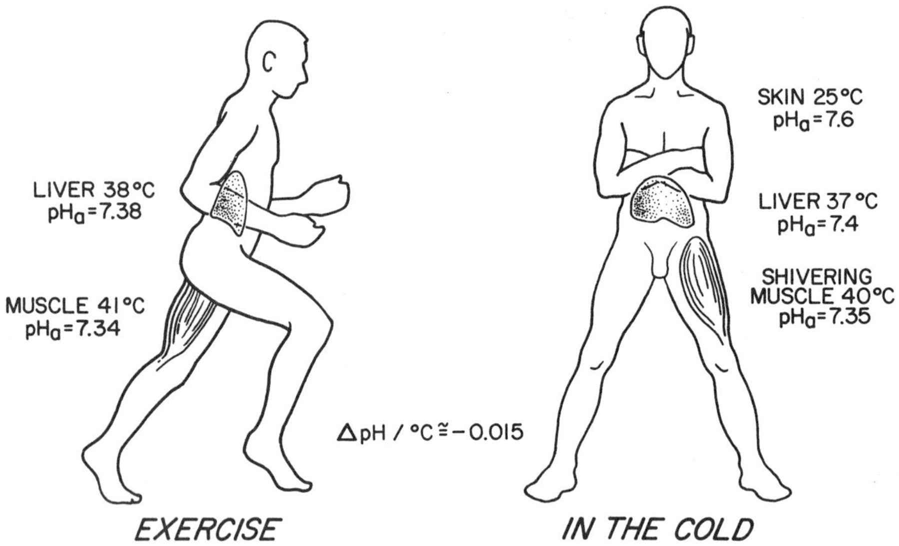

Figure 14.2. Heterogeneous pHa of man. Arterialized blood in man may represent a spectrum of pHs, depending on the tissue temperature with which the precapillary blood equilibrates.

about the acid-base state of perfusates of hypothermic tissues.

Change of body temperature, as a function of environmental temperature, is the *sine qua non* of the ectotherm. What patterns of acid-base homeostasis characterize this thermal heterogeneity? Over the past decade, numerous studies have demonstrated that the normal acid-base pattern of various invertebrates and vertebrates[4–9] is characterized by a direct relationship between body temperature and $[H^+]$ (Fig. 14.3). The slope of pH against body temperature exhibited by this broad spectrum of animals bears a remarkable similarity to the *in vitro* behavior of blood described by Rosenthal. Rahn and his associates[10] have emphasized that the pH-temperature slope exhibits a remarkable parallelism with the neutral pH of H_2O (pN_{H_2O}). When the pOH is calculated it is seen that these animals exhibit a near constancy of $[OH^-]/[H^+]$ across the great spectrum of temperatures. In other words, they exhibit constant blood alkalinity relative to the pH of neutrality of water. It should also be noted that the spectrum of these values includes pH 7.4 at 37°C. We are left with the conclusion that all these animals behave *as if* they were closed systems, at constant CO_2 content, and referenced

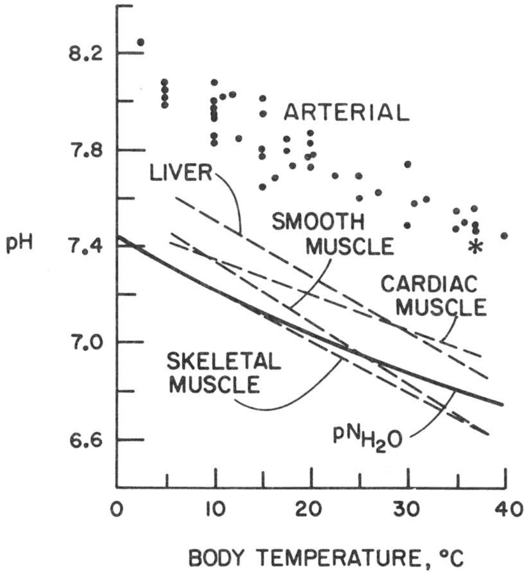

Figure 14.3. Arterial pH as a function of body temperature in a variety of ectothermic invertebrates and vertebrates. *Asterisk* indicates normal human value. The arterial pHs exhibit a slope similar to the neutral pH of H_2O (pN_{H_2O}). Intracellular pHs of various tissues of the turtle are displaced to the acid-side of extracellular pH and also exhibit slopes similar to pN_{H_2O}. (pH_i data from A. Malan et al.[18])

to pH of around 7.4 at 37°C. However, they are clearly open systems. It can be demonstrated that such organisms must institute regulations involving the variables within the Henderson-Hasselbalch relationship to achieve constant $[OH^-]/[H^+]$ of the blood perfusing their tissues.

The Henderson-Hasselbalch relationship,

$$pH = pK + \log \frac{[HCO_3^-]}{\alpha CO_2 \cdot P_{CO_2}},$$ contains two important thermal variables, pK and αCO_2. Severinghaus et al. have evaluated[11, 12] these variables and their monogram for pK and table of solubility factors for CO_2 are of immense use in evaluating the effects of temperature on this important blood buffer system. When the *in vivo* arterial pH values of lower vertebrates are related to this equation, it can be shown that in progressing from low to high temperature, either the $[HCO_3^-]$ must fall or P_{CO_2} must rise. Pa_{CO_2} of a lung breather is governed by the gas equilibrium conditions across the respiratory exchange surfaces. The strategy of altering the ratio of pulmonary ventilation to CO_2 production as a function of body temperature has been shown to be the major factor in guarding the constant CO_2 content and relative alkalinity of the blood of such forms. Blood gas data for a number of ectothermic lung breathers reveals that $[HCO_3^-]_a$ is maintained at a relatively constant level while Pa_{CO_2} is a direct function of temperature (Table 14.1). For each of the reptilian species in the table, measurements of oxygen consumption and ventilation allow the assessment of ventilatory intensity *relative* to metabolic intensity. This relationship may be expressed in terms of $\dot{V}E/\dot{V}O_2$. In each of the cases in Table 14.1, there is an inverse relationship between this ratio and temperature. The relative underventilation accompanying increased body temperature (and metabolism) accounts for the adjustment in Pa_{CO_2} which is necessary to maintain constant C_{CO_2}, pH parallel to the pN_{H_2O}, and $[OH^-]/[H^+]$ constant. Exemplary of this regulatory pattern are data for the semiaquatic turtle *Pseudemys floridana* (Fig. 14.4). The inverse relationship between $\dot{V}E/\dot{V}O_2$ would appear paradoxical since increasing oxygen demands are met by relatively lower ventilatory intensity. However, when animals exercise, $\dot{V}E/\dot{V}O_2$ remains at the resting level at any given

Table 14.1
Arterial Acid-Base Parameters in Lung Breathing Vertebrates

Literature Source (Ref.)		Temperature Range (°C)	P_{CO_2} range (torr) (Low to High Temperature)	$[HCO_3^-]$mEq/liter	ΔpH/°C
2	*Rana catesbeiana* (bullfrog)	5–34	7.0–23.1	22.6 ± 1.27*	−0.016
49	*A. mississippiensis* (alligator)	15–35	11.8–23.2	15.1 ± 0.95	−0.013
6	*Pseudemys scripta* (turtle)	10–30	14.1–31.9	33.3 ± 1.46	−0.010
7	*P. floridana* (turtle)	22–37	20.8–34.8	29.6 ± 1.43	−0.013
47	*Sauromalus obesus* (lizard)	16–40	11.0–40.0	14.1 ± 1.63	−0.017
48	*Dipsosaurus dorsalus* (lizard)	17–42	9.9–32.0	19.5 ± 1.20	−0.014

* Mean ± SD.

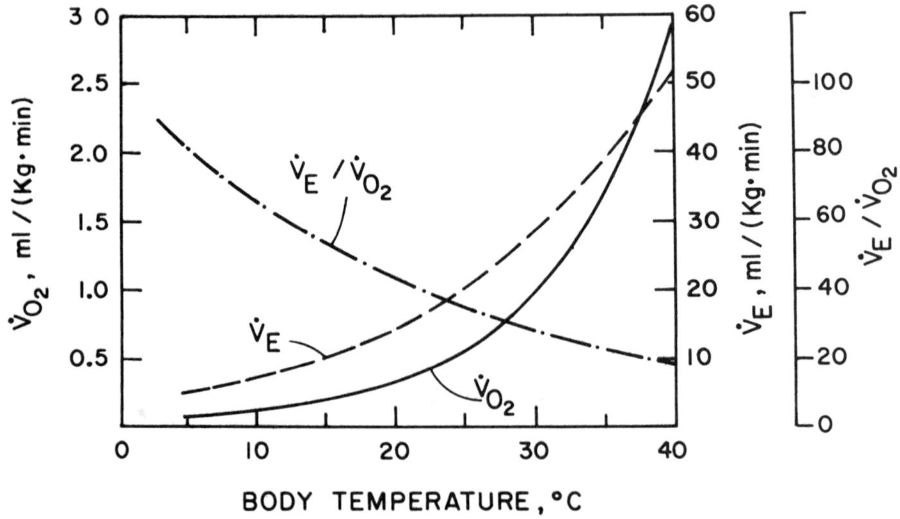

Figure 14.4. Relationships between ventilation and oxygen consumption at various body temperatures in the turtle *Pseudemys floridana*. The ratio of ventilation to oxygen consumption is inverse to temperature (Data from J. L. Kinney et al.[7])

temperature. This pattern of meeting variable oxygen requirements is similar to that of man. Expressing $\dot{V}E/\dot{V}O_2$ as an *air convection requirement* (liters of air ventilated/mmol O_2 consumed) allows comparisons of diverse organisms. While the figures for the turtle are quite large at low temperatures, the convergence of man and turtle, when at a common temperature of 37°C, is striking (turtle, 0.5 liters/mmol O_2; man, 0.56 liters/mmol O_2). The respiratory poise of both turtle and man achieve a similar P_{CO_2} and pH_a only at a common temperature! The pattern of CO_2 regulation of man would appear to be an isothermal case of the general pattern of regulation of ectotherms—a pattern of long evolutionary standing.

The heterogeneous nature of the thermal world of many ectotherms presents a regulatory challenge which endotherms seldom encounter, and we have established rather sharply defined norms for acid-base and ventilatory parameters in healthy normothermic humans. The marine iguana of the Galapagos Islands experiences diurnal variations in body temperature exceeding 20°C. Such thermal variation is met with a new set of acid-base and respiratory parameters specific to each temperature experienced (Fig. 14.5). Common to man and such ectotherms is the convergence of the arterial pH at around 7.4 and 37°C.

Because of the relationship of the respiratory medium to the gills of fishes (a flow-through system), water represents a constant "sink" for CO_2. Consequently, the arterial blood characteristically exhibits a low partial pressure of CO_2, a few torr at most. Studies on trout, acclimated to various temperatures, revealed that it is the regulation of the $[HCO_3^-]$ (inverse to temperature) via active transport mechanisms which is responsible for the maintenance of constant $[OH^-]/[H^+]$.[8, 13]

We are beginning to see a pattern of an $[H^+]$-temperature relationship which is rather ubiquitous in its distribution among living forms. There is an exception which warrants attention. Hibernating mammals appear to maintain arterial pH near the typical normo-

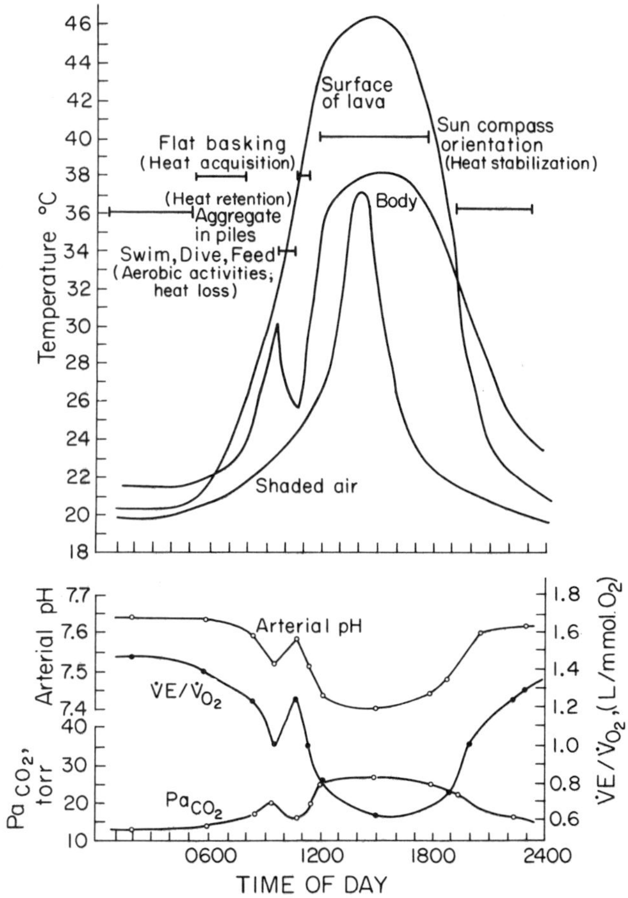

Figure 14.5. Behavior and temperature relations for the Galapagos marine iguana *Amblyrhynchus cristatus* during a typical day in the Galapagos Islands. Ventilatory and acid-base parameters calculated from laboratory studies extending over the range of thermal conditions experienced by animals in nature. (Data from R. A. Ackerman and F. N. White.[45, 46])

thermic value of 7.4 while body temperatures fall to around 5°C.[14, 15] Thus, they do not conform to the common ectothermic pattern which would predict an arterial pH of around 7.9 at the hibernating body temperature. The full implications of this "acidotic" state for overall energy requirements, oxygen transport, and function and structure of proteins are not clear.

INTRACELLULAR pH AND TEMPERATURE

The measurement of intracellular pH (pH_i) is technically difficult, and most available measures are based on the dimethyl-2,4-oxazeolidinedione (DMO) method, a technique thought to evaluate "overall" pH_i. The estimates represent some mix of cytosol and mitochondrial values, the latter being a few tenths of a pH unit higher than the cytosal. A useful discussion of methods and limitations of pH_i measurements is supplied by Poole-Wilson.[16, 17]

Malan *et al.*[18] studied temperature-pH_i relationships in the frog and turtle and reported that pH_i of several tissues varied inversely with temperature along a slope rather parallel to but displaced to the acid side of the extracellular fluid. The pH_i values reported are near the neutral pH of water (Fig. 14.3). The concentration of the imidazole residue and its characteristic pK of around 7 and $\Delta H°$ of 7 kcal/mole allows its pK to change with temperature along with pN_{H_2O}. This feature maintains the fractional dissociation of titratable imidazole groups at a rather constant level at constant CO_2 content (see Reeves[19] for a detailed analysis). Thus, enzymatic reactions requiring protonated histidine for ligand binding to facilitate the reaction in one direction may occur in the reverse direction when binding requires uncharged imidazole. An enzyme known to involve a histidine residue in substrate binding is lactate dehydrogenase.[20] LDH functions both as a pyruvate reductase and a lactate oxidase. Yancey and Somero[21] have examined the pyruvate reductase behavior of this enzyme in a variety of ectothermic muscles and the rabbit. The effect of temperature on the Michaelis constant (K_m) of substrate was determined under conditions of constant pH and $\Delta pH/°C$ equals −0.017 along the pH curve for pN_{H_2O}. It should be noted that optimal enzyme function is preserved when K_m of substrate is held to a narrow range such that the capacity of enzyme to regulate its rate of catalysis is preserved.[22, 23] In the case of the M_4-LDHs under consideration, the K_m of pyruvate must be stabilized at values allowing the enzyme to increase its activity as pyruvate concentration rises during muscular work. The regulatory advantages of conserving K_m values around a narrow range are discussed by Atkinson[24] and Fersht[22] (Fig. 14.6) illustrates the steep slopes of of K_m against temperature when pH was held constant at 7.4. The marked conservation of K_m found at pH's of neutral water illustrate that the enzyme function is more optimally maintained under these conditions. It is noteworthy that this is true for an endotherm, the rabbit, as well as the various species of fishes utilized in the study.

It may be inferred that enzymes which display the type of temperature-pH relationship shown for LDH, but for which the active site sequences are not yet known, are likely to have histidine residues in their active sites. The data for Na-K-ATPase of toad skin is interesting in this regard. Park and Hong[25] demonstrated that when $[OH^-]/[H^+]$ of the *in vitro* medium was held constant, the K_m of

Figure 14.6. *Upper panel*, effect of temperature on apparent Michaelis constant (K_m) for pyruvate of M_4-lactate dehydrogenases of various vertebrates. Assays conducted in phosphate buffer (pH 7.4) at all temperatures. *Solid lines* represent approximate temperature ranges for the species. *Error bars* represent 95% confidence intervals around K_m values. *Lower panel*, effect of temperature on K_m for pyruvate of M_4-LDHs determined under conditions of temperature-dependent pH (pH regime used is shown by *heavy line* in small graph; *upper* and *lower lines* are limits of skeletal muscle pH_i measured in animals acclimated to different temperatures). (Modified from R. B. Reeves.[21])

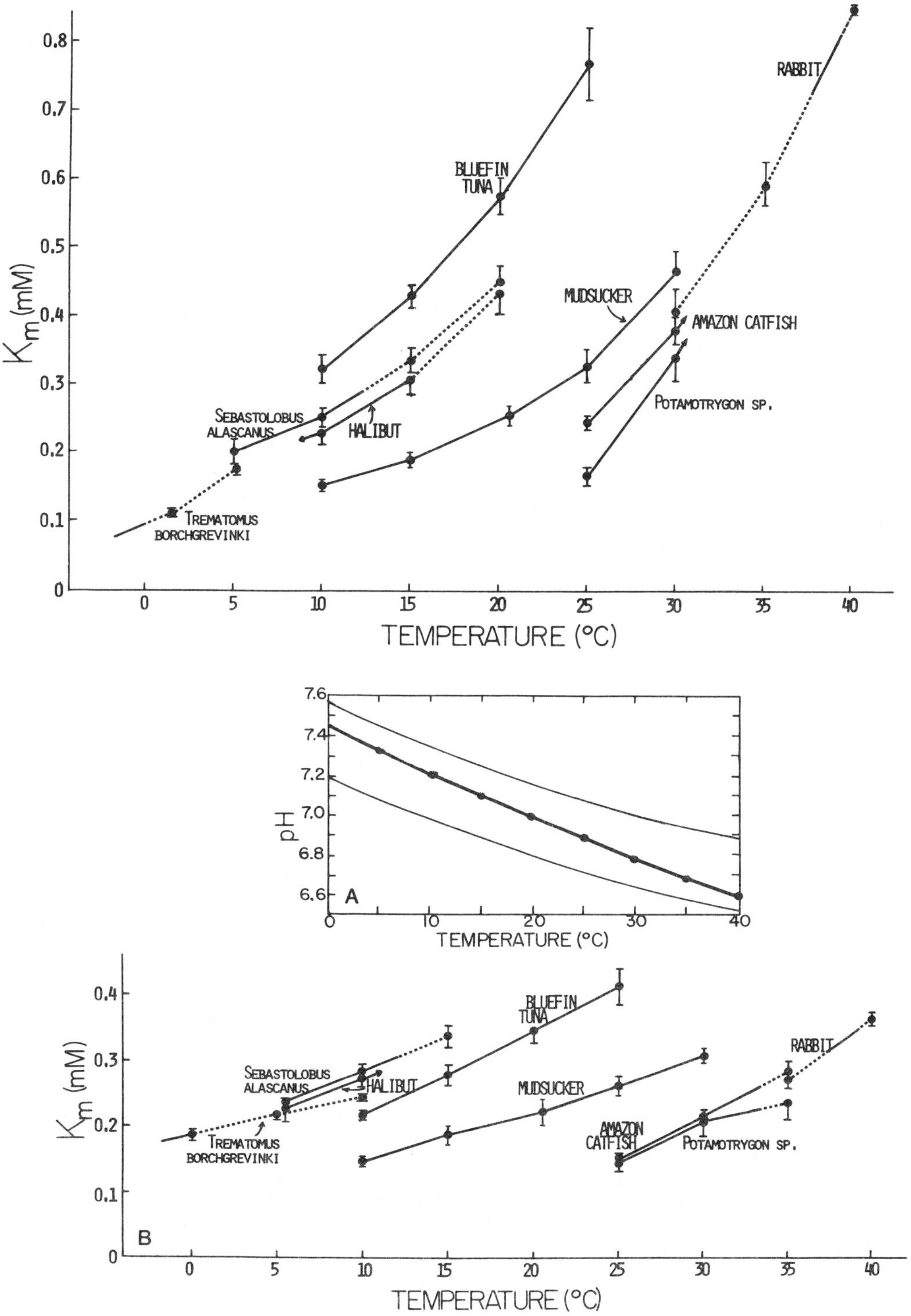

K_m(mM)
0.8
0.7
0.6
0.5
0.4
0.3
0.2
0.1
0
BLUEFIN TUNA
RABBIT
MUDSUCKER
AMAZON CATFISH
POTAMOTRYGON SP.
SEBASTOLOBUS ALASCANUS
HALIBUT
TREMATOMUS BORCHGREVINKI
0
5
10
15
20
25
30
35
40
TEMPERATURE (°C)
7.6
7.4
7.2
7.0
6.8
6.6
pH
A
0
10
20
30
40
TEMPERATURE (°C)
K_m (mM)
0.4
0.3
0.2
0.1
0
B
BLUEFIN TUNA
SEBASTOLOBUS ALASCANUS
HALIBUT
MUDSUCKER
RABBIT
TREMATOMUS BORCHGREVINKI
AMAZON CATFISH
POTAMOTRYGON SP.
0
5
10
15
20
25
30
35
40
TEMPERATURE (°C)

Figure 14.6

ATP remained constant over the range of 8–37°C. Catalytic rates are also closely related to pH, and the change in pH optimum for peak activity of the enzyme is −0.017 units/°C between 2 and 37°C. These results probably reflect the responses of the mammalian Na-K-ATPase since Park and Hong[25] found that the interactions of pH and temperature are similar, regardless of the species source of the enzyme. A number of other enzymes also exhibit higher pH optima with decreasing assay temperature: acetyl CoA carboxylase, fatty acid synthetase, NADH-cytochrome c reductase and, succinate-cytochrome c reductase.[26]

An additional effect of maintaining a constancy of $[OH^-]/[H^+]$ is the stabilization of Donnan ratios. The influence of this stratagem on Cl ratio in blood is demonstrated by the work of Reeves.[27] Figure 14.7 contrasts the well-known influence of pH on the Donnan ratio at 37°C with the findings of Reeves. Not only is Cl_c/Cl_s stabilized under the regime of ΔpH/°C equaling −0.017 but also cell volume is stabilized.[28]

The maintenance of cytosol pH near the neutral pH of water has the consequence of maintaining the imidazole charge state constant while also creating an environment in which low molecular weight water soluble biosynthetic intermediates with pKs near neutrality will remain ionized. Davis[29] has argued that the maintenance of such an "ionization window" prevents such ionized intermediates from escaping across the membrane owing to charge repulsion.

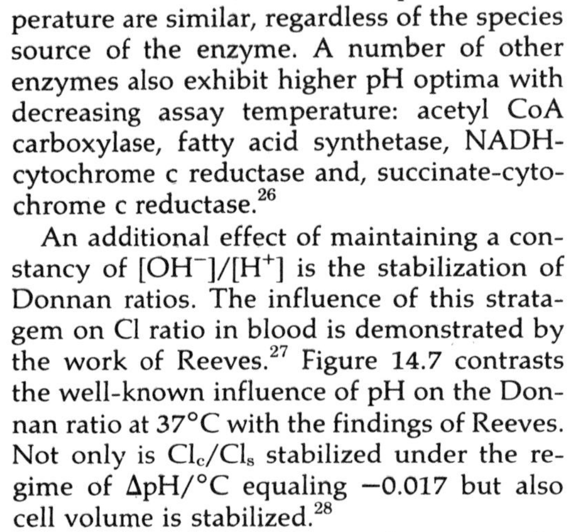

Figure 14.7. Donnan ratio for Cl^- in mammalian red blood cells when plasma pH is varried at 37°C and when pH is maintained at a constant alkalinity relative to pN_{H_2O} as temperature is changed. In the latter case, both the Cl^- ratio and red cell volume are stabilized. (Modified from R. B. Reeves[27] and D. B. Dill et al.[28])

In assessing the virtues of alpha-imidazole regulation, several fundamental types of processes have been stressed. Extracellular regulation, through respiratory adjustments in Pa_{CO_2} or active transport of $[HCO_3^-]_a$, tends to hold the total CO_2 content of the blood at a constant level and allow imidazole buffering to dominate the slope of pH against temperature to the alkaline side and parallel to the neutral pH of water. We have seen that this strategy results in stabilization of the Donnan ratio and cell volume as well. A similar pH-temperature slope to the acid-side of the extracellular fluid characterizes the intracellular fluids, and the cytosol pH appears to track the neutral pH of water rather closely. Maintenance of proton concentration in such a manner conserves the charge state of imidazole and for a number of enzymes creates the condition for conservation of K_m values near optimal levels while at the same time promoting retention of small molecular weight water-soluble intermediates with pKs near the neutral pH of water. That this acid-base regulatory pattern, dominated by the ubiquitous imidazole buffer, should occur in such diverse animals as crabs, fishes, amphibians, reptiles, and mammals speaks to the fundamental importance this regulatory strategy has played in evolution of such regulatory systems as respiration, active transport of $[HCO_3^-]$ by both gills and kidneys, and the evolution of enzyme structure and function. The convergence of the extracellular pH at around 7.4 at 37°C by ectotherms and endotherms suggests that these groups share greater similarity than differences in their acid-base poise when at a common temperature. The heterogeneity of arterial pH of such tissues as working muscle (41°C, pH = 7.3), cool skin (25°C, pH = 7.6), and liver (37°C, pH 7.4) illustrates that human tissues experience the dominant influence of imidazole buffering under conditions of constant CO_2 content of the blood—the precise acid-base environment achieved by ectothermic lung breathing vertebrates through ventilatory regulation of the CO_2 content of the blood.

An interesting exception to the general pattern of maintaining arterial pH such that ΔpH/°C equals >0.017 is the case of hibernating mammals. The hibernating ground squirrel exhibits an arterial pH of near 7.4 while at 5°C.[14] Wilson[30] has suggested that the significance of maintaining the "wrong" pH during hibernation may be in the depression of enzymatic (metabolic) activity due to the combined effects of reduced temperature (Q_{10} effect) and a cellular environment acid to the pH optima for maximum enzymic activity.

Thus, animals exhibit at least two strategies of regulation. Ectotherms exhibit the strategy of preserving temperature-insensitive enzymatic relationships while the hibernating mammals appear to have opted for an acid-base strategy in which metabolic activity is suppressed.

WHAT IS AN APPROPRIATE ACID-BASE STRATEGY FOR HYPOTHERMIA?

It is too early to offer a definitive answer to this question. We can expect, with certainty, that the functional characteristics of mammalian tissues will differ, say, at 22°C, when perfused with blood at pH 7.66 and 7.4. The choice between these two strategies is one which must depend on considerable experimental work and careful definition of the desired metabolic state of the hypothermic tissues or organs in question. There has been relatively little experimental work done to specifically evaluate the consequences of the two acid-base strategems; yet, the comparative observations cited above would appear to offer the rudiments of a rationale whereby the role of the acid-base status during and following hypothermia may be evaluated.

If the objective, during hypothermia, is to maintain enzyme functions at optimal levels, stabilize Donnan ratios, maintain a constant net charge of imidazole, and maintain cellular volume, the experimental strategy is to play the ectotherm's game, i.e., make the necessary P_{CO_2} adjustments to maintain CO_2 content constant, i.e., to achieve ΔpH/°C equal to −0.017. This approach has been suggested by Rahn *et al.*[5] In practice the procedure is quite straightforward: from the Rosenthal curve it is expected that a sample of blood taken at any low temperature will be characterized by constant CO_2 content if its pH is 7.4 when measured at 37°C. Such a sample should exhibit a pH at the cold temperature predicted from the formula ΔpH/°C = −0.014. We have seen that in an open system this requires an inverse relationship between P_{CO_2} and temperature which mimics the *in vitro* behavior of blood at constant CO_2 content. That level of P_{CO_2} which produces pH equaling 7.4 when measured in a 37°C electrode system is the appropriate P_{CO_2} to achieve constant relative alkalinity of the blood. An approximation of the appropriate P_{CO_2} for gassing the blood at a specific temperature can be calculated and is given in Fig. 14.8. It should be emphasized that correcting

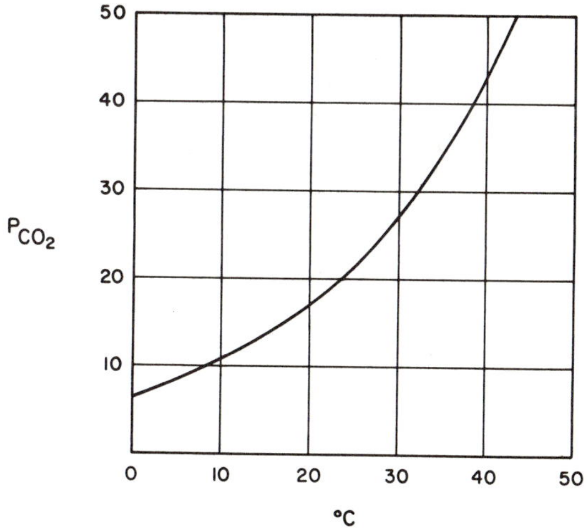

Figure 14.8. The relationship between P_{CO_2} and temperature for human blood when CO_2 content remains constant. When normal blood gas and acid-base conditions exist at 37°C, adjusting P_{CO_2} of gas mixtures with which blood is equilibrated, as indicated in the graph, will achieve ΔpH/°C ≅ −0.014. (Modified from R. B. Reeves.[27])

the P_{CO_2} (rather than $[HCO_3^-]$) has the advantage of rapid reversal when normothermia is achieved. Furthermore, Poole-Wilson and Langer[31] have reported that alterations in pH due to $[HCO_3^-]$ are largely restricted to the extracellular compartment of the mammalian myocardium while P_{CO_2} effects are expressed in both compartments.

McConnell *et al.*[32] have evaluated function of the canine heart during cardiopulmonary bypass at 28°C and made comparisons at pH 7.4 and pH 7.7. The results are seen in Table 14.2. Under the ectothermic acid-base regime, there were significant elevations in coronary blood flow, left ventricular oxygen consumption, and lactate utilization by comparison to pH 7.4. There was also a significant increase in peak ventricular pressure when a standard preload was applied. The generally expected Q_{10} of around 2 for metabolism was expressed at pH 7.7 while a Q_{10} of 4 characterized the pH 7.4 regime. Interestingly, the ratio of total blood flow to oxygen consumption (blood convection requirement, expressed as liters/mmol O_2 consumed) was similar in both instances (pH 7.4: 0.47 liters/mmol O_2; pH 7.4: 0.43 liters/mmol O_2). Thus, the capacity for autoregulation of blood flow to match extant oxygen consumption appears to have been preserved in the two instances. This appears to be true regionally since the differences between total blood flow and subendocardial blood flow are proportional. The decrease in lactate consumption by the heart at pH 7.4 (expressed as mg/(100 gm · min) · mmol O_2 consumed) is striking in this study (pH 7.4 = 0.7; pH 7.7 = 1.45). Reduction in lactate utilization has long been associated with depressed mechanical function during cardiac ischemia in man[33] and animals[34, 35] (Fig. 14.9). The reduction observed at pH 7.4 is suggestive of a serious alteration in the metabolic pathways—one which is associated with decreased mechanical performance. The contractile and ion pump functions are dependent on the electron transport system for their high energy requirements.[36]

A recent study by Becker *et al.*[50] extends the observations of McConnell *et al.*[32] Using surface cooling hypothermia, they report that maintenance of pH 7.4 (CO_2 management) was associated with marked arterial hypotension, low cardiac output, systemic lactic acidosis, and a fall in renal and cerebral blood flow (26 to 10 ml/(100 gm · min)). There was a net production of lactic acid by the heart. Management of arterial pH by lowering P_{CO_2} to achieve an "ectothermic" pH resulted in improvement in arterial pressure, a doubling of cerebral blood flow, net extraction of lactate by the heart, and normal systemic lactate metabolism. Cardiac output was 25% greater than with the pH 7.4 regime. These workers also report that, following cardioplegia in puppies at 17°C, postischemic myocardial performance was depressed 50% at pH 7.4 and was normal when pH was varied appropriately during cooling and rewarming.

Poole-Wilson and Langer[37] evaluated the performance of hypothermic isolated perfused papillary muscle and found that pHs of perfusate to the alkaline side of pH 7.4 re-

Table 14.2
Myocardial Function of the Hypothermic Canine Heart*, †

Arterial pH	Coronary Blood Flow in Left Ventricle (LV): Total (ml/(100 g·min))	Coronary Blood Flow in Left Ventricle (LV): Subendocardium (ml/(100 g·min))	Oxygen Consumption in LV: ml/(100 g·min)	Oxygen Consumption in LV: ml/(100 g·beat)	LV Lactate Consumption: mg/(100 g·min)	LV Function (25 ml Preload Peak Pressure in mm Hg)
7.39 ± 0.02	65	60	3.1	0.036	1.9	200
(n = 6)	±22	±12	±0.6	±0.01	±1.4	±17
7.72 ± 0.03‡	107	91	5.6	0.073	5.9	330
(n = 6)	±17	±19‡	±0.9‡	±0.014‡	±1.2‡	±26‡

* Modified from D. H. McConnell et al.[32]
† Temperature 28°C at pHs 7.4 and 7.7 (ΔpH = 0.017).
‡ $p < 0.01$, mean ± SEM.

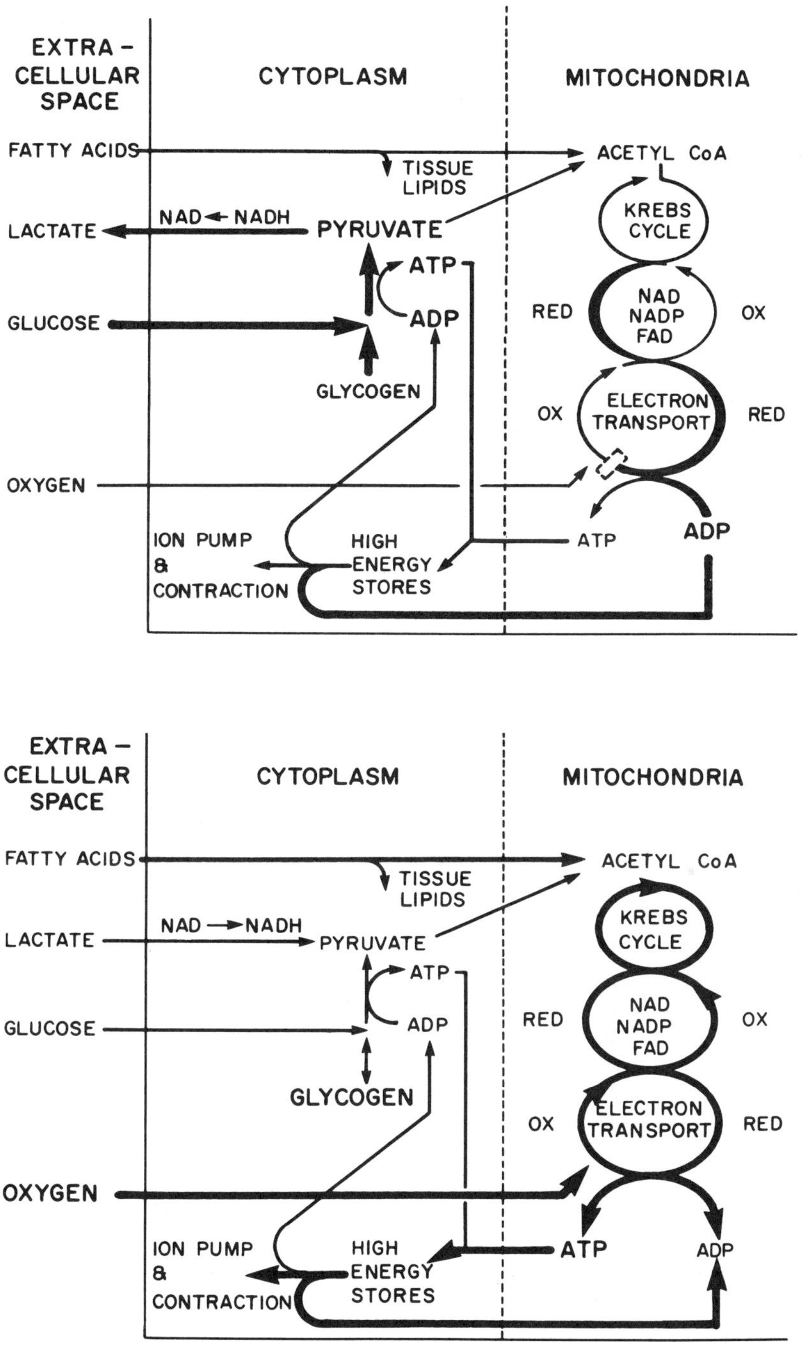

Figure 14.9. Energy pathways in well-oxygenated and hypoxic myocardium. (Modified from J. Scheuer.[36])

sulted in the preservation of greater contractility. These same workers later reported that acidosis, caused by increasing perfusate P_{CO_2}, was associated with a rapid fall in myocardial tension development as well as an inhibition of the efflux of slow exchanging $^{45}Ca^{2+}$ and uptake of $^{47}Ca^{2+}$.[31]

The central nervous susceptibility to ischemia has been evaluated by measuring the extent of no-flow lesions (NFL) following circulatory arrest or perfusion with anoxic blood at normothermia and hypothermia (20°C) in dogs.[38] It was reported that maintenance of higher pHs by reduction in P_{CO_2} and elevation of $[HCO_3^-]$ of an anoxic perfusate, while not preventing NFL, clearly ameliorated the appearance of NFL during hypothermia. An acidic perfusate was shown to enhance the extent of the lesion.

A traditional approach to perfusional preservation of organs, such as the kidney, is an attempt to provide a physiological environment at hypothermia in order to permit the longest survival with the least injury. In the design of this environment there is an attempt, in a cold setting, to mimic as closely as possible the usual circumstances of normothermia.[39] A recent study of creatinine clearances following cold preservation and retransplantation of rabbit and canine kidneys showed a positive correlation between function and preservation pHs at low temperature to the alkaline side of pH 7.4.[40] A previous study from this group demonstrated that maintenance of pH to the alkaline side of pH 7.4 during cold perfusion of the kidney resulted in lower vascular resistance and reduced lysosomal enzyme release.[41]

CONCLUSION

I have examined the general pattern by which ectotherms regulate the acid-base status as a function of temperature. The maintenance of constant $[OH^-]/[H^+]$ preserves the charge state of the dominant protein buffer, imidazole. Since animals are open systems, the regulation of either the $[HCO_3^-]$ or the P_{CO_2} is required to achieve this "goal." A number of enzymes appear to exhibit optimal function, in terms of preservation of K_m values or activity optima, under these conditions. Preservation of Donnan ratios and cell volume is another result.

Hibernating mammals exhibit a pattern of a relatively constant arterial pH and are far to the acid side of the pH-temperature slope exhibited by ectotherms. There is little known concerning the role of extracellular pH and its interactions with enzyme kinetics, structure, and function during hibernation. This is an area where much remains to be learned. Do hibernators minimize metabolic intensity by altering the activity level of key energy-consuming systems by selecting the "wrong" pH? Or, are hibernators served by key isoenzymic systems which function more optimally when pH is held constant in the face of a wide spectrum of temperatures?

Animals in nature would thus appear then to offer two possible strategies for acid-base management of hypothermic tissues—and a range of options within the extremes exhibited. A few recent studies indicate that the ectothermic strategy of preserving $[OH^-]/[H^+]$ constant during hypothermia is more efficacious in "normalizing" the function of heart and kidney than is the practice of holding pH at 7.4 at reduced temperatures. We might ask, through experimentation on appropriate animal models, whether the safe lower limits of temperature may be further extended by maintaining the CO_2 content of the blood constant, as in ectotherms. Clearly, the paucity of extant studies which specifically address the question of acid-base management during and following hypothermia place this subject in a provocative rather than in a definitive stage relevant to practice. Comparative physiology and biochemistry do, however, provide a rationale by which to approach the important question of acid-base management during altered thermal states in man.[10, 42, 43]

A pioneer in hypothermia, Henry Swan[44] has stated: "In the light of current variables in the management of induced hypothermia, the acknowledged presence of extensive thermal gradients, *and the unsettled status of the relationship of acid-base to H^+ concentration and the resultant effect on enzyme function, we can only conclude that this is an area for intensive and long investigation and constructive thinking*." (Italics added.) Comparative physiology, by searching for fundamental rules of similarity among diverse species, attempts to develop unitary concepts which, in the case of acid-base homeostasis, offers those involved in the welfare of hypothermic human tissues an additional avenue for responding to Dr. Swan's call for further investigation and constructive thinking.

References

1. Rosenthal TB: The effect of temperature on the pH of blood and plasma *in vitro*. J. Biol. Chem. 173:25, 1948.
2. Reeves RB: An imidazole alphastat hypothesis for vertebrate acid-base regulation: Tissue carbon dioxide content and body temperature in bullfrogs. Resp Physiol 14:219, 1972.
3. Rahn H: Body temperature and acid-base regulation. Pneumonologie 151:87, 1974.
4. Howell BJ, Rahn H, Goodfellow D, Herreid C: Acid-base regulation and temperature in selected invertebrates as a function of temperature. Am Zool 13: 557, 1973.
5. Rahn H, Reeves RB, Howell BJ: Hydrogen ion regulation, temperature and evolution. Am Rev Respir Dis 112:165, 1975.
6. Jackson DC: Respiratory control in air-breathing ectotherms. In *Regulation of Ventilation and Gas Exchange*, edited by DG Davies and CD Barnes. New York, Academic Press, 1978, p 93.
7. Kinney JL, Matsuura DT, White FN: Cardiorespiratory effects of temperature in the turtle, *Pseudemys floridana*. Resp Physiol 31:309, 1977.
8. Randall DJ, Cameron JN: Respiratory control of arterial pH as temperature changes in rainbow trout, *Salmo gairdneri*. Am J Physiol 225:997, 1973.
9. Truchot JP: Temperature and acid-base regulation in the shore crab, *Carcinus maenas*. Resp Physiol 17: 11, 1973.
10. Rahn H, Reeves RB: *Protons, Proteins and Claude Bernard's "Fixité du Milieu Intérieur."* (Colloque Claude Bernard, Fondation Singer-Polignac), edited by ED Robin. Paris, Masson et Cie, 1980, p. 263.
11. Severinghaus JW, Stupfel M, Bradley AF: Variation of serum carbonic acid pK′ with pH and temperature. J Appl Physiol 9:197, 1956a.
12. Severinghaus JW, Stupfel M, Bradley AF: Accuracy of blood pH and P_{CO_2} determinations. J Appl Physiol 9: 189, 1956b.
13. Cameron JN: Branchial ion uptake in arctic grayling: Resting values and effects of acid-base disturbance. J Exp Biol 64:711, 1976.
14. Lyman CP, Hastings AB: Total CO_2, plasma pH and pCO_2 of hamsters and ground squirrels during hibernation. Am J Physiol 167:633, 1951.
15. Kreienbühl G, Strittmatter J, Ayim E: Blood gas analyses of hibernating hamsters and dormice. Pflügers Arch 366:167, 1976.
16. Poole-Wilson PA: Measurement of myocardial intracellular pH in pathological states (editorial). J Mol Cell Cardiol 10:511, 1978.
17. Poole-Wilson PA: The kinetics of efflux of 5,5-dimethyl-2,4-oxazolidinedione (DMO) from the myocardium. Clin Sci Mol Med 51:197, 1976.
18. Malan A, Wilson TL, Reeves RB: Intracellular pH in cold-blooded vertebrates as a function of body temperature. Resp Physiol 28:29, 1976.
19. Reeves RB: Temperature-induced changes in blood acid-base status: pH and P_{CO_2} in a binary buffer. J Appl Physiol 40:752, 1976.
20. Everse J, Kaplan NO: Lactate dehydrogenase: Structure and function. Adv Enzymol 37:61, 1973.
21. Yancey PH, Somero GN: Temperature dependence of intracellular pH: Its role in the conservation of pyruvate apparent K_m values of vertebrate lactate dehydrogenase. J Comp Physiol 125:129, 1978.
22. Fersht A: *Enzyme structure and mechanism.* San Francisco, Freeman, 1977, p. 371.
23. Somero GN: Temperature adaptation of enzymes: Biological optimization through structure-function compromises. Ann Rev Ecol Syst 9:1, 1978.
24. Atkinson DE: *Cellular Energy Metabolism and its regulation.* New York, Academic Press, 1977, p. 283.
25. Park YS, Hong SK: Properties of toad skin Na-K-ATPase with special reference to effect of temperature. Am J Physiol 231:1356, 1976.
26. Hazel JR, Garlick WS, Sellner PA: The effects of assay temperature upon the pH optima of enzymes from poikilotherms: A test of the the imidazole alphastat hypothesis. J Comp Physiol 123:97, 1978.
27. Reeves RB: Temperature-induced changes in blood acid-base status: Donnan r_{cl} and red cell volume. J Appl Physiol 40:762, 1976.
28. Dill DB, Edwards HT, Florkin M, Campbell RW: Properties of dog blood. J Biol Chem 95:143, 1932.
29. Davis BD: On the importance of being ionized. Arch Biochem Biophys 78:497, 1958.
30. Wilson T: Theoretical analysis of the effects of two pH regulation patterns on the temperature sensitivities of biological systems in nonhomeothermic animals. Arch Biochem Biophys 182:409, 1977.
31. Poole-Wilson PA, Langer GA: Effects of acidosis on mechanical function and Ca^{2+} exchange in rabbit myocardium. Am J Physiol 236:H525, 1979.
32. McConnell DH, White F, Nelson RL, Goldstein SM, Maloney JV Jr, DeLand EC, Buckberg GD: Importance of alkalosis in maintenance of "ideal" blood pH during hypothermia. Surg Forum 26:263, 1975.
33. Cohen LS, Elliott WC, Klein MD, Gorlin R: Coronary heart disease: Clinical, cinearteriographic and metabolic correlations. Am J Cardiol 17:153, 1966.
34. Case RB, Nasser MG, Crampton RS: Biochemical aspects of early myocardial ischemia. Am J Cardiol 24:766, 1969.
35. Nasser MG, Case RB: Early changes in lactate metabolism in myocardial ischemia. Fed Proc 27:632, 1968.
36. Scheuer J: Myocardial metabolism in cardiac hypoxia. Am J Cardiol 19:385, 1967.
37. Poole-Wilson PA, Langer GA: Effect of pH on ionic exchange and function in rat and rabbit myocardium. Am J Physiol 229:570, 1975.
38. Norwood WI, Norwood CR, Castaneda AR: Cerebral anoxia: Effect of deep hypothermia and pH. Surgery 86:203, 1979.
39. Halasz NA, Collins GM, White FN: *The Right pH for Preservation? Organ Preservation*, Ed. 2, edited by D. E. Pegg and IA Jacobsen. Churchill-Livingstone, 1979, p. 259.
40. Carter JN, White FN, Collins GM, Halasz NA: Studies of the ideal $[H^+]$ for perfusional preservation. Transplantation 30:409, 1980.
41. Romolo, JL, Ariyan S, Halasz NA: Evaluation of perfusion techniques in renal preservation. Cry-

obiology 8:407, 1971.
42. Reeves, RB: The interaction of body temperature and acid-base balance in ectothermic vertebrates. Annu Rev Physiol 39:559, 1977.
43. White FN: Comparative aspects of vertebrate cardiorespiratory physiology. Annu Rev Physiol 40:471, 1978.
44. Swan H: *Thermoregulation and Bioenergetics—Patterns for Vertebrate Survival.* New York, American Elsevier, 1974.
45. Ackerman RA, White FN: The effects of temperature on acid-base balance and ventilation of the marine iguana. Resp Physiol 39:133, 1980.
46. White FN: Temperature and the Galapagos marine iguana. Insights into reptilian thermoregulation. Comp Biochem Physiol 45A:503, 1973.
47. Crawford EC Jr, Gatz RN: Carbon dioxide tension and pH of the blood of the lizard *Sauromalus obesus* at different temperatures. Comp Biochem Physiol 47A:529, 1974.
48. Bickler P: Personal communication.
49. Davies DG, Kopetzky MT: Effect of body temperature on the ventilatory response to hypercapnia in the awake alligator. Fed Proc 35:840, 1976.
50. Becker H, Lazar H, Manganaro AM, Buckberg GD: Myocardial damage caused by keeping pH 7.4 during systemic deep hypothermia, personal communication from G. D. Buckberg.

CHAPTER 15

CARDIOPULMONARY BYPASS AND DEEP HYPOTHERMIA WITH CIRCULATORY ARREST IN INFANTS

John J. Lamberti, M.D.
Mary Hartley-Winkler, R.N., C.C.P.
J. Deane Waldman, M.D.
Jordan Waldman, M.D.

Corrective heart surgery began in 1939, when Dr. Robert Gross of Boston performed the first successful ligation of a patent ductus arteriosus.[1] Corrective surgery of coarctation of the aorta followed soon thereafter.[2] At about the same time, palliative systemic-to-pulmonary artery shunt operations for children born with cyanotic congenital heart disease were introduced.[3] In 1952, pulmonary artery banding allowed palliation of children with intractable congestive heart failure caused by increased pulmonary blood flow.[4] The modern era of open heart surgery began when Gibbon[5] repaired an atrial septal defect using a pump oxygenator. From 1955 to 1965, many innovations were made in pump oxygenator technology and surgical instrumentation. During that decade, great advances were made in the general understanding of congenital heart disease, including the anatomic location of the cardiac conducting system. By the year 1965, many congenital heart defects could be safely repaired in larger infants and children, but mortality and morbidity were high for open heart surgery during the 1st year of life. For lesions which were amenable to palliative surgery, delay of operation until age 2 years or older was reasonable (Table 15.1). In many cases, the two-stage approach is still applicable today. Unfortunately, there exists a group of congenital heart defects for which no palliative operation operation is available (Table 15.2).

The technique of deep hypothermia and circulatory arrest was developed in response to the need for a safe method for correction of complex intracardiac congenital heart defects in infants. The first successful open intracardiac operation had been performed using the technique of surface-induced hypothermia when F. John Lewis of the University of Minnesota repaired an atrial septal defect during a brief period of circulatory arrest.[6] With the development of safe cardiopulmonary bypass, the technique of hypothermia and circulatory arrest was generally ignored except by a few centers. In 1963, Horiuchi et al.[7] of Japan and in 1966, Mohri et al.[8] of the United States reported success using the technique of deep hypothermia and circulatory arrest for the correction of congenital heart defects during infancy. Initial experience with the technique utilized ether anesthesia and avoided the use of a pump

Table 15.1
Congenital Heart Defects Suitable for Early Primary Repair or Initial Palliation with Later Correction

Tetralogy of Fallot
Ventricular septal defect
Truncus arteriosus
Transposition of the great arteries +/− VSD
Pulmonary atresia +/− VSD
Complete atrioventricular canal

Table 15.2
Congenital Heart Defects which Require Correction only at any Age (Defects Requiring Open Heart Surgery)

Aortic stenosis
Pulmonary stenosis with intact ventricular septum
Total anomalous pulmonary venous connection
Cor triatriatum
Anomalous origin of left coronary artery
Atrial septal defect

oxygenator. In 1971, Barratt-Boyes et al.[9] described the combination of surface cooling and core cooling with a pump oxygenator followed by core rewarming for the correction of congenital heart defects. His report heralded the era of early total repair of many congenital heart defects.

The purpose of surface cooling was to gradually reduce core temperature while avoiding peripheral acidosis. In recent years, there has been a trend away from prolonged surface cooling. Kunkel et al.[10] at the Deutsches Herzzentrum in Munich, Germany, compared a group of infants undergoing corrective cardiac surgery utilizing core cooling only with a group of infants utilizing surface cooling followed by core cooling. They measured acid base status, oxygen consumption, serum lactate concentrations, and serum electrolytes, as well as various serum enzymes. The serum creatinine phosphokinase, alpha-hydroxybuteric dehydrogenase, lactic dehydrogenase, glutamic oxaloacetic transaminase, and serum glutamic pyruvate transaminase were all monitored. No significant difference between the two methods of cooling to 20°C could be detected. As might be expected, total cooling time was shorter in patients undergoing core cooling only. Total cardiopulmonary bypass time was greater in patients who underwent core cooling only. The rewarming time was equal in both groups. Serum glucose concentrations were lower in patients who were core-cooled, but the differences did not seem to have any clinical significance. The surgical approach at most centers today utilizes minimal surface cooling in conjunction with central or core cooling.

INDICATIONS

The technique of deep hypothermic circulatory arrest is particularly useful in the critically ill infant who requires open heart surgery in the first few months of life.[9] In addition, deep hypothermia and circulatory arrest allows primary correction of certain defects during early infancy, thereby avoiding the increased morbidity and mortality of a two-stage repair.[11] Ischemic cardiac arrest protected by cardioplegia and topical cooling provides a flaccid heart but does not eliminate pulmonary venous return unless low pump flow is utilized. When the technique of deep hypothermia and circulatory arrest is combined with cardioplegic arrest of the heart, the operative field is completely bloodless, and there are no cannulae to interfere with the intracardiac procedure. In general, we utilize the technique of hypothermia and circulatory arrest for the repair of all complex intraatrial defects in infants weighing less than 7 kg. The Senning or Mustard procedure is performed using this technique, and any form of total anomalous pulmonary venous connection can be corrected during a relatively short circulatory arrest interval.

Additional indications for circulatory arrest involve almost any intracardiac defect requiring operation in an infant weighing less than 4 kg. Cannulation of the inferior and superior vena cava may be technically difficult in small infants with tetralogy of Fallot or ventricular septal defects. Although these operations may not require intraatrial surgery, the heart may be small and the technical aspects of operating during continuous cardiopulmonary bypass may be formidable. In general, it would not seem necessary to use circulatory arrest for the repair of tetralogy of Fallot in a child greater than 4 kg. The right atrium is usually quite large in children born with complete common atrioventricular canal, and operation can be performed during continuous conventional low-flow, hypothermic cardiopulmonary bypass, if the right atrial cannulae are placed posteriorly along the crista terminalis. We have also performed transatrial repair of a large perimembranous ventricular septal defect in a 4-kg infant using low-flow cardiopulmonary bypass. Hypothermia and circulatory arrest may not be necessary for aortic or pulmonary valvotomy, since these operations can be performed using the technique of inflow occlusion at normothermia or moderate hypothermia.

TECHNICAL ASPECTS OF THE TECHNIQUE (Fig. 15.1)

During induction of anesthesia, we routinely monitor the electrocardiogram, radial arterial pressure, central venous pressure, and urine output, as well as nasopharyngeal, esophageal, and rectal temperatures. The electroencephalogram can also be continuously monitored throughout the procedure. The end-tidal pCO_2 is continuously monitored. In addition to the electronic monitoring devices, an esophageal stethoscope is always inserted. Anesthetic premedication depends upon the age and cardiovascular stability of the infant. In older, stable infants, Innovar (0.04 ml/kg) and atropine (0.01 mg/kg) are administered 45 minutes prior to induction. Anesthesia is induced by a combination of parenteral ketamine or halothane by mask. Prior to operation, and during cardiopulmonary bypass, Pavulon is utilized as a muscle relaxant, and morphine sulfate is administered for analgesia. During the induction of anesthesia and insertion of monitoring lines, the baby is left uncovered and the rectal temperature will be noted to drift downward. When the child is positioned for prepping, the head is packed in ice bags and the hypothermia mattress is adjusted for surface cooling. As the rectal temperature decreases, the respiratory minute volume is decreased to maintain end-tidal pCO_2 between 30 and 40. Morphine sulfate is administered in small doses until the total dose is approximately 0.5 mg/kg.

The extracorporeal circuit consists of a bubble oxygenator with an efficient heat ex-

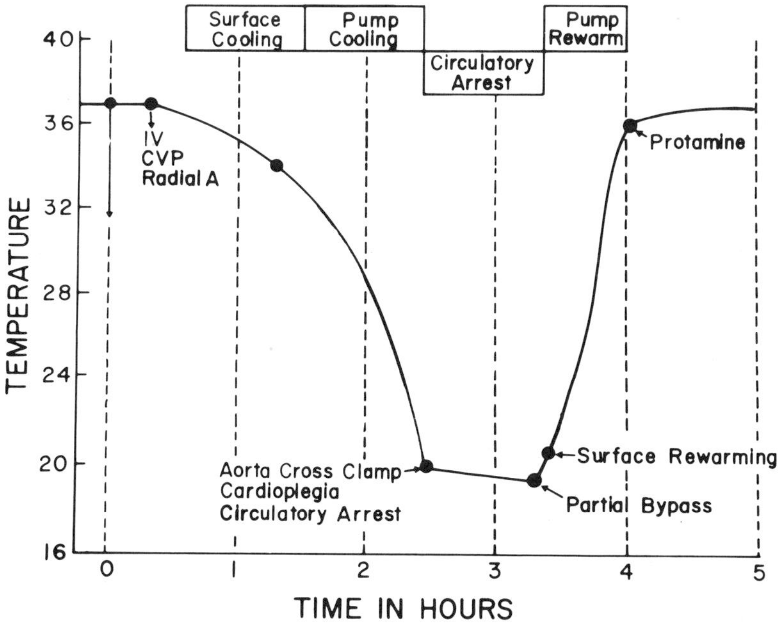

Figure 15.1. Graphic depiction of time course of events during the technique of deep hypothermia and circulatory arrest. For complete explanation see text.

changer, a cardiotomy reservoir with an integral filter, ¼ inch tubing, and an arterial filter. We do not believe that the membrane oxygenator offers any advantage for these operations, since the total cardiopulmonary bypass time is generally less than 2 hours. The circuit is primed with packed red cells and a balanced electrolyte solution to create a hematocrit of 23–25% during bypass. This degree of hemodilution should improve peripheral perfusion while maintaining adequate oxygen delivery. Heparin, methyl prednisolone (30 mg/kg), and 12.5 gm of albumin are routinely utilized. Bicarbonate is added to adjust the pH to normal. During core cooling, Lasix (up to 1 mg/kg) is administered if urine flow is less than 1 ml/kg/30 minutes. No mannitol is given during cooling.

A standard median sternotomy is utilized. We avoid entering the pleural space if possible. A portion of the thymus gland may need to be resected for exposure. The aorta is encircled with a tape, and purse string sutures are placed in the right atrial appendage and the ascending aorta. A single venous cannula is inserted in the right atrial appendage, and the aorta is cannulated with a small metal tip Sarn's cannula. The inferior and superior vena cava are not usually encircled with tapes. Cardiopulmonary bypass is instituted, and perfusate temperature is gradually lowered, maintaining a 10°C temperature gradient between the water bath and the blood. A 10°C gradient between the blood, nasopharyngeal, and rectal temperatures is not exceeded. We prefer slight metabolic alkalosis during cooling. Flow rates are adjusted to obtain 120 ml/kg/minute in a newborn, or 2.4 liters/m^2/minute in older infants. Steroids are added to the pump prime prior to the circulatory arrest interval for their potential usefulness in the protection of lysosomal integrity and in the prevention of cellular edema.[12] The rectal temperature desired for the circulatory arrest interval is usually 20°C. Total anomalous pulmonary venous connection may require between 25 and 40 minutes of circulatory arrest. A ventricular septal defect may require 30 to 40 minutes of circulatory arrest. The Senning procedure requires between 45 and 55 minutes, and more complex defects will require more time. If we anticipate more than 60 minutes of circulatory arrest, rectal temperature is lowered to 18°C. In addition, a venous cannulation technique can be utilized which will allow reinstitution of cardiopulmonary bypass prior to completion of the intracardiac operation (i.e., innominate vein or main pulmonary artery cannula).

When the desired rectal temperature is achieved, the aorta is cross-clamped, and 10 ml/kg of 4° C glucose-insulin-potassium cardioplegic solution[13] is infused into the proximal ascending aorta. Myocardial septal temperature is continuously monitored with a thermocouple. The cardioplegic solution is collected by the venous cannula and returned to the pump. With cessation of cardiac activity, the pump is turned off, and the aortic perfusion line is clamped. The venous line is left open to allow complete drainage of the patient. When venous return is decreased to a minimum, the venous cannula is clamped and removed. Operation may now be performed in a bloodless, flaccid heart.

When the surgical procedure is completed, the venous cannula is reinserted in the right atrium, and the pump is slowly restarted. As venous return commences, pump flow can be increased. A pulmonary artery catheter may be used for supplemental venous return after operation for transposition of the great vessels when the right atrial appendage cannula is now in the physiologic left atrium. An alternative to a pulmonary artery catheter is a second venous catheter placed in the innominate vein or superior vena cava. Rewarming is carried out at approximately 2.4 liters/m^2/minute. A maximal 10°C gradient is maintained among rectal temperature, blood temperature, and heat exchanger. During rewarming, blood pH is maintained as close to 7.4 as possibly by adjusting gas flow rates, blood flow rates, and adding sodium bicarbonate when necessary. If urine flow is less than 1 ml/kg/30 minutes, Lasix, 1 mg/kg, is administered and mannitol (1 mg/kg) can be given. We do not administer mannitol prior to circulatory arrest in order to avoid the potential for crystal formation. At the completion of rewarming, the patient is gradually weaned from cardiopulmonary bypass. Calcium chloride (100 mg/kg) is administered prior to termination of bypass for its inotropic effects and to increase the blood calcium level. Calcium is not added to the circuit during priming. A left atrial line is often inserted for monitoring filling pressure of the systemic ventricle. After cessation of bypass, superior vena cava and pulmonary artery saturation are measured, and pressure in the various cardiac chambers is recorded to ensure satisfactory postrepair hemodynamics. Decannulation is performed, and heparin is reversed slowly with protamine. Protamine dosage is predicted on the basis of ACT testing during bypass. Platelets are generally necessary and are routinely administered. The platelet count during cardiopulmonary bypass for deep hypothermia and circulatory arrest ranged from 38,000 to 110,000 (average, 52,000). The cell-saver device is utilized to harvest all red cells in the pump. During opening of the chest, 50 ml of pump prime is withdrawn from the oxygenator and given to the anesthesiologist for use should volume replacement be necessary. At the completion of operation, a similar syringe of buffered pump prime is used for volume replacement until heparin is reversed with protamine and the oxygenator prime has been washed and prepared as packed cells. When there is no postoperative bleeding, the total volume of blood replacement required is quite small, and we find it generally unnecessary to utilize more than the washed packed red cells harvested from the oxygenator. Platelets are administered to maintain the platelet count greater than 100,000 during the first 6 to 12 hours after operation. Dopamine (1–2 mg/kg/minute) is routinely administered unless marked tachycardia is present. This drug is utilized for its potential benefit in terms of renal blood flow and for a mild inotropic effect.

PATHOPHYSIOLOGIC ALTERATIONS

Hypothermia causes a significant reduction in oxygen consumption which is directly related to the magnitude of the decrease in temperature. In addition, the oxyhemoglobin dissociation curve shifts to the left with cooling.[14] As blood is cooled, there is a slight increase in the solubility of oxygen in the plasma.[15] The various effects counterbalance, and a delicate homeostasis is maintained despite the reduction in systemic oxygen delivery. Acid base status is generally maintained if cooling proceeds in a gradual fashion. There has been some controversy regarding the optimal arterial pCO_2 during cooling.[14] We prefer to maintain the pCO_2 at 35–40 mm Hg and the arterial pH in the high normal range. It is important to remember that the volume of CO_2 generated is decreased with cooling and the ventilator must be adjusted to compensate for this to avoid marked hypocarbia.

Other metabolic abnormalities reported include elevation of serum glucose associated with hypothermia.[14] The increase in serum glucose is accompanied by a decrease in plasma insulin levels.[16] Thus, there is probably decreased systemic utilization of glucose plus inhibition of release of insulin secondary to hypothermia. No significant alterations in serum electrolytes have been attributed to hypothermia itself.[10, 14] Increases in circulating catecholamines have been recorded in response to hypothermia.[17] Free fatty acids are increased, probably due to central nervous system activation of the sympathetic nervous system.[18] The increase in glucose and free fatty acids might provide additional substrate for the heart and brain during the arrest interval.

In 1978, Lamberti et al.[19] reported reversible derangement of renal function in patients undergoing hypothermia and circulatory arrest. Sequential changes in BUN and creatinine levels were analyzed in a relatively homogeneous group of patients undergoing repair of ventricular septal defect. The elevation of BUN was noted, despite the presence of adequate cardiac output by clinical assessment and a stable postoperative course. Experimental data suggest that renal blood flow is substantially reduced during surface or core cooling.[20] The decrease in cardiac output and increase in systemic vascular resistance detected during cooling[19] may be chiefly responsible for the renal dysfunction. We believe that the kidney is more vulnerable to insult in the early postoperative interval in these patients. Refinement of our technique, including continuous core cooling rather than surface cooling, seems to have improved the postoperative renal function. In the last 3 years, we have not seen unexpected elevation in the blood urea nitrogen in any patient undergoing an uncomplicated recovery from surgery. We believe that adequate urine flow must be maintained during cooling and rewarming, as well as in the early postoperative interval. Low dose dopamine therapy is recommended, and prompt use of small doses of Lasix are appropriate. Cessation of urine flow may result in rapid rise of the serum potassium which can be difficult to treat.

In 1978, Lamberti et al.[19] reported the results of a clinical study comparing cardiac function at 21°C (before repair) with cardiac function at 37°C (after repair). In a group of 10 patients undergoing repair of ventricular septal defect, surface cooling only was utilized. This approach allowed measurement of cardiac output at 21°C prior to circulatory arrest. An electromagnetic flow probe was placed around the ascending aorta, and a catheter with a microtransducer on its tip was placed in the left ventricle for pressure measurements. Heart rate, left ventricular systolic pressure, left ventricular systolic ejection time, stroke work index, dp/dt max, and cardiac index were measured. Oxygen consumption was calculated after measuring arterial and venous oxygen content and cardiac output. The systemic vascular resistance was also calculated. Heart rate was significantly reduced at 21°C, as was left ventricular systolic pressure, systolic ejection time, and the stroke work index. Dp/dt max was also reduced significantly. The cardiac index was 0.45 liters/minute/m^2 at 21°C and 2 liters/minute/m^2 at 37°C. The reduction in cardiac index was accompanied by a significant reduction in oxygen consumption from 95.5 ml/minute/m^2 at 37°C to 14.6 ml/minute/m^2 at 21°C. Systemic vascular resistance was significantly increased. The data indicated reversible depression of myocardial function. The calculated oxygen consumption of the infant was substantially reduced; however, acidosis did not occur. The low output state noted during hypothermia appears adequate to meet the reduced metabolic needs of the infant. Other investigators have reported similar changes in heart rate and left ventricular function in response to hypothermia.[14]

Neurologic abnormalities have not been detected in most survivors.[11,19,21] Children who have recovered from successful operation with an uncomplicated postoperative course have generally not experienced seizures or any apparent neurologic deficit. No specific abnormality of cerebral function has been detected in children subjected to 1 hour of circulatory arrest at a rectal temperature of 20°C or lower. Long-term follow-up studies of children undergoing correction under circulatory arrest have shown no definite residual neurologic abnormalities attributable to the technique. Of course, isolated examples of cerebral damage have been detected, but usually in patients who have had a stormy postoperative course and/or sustained cardiac arrest at one time or another. It is difficult in such individual cases to identify the exact causal factors of neurologic injury.

The only consistent hematologic abnormality detected after operation is thrombocytopenia. It is known that the platelet count decreases immediately after institution of cardiopulmonary bypass.[22] This decrease is aggravated by hypothermia. Platelet transfusions are administered to all infants at the completion of operation and repeated later should there be continued bleeding or marked reduction in platelet count (below 60,000). The etiology of the platelet decrease in response to cardiopulmonary bypass is thought to be caused by adherence of platelets to the components of the extracorporeal circuit. This platelet reduction is not avoided by the use of a membrane oxygenator.[23] Coating the extracorporeal circuit with albumin may decrease platelet adhesion to the circuit components.

CLINICAL EXPERIENCE

During the past 30 months deep hypothermia and circulatory arrest were utilized in 12 infants. Five infants less than 1 year of age underwent repair using the technique of inflow occlusion at normothermia. The remaining 22 patients less than 1 year of age were operated upon using the technique of continuous cardiopulmonary bypass and moderative hypothermia. The overall mortality for open heart surgery in the 1st year of life was 10%. There were no deaths in the inflow occlusion group (three pulmonary valvotomies, one aortic valvotomy, and one atrial septectomy). There were two deaths in the cardiopulmonary bypass group (9%); both patients underwent complete repair of tetralogy of Fallot with absent pulmonary valve syndrome. The patients undergoing deep hypothermia and circulatory arrest are described in detail below (Table 15.3).

There were three types of congenital heart defects represented in the group of patients requiring deep hypothermia and circulatory arrest. Two infants underwent repair of large ventricular septal defect. They were 6 and 7 weeks old and weighed 3.5 and 3.4 kg, respectively. Both patients have done well.

Six infants required operation during the 1st year of life. In our experience, 23% (6 of 26) of patients presenting with ventricular septal defect (VSD) will require operation during the 1st year of life, and approximately one-third of these infants will require the use of hypothermia and circulatory arrest. We have been able to perform transatrial patch closure of a large ventricular septal defect in an infant as small as 4 kg using conventional cardiopulmonary bypass with moderate hypothermia if the caval cannulae are inserted posteriorly along with crista terminalis. There were no operative deaths or episodes of heart block in these patients. During the same period, three patients underwent repair of total anomalous pulmonary venous connection. Two infants, ages 5 weeks and 12 weeks, required deep hypothermia and circulatory arrest for repair. The postoperative course was unremarkable, and both patients are well at the present time.

Eight infants have undergone repair of d-transposition of the great arteries using the technique of deep hypothermia and circulatory arrest. This represents 50% of our total experience with d-transposition of the great arteries. There were two operative deaths in this group. One was a patient presenting with severe hyperdynamic muscular subvalvular pulmonary stenosis, and one was a patient with severe asthma and dextrocardia. The infant presenting with severe subpulmonary stenosis died in a low output state 36 hours after Mustard procedure. This patient was moribund due to severe, prolonged hypoxia and acidosis prior to emergency operation. The asthmatic infant died 16 days after the Mustard procedure in respiratory failure. The other six patients underwent the Senning procedure. Three patients had transatrial patch closure of large ventricular septal defect in addition to the Senning procedure. All six infants undergoing the Senning procedure survived operation. The only neurologic complication in our entire series occurred in a 5-month-old female infant who underwent the Senning repair for d-transposition of the

Table 15.3
Open Heart Surgery during the First Year of Life at the Children's Hospital of San Diego*

Operation	Total		CPB		IO		DH/CA	
	N.	Mort	No.	Mort	No.	Mort	No.	Mort
Aortic valvotomy	1	0			1	0		
Pulmonary valvotomy	6	0	3	0	3	0		
Atrial septectomy	1	0			1	0		
Patch closure VSD	6	0	4	0			2	0
Repair CAVC	3	0	3	0				
Mustard or Senning	11	2	3	0			8	2
Repair TAPVC	2	0					2	0
Repair TOF	5	0	5	0				
Repair TOF + absent pul. valve	2	2	2	2				
ASD secundum	2	0	2	0				
Total	39	4	22	2	5	0	12	2

* Abbreviations used are: CPB, cardiopulmonary bypass; IO, inflow occlusion; DH/CA, deep hypothermia and circulatory arrest; Mort, mortality; CAVC, complete common atrioventricular canal; TAPVC, total anomalous pulmonary venous connection; TOF, tetralogy of Fallot; ASD, atrial septal defect.

great arteries with intact ventricular septum. The operation was uncomplicated, and the circulatory arrest interval was 57 minutes at 19°C rectal. Approximately 20 hours after repair, she developed supraventricular tachycardia at a rate of 210 beats per minute. The tachycardia caused a secondary low cardiac output state and acute renal failure. The postoperative course was prolonged due to respiratory and renal failure. Three weeks after repair, she was extubated and noted to have a focal seizure disorder. This was associated with marked problems with deglutition. The etiology of the neurologic defect was not clear since there was no seizure disorder noted in the immediate postoperative interval. In our series, the circulatory arrest interval ranged from 35 to 37 minutes for repair of ventricular septal defect and from 33 to 44 minutes (mean, 38.5 minutes) for repair of total anomalous pulmonary venous connection. The circulatory arrest interval for Mustard or Senning procedure ranged from 48 to 57 minutes (mean 52 minutes). The arrest interval for Senning plus ventricular septal defect repair was 70 to 81 minutes (mean, 75.5 minutes). Circulatory arrest intervals greater than 60 minutes were carried out at rectal temperatures of 18°C. It is of interest to note that the only infant who developed a neurologic abnormality had a circulatory arrest interval within generally accepted limits[10] at a rectal temperature of 19°C. This patient did not suffer a cardiac arrest but did have a prolonged period of low cardiac output due to supraventricular tachycardia and associated cardiac failure. No evidence of hemodynamic abnormality has been detected at follow-up in this infant, and she has shown some neurologic improvement within 5 months of operation. In view of our general experience and the reported experience of others,[9-11,19] it is difficult to implicate deep hypothermia with circulatory arrest as the only causal factor in this patient. Since we have had no neurologic abnormality in any other patient in our entire series it is also difficult to exclude hypothermia with circulatory arrest as a potential causal factor. It is possible that hypothermia and circulatory arrest predispose the infant to cerebral injury should significant complications occur during the early postoperative interval.

SUMMARY

The technique of deep hypothermia with circulatory arrest provides a safe and effective means for treating infants and small children born with congenital heart defects which are not amenable to palliation. The success and safety of this technique has led to an increasing emphasis upon early primary repair of congenital heart defects. For example, we have not performed pulmonary artery banding in any symptomatic infant with a ventricular septal defect. We continue to advocate two-stage repair in circumstances where early primary repair has not been proven to be superior to the two-stage approach. In our experience, approximately one-quarter of all children requiring corrective open heart surgery will come to operation during the 1st year of life. In this subset of patients, approximately 30% will require the technique of deep hypothermia and circulatory arrest. The advantages of early primary repair are obvious, and we agree with most authors in this regard. We have found that many infants with tetralogy of Fallot or ventricular septal defect can be repaired using conventional cardiopulmonary bypass. However, for infants less than 4 kg or for infants requiring complex intraatrial surgery, deep hypothermia and circulatory arrest is the procedure of choice. There is a small risk of neurologic abnormality in patients who develop significant complications before or after operation. Since the technique is utilized only for high risk procedures, the morbidity and mortality rates are acceptable.

References

1. Gross RE, Hubbard JP: Surgical ligation of a patent ductus arteriosus: Report of first successful case. JAMA 112:729, 1939.
2. Gross RE, Hufnagel CA: Coarctation of the aorta. Experimental studies regarding its surgical correction. N Engl J Med 233:287, 1945.
3. Blalock A, Taussig H: Surgical treatment of malformation of the heart in which there is pulmonary stenosis or pulmonary atresia. JAMA 128:189, 1945.
4. Muller WH Jr, Dammann JF Jr.: The treatment of certain congenital malformations of the heart by the creation of pulmonic stenosis to reduce pulmonary hypertension and excessive pulmonary blood flow: A preliminary report. Surg Gynecol Obstet 95:213, 1952.
5. Gibbon JH Jr: Application of a mechanical heart and

lung apparatus to cardiac surgery. Minn Med 37: 171, 1954.
6. Lewis FJ, Taufic M: Closure of atrial septal defects with the aid of hypothermia. Experimental accomplishments and the report of one successful case. Surgery 33:52, 1953.
7. Horiuchi T, Koyamada K, Matano I, Mohri H, Komatsu T, Honda T, Abe T, Ishitoya T, Sagawa Y, Matsuzawa K, Matsumura M, Tsuda T, Ishizawa E, Ishikawa S, Susuki H, Saito Y: Radical operation for the ventricular septal defect in infancy. J Thorac Cardiovasc Surg 46:180, 1963.
8. Mohri H, Hessel EA, Nelson RJ, Matano I, Anderson HN, Dillard DH, Merendino KA: The use of Rheomacrodex and controlled hypoventilation in prolonged circulatory arrest under deep hypothermia induced by surface cooling: A method for open heart surgery in infants. Am J Surg 112:241, 1966.
9. Barratt-Boyes BG, Neutze JM, Seelye ER, Simpson M: Complete correction of cardiovascular malformations in the first year of life. Prog Cardiovasc Dis 15:229, 1972.
10. Kunkel R, Hagl S, Richter JA, Habermeyer P, Sebening F: The effects of deep hypothermia and circulatory arrest on systemic metabolic state of infants undergoing corrective open heart surgery: A comparison of two methods. Thorac Cardiovasc Surg 27:168, 1979.
11. Castaneda AR, Lamberti J, Sade RM, Williams RG, Nadas AS: Open-heart surgery during the first three months of life. J Thorac Cardiovasc Surg 68:719, 1974.
12. Fecht DC, Magovern GJ, Park SB, Merkow LP,Dixon CM, Dosios T, Pardo M: Beneficial effects of methylprednisolone in patients on cardiopulmonary bypass. Circ Shock 5:415, 1978.
13. Roe BB, Hutchinson JC, Fishman NH, Ullyot DJ, Smith DL: Myocardial protection with cold, ischemic, potassium-induced cardioplegia. J Thorac Cardiovasc Surg 73:366, 1977.
14. Black PR, Van Devanter S, Cohn LH: Effects of hypothermia on systemic and organ systemic metabolism and function. J Surg Res 20:49, 1976.
15. Fairley HB: Metabolism in hypothermia. Br Med Bull 17:52, 1961.
16. Baum D, Dillard DH, Porte D Jr: Inhibition of insulin release in infants undergoing deep hypothermic cardiovascular surgery. N Engl J Med 279:1309, 1968.
17. Brown TG, Jr, Cotten Med V: Evaluation of factors enhancing cardiac force during hypothermia. Fed Proc 15:405, 1956.
18. Nesbakken R: Aspects of free fatty acid metabolism during induced hypothermia. Scand J Clin Lab Invest 131 31(Suppl 131):1, 1973.
19. Lamberti JJ, Lin C-Y, Cutilletta A, Anagnostopoulos CE, Arcilla RA, Replogle RL: Surface cooling (20°C) and circulatory arrest in infants undergoing cardiac surgery. Arch Surg 113:822, 1978.
20. Zarins CK, Skinner DB. Hemodynamics and blood flow distribution following prolonged circulation at 5°C. Am J Physiol 229:275, 1975.
21. Rein JG, Freed MD, Norwood WI, Castaneda AR: Early and late results of closure of ventricular septal defect in infancy. Ann Thorac Surg 24:19, 1977.
22. de LeVal, M, Hill JD, Mielke H, Bramson ML, Smith C, Gerbode F: Platelet kinetics during extracorporeal circulation. Trans Am Soc Artif Intern Organs 18: 355, 1972.
23. Dutton RC, Edmunds LH Jr, Hutchinson JC, Roe BB: Platelet aggregate emboli produced in patients during cardiopulmonary bypass with membrane and bubble oxygenator and blood filters. J Thorac Cardiovasc Surg 67:258, 1974.

CHAPTER 16

PHARMACOLOGIC INTERVENTIONS DURING CARDIOPULMONARY BYPASS

BARRY L. ZIMMERMAN, M.D.

There have been few systematic studies of pharmacology during total cardiopulmonary bypass (CPB), although the behavior of individual drugs has been studied in detail. This chapter is designed to accomplish several objectives. First, a basic review of fundamental principles of clinical pharmacology will lead into a general discussion of how CPB may affect the actions of drugs. Second, the pharmacology of drugs used commonly in patients undergoing cardiac operations will be discussed from two perspectives. One perspective is how CPB will affect the action of the specific drug. The other perspective is how the drug will affect the process of CPB.

PRINCIPLES OF PHARMACOLOGY

Drugs exert a pharmacologic effect when they achieve an effective concentration at a particular site of action. The science of pharmacology is traditionally divided into two disciplines. First, *pharmacokinetics* is the study of the dispersion of a drug in the body and defines the concentration that will be achieved by a given drug in a given tissue under defined circumstances. This is further subdivided into the studies of *uptake, distribution*, and *elimination*. Secondly, *pharmacodynamics* is the study of the pharmacologic effect that is produced by a given concentration of a drug at a site of action. This is usually approached as a study of *dose-response* relationships. While these two disciplines can be studied separately, they are obviously interdependent in clinical medicine.

Since the effect at the site of action is more or less passively dependent upon the concentration of drug delivered to it, pharmacokinetics often receives more attention than dynamics. This discussion will therefore concentrate on pharmacokinetics, and concepts of pharmacodynamics will be introduced where appropriate.

Figure 16.1 illustrates a simple two-compartment model that is commonly used when discussing principles of pharmacokinetics.[1] The *dose* of drug enters the body via the process of *uptake*. When the drug is administered by any route other than intravenous, the study of uptake is a very important part of the overall study of the drug's kinetics. Many studies of drug *bioavailability* have dealt specifically with drug uptake. Intravenous administration bypasses the problem of uptake, and the entire dose is considered to enter the *central compartment* (V_1). This compartment is more theoretical than real, but under most circumstances corresponds fairly closely to the circulating blood volume. From the central compartment the drug is *distributed* to the *peripheral compartment* (V_2), which usually corresponds to the body tissues.

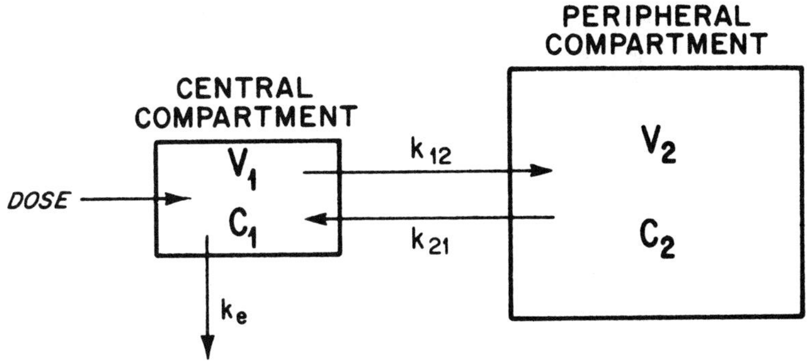

Figure 16.1. Two compartment open pharmacokinetic model, illustrating the central and peripheral compartments (V_1 and V_2) and the drug concentrations in them (C_1 and C_2), and the processes of uptake ("dose"), distribution (k_{12} and k_{21}), and elimination (k_e). (Reproduced with permission from: D. J. Greenblatt, and J. Koch-Weser.[1])

At the same time that the drug is being distributed, some of it is being *eliminated* from the body by active or passive processes. These would include glomerular filtration, hepatic microsomal degradation, pulmonary excretion, etc.

It must be recognized that such a two-compartment model is too oversimplified to describe the actual kinetic behavior of most drugs. However, it serves to illustrate certain basic principles. First of all, the processes of *uptake* and *elimination* are considered to apply to drug in the central compartment only. A drug is administered into the central compartment and is eliminated from it. On the other hand, the site of pharmacologic action is usually considered to be in the peripheral compartment and depends on the process of *distribution* from the central compartment.

The concentration of drug measured in the central compartment (C_1) after intravenous bolus administration will depend on the rate of diffusion into the peripheral compartment (k_{12}), the rate of back-diffusion out of the peripheral compartment (k_{21}), and the rate of elimination (k_e). With acute administration, k_{21} is usually insignificant, and k_{12} is initially faster than k_e. The central concentration (C_1) initially will fall rapidly due to peripheral distribution (Fig. 16.2). The magnitude of this distribution phase, or alpha-phase, is determined by the total volume into which the drug appears to be distributed after acute administration. The phrase "*appears* to be distributed" is important, since this volume often does not correspond to an actual volume of a body fluid or tissue, but rather reflects the extent of tissue uptake of the drug. This *apparent volume of distribution* (V_d) is the sum total of V_1 and V_2. Values for V_d range from the low of, for instance, heparin (0.06 liters/kg of body weight, or essentially just the circulating blood volume) to drugs such as digoxin or propranolol, whose V_d's are several times larger than the total body water, and which will therefore have a very long alpha-phase.[2]

As distribution slows, the rate of fall of C_1 will depend more on the speed of elimination (k_e) and the rate of diffusion back into the central compartment (k_{21}). This elimination phase, or beta-phase, may be as short as seconds or as long as years. It depends on the extent of body stores of the drug ($V_2 \times C_2$) and the magnitudes of k_{21} and k_e. When V_2 and/or C_2 are large, and k_{21} is slower than k_e (e.g., digoxin), tissue drug levels will be higher than blood levels, and very low blood levels may persist for long times. The slope of the beta-phase will be very flat, and the *elimination half-life*, or the time for C_1 to be reduced by one-half, will be long. If k_{21} is fast and k_e is slow, the curve illustrated in Figure 16.2 will appear the same, but blood levels (C_1) will approximate tissue levels (C_2). If k_e is very fast, the beta-phase slope will be steep, and plasma levels may become undetectable fairly quickly. However, pharmacologic effect may continue after the disappearance of drug from the plasma for two reasons. First, if k_{21} is slow, drug may persist at the site of action for a period of time after plasma

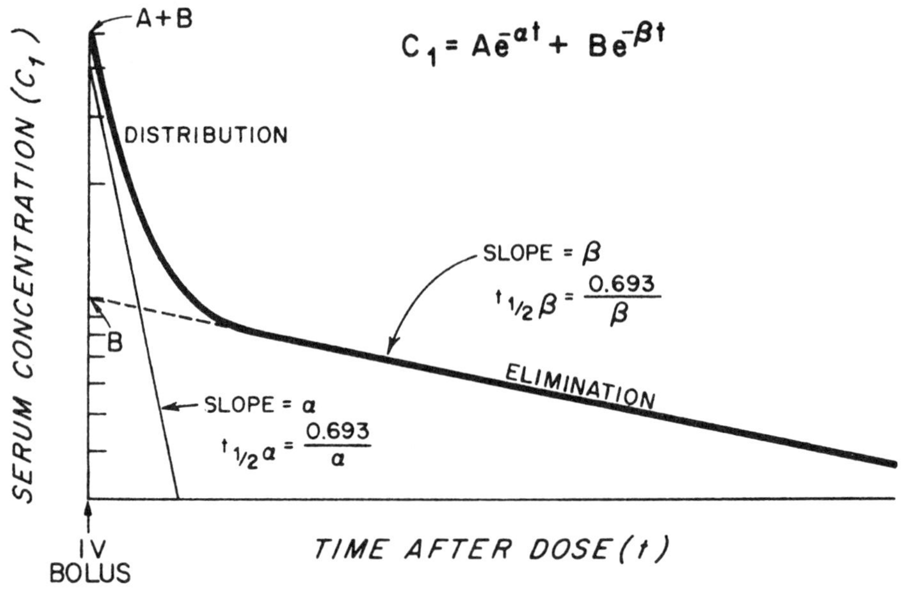

Figure 16.2. Semilogarithmic plot of concentration of drug in central compartment (C_l) *vs.* time, illustrating first-order kinetics for both the alpha-phase ("distribution") and beta-phase ("elimination"). (Reproduced with permission from D. J. Greenblatt and J. Koch-Weser.[1])

levels have disappeared. This mechanism may help to account for some of the apparent continued action of a drug such as propranolol in the absence of detectable blood levels.[3] Secondly, metabolites may be created that also possess pharmacologic activity, but are not measured by the assay technique being used. For instance, propranolol is metabolized to 4-hydroxypropranolol, which is an active, though short-lived compound.[4]

Both distribution and elimination in this model conform to "first-order kinetics," meaning that the rate of change of drug concentration (C_1 in Fig. 16.1) is proportional to the concentration at that time. C_1 is defined at any time after acute administration by the biexponential equation shown in Figure 16.2, solving for both the alpha-phase and beta-phase slopes simultaneously. For a more thorough discussion of this model and the science of pharmacokinetics in general, the reader is referred to the review of Greenblatt and Koch-Weser.[1]

EFFECTS OF CPB ON PHARMACOLOGY

Although there are few systematic discussions of the effects of CPB on pharmacology in general, various features of CPB are known to affect drug handling in their own right. Some of these are listed in Table 16.1.

Hemodilution

The concentrations of most drugs in plasma fall immediately upon initiation of CPB. The most commonly cited explanation for this observation is the sudden dilution of the blood volume by the addition of the prime volume from the heart-lung machine.[5, 6]

However, even this apparently simple phenomenon is the subject of some disagreement. The concentrations of some drugs, particularly those widely distributed in body tissues such as propranolol and the narcotic fentanyl, may fall more than can be accounted for by simple hemodilution.[7, 8] This would imply an increase in apparent volume of distribution for the drug, possibly caused by one of the other factors discussed below such as alterations in protein binding, or changes in peripheral flow due to nonpulsatile perfusion. On the other hand, McAllister et al.[9] found a decrease in the apparent V_d for propranolol during hypothermia, causing elevated plasma levels despite hemodilution.

The subject requires further study, but

Table 16.1
Features of Cardiopulmonary Bypass That Affect Pharmacology

1. Hemodilution
2. Hypothermia
3. Nonpulsatile perfusion
4. Exclusion of lungs from circulation
5. Alterations in protein binding

serves to illustrate the complex nature of CPB effects on pharmacology. It is obviously too simplistic to say that the plasma concentration of a drug will invariably fall during CPB, and that this fall will be the result of acute hemodilution. In fact, of the features listed in Table 16.1, hemodilution may be the least important in terms of the effects of CPB on overall pharmacokinetics.

Hypothermia

Activity of enzyme systems decreases at reduced temperature, and *in vitro* metabolism of most drugs is delayed by hypothermia. Similarly, the *in vivo* elimination of drugs during hypothermic CPB is usually, but not invariably, prolonged. As is true with hemodilution, other factors may have more influence on total drug kinetics. For instance, the *in vitro* metabolism of propranolol by hepatic microsomal enzymes is slowed by hypothermia.[10] However, *in vivo* elimination of propranolol during hypothermic CPB may be relatively efficient.

McAllister et al.[9] actually found an increase in the elimination rate constant (k_e) for propranolol during hypothermia, possibly because of redistribution of total cardiac output away from the periphery and towards visceral organs. The relative increase in hepatic blood flow might deliver more propranolol for metabolism, resulting in enhanced elimination.

Nonpulsatile Perfusion

The significant differences between pulsatile and nonpulsatile flow on organ perfusion are discussed elsewhere (Chapter 3). In general, nonpulsatile flow has more profound effects on renal filtration than on hepatic metabolism.[11] Elimination of drugs that are cleared by glomerular filtration may decrease in parallel with the creatinine clearance during CPB, but clearance by the liver may remain efficient.

Exclusion of the Lungs from the Circulation

The lungs are highly selective in their handling of small and medium-sized molecules in artery pulmonary-blood. Some endogenous molecules are very rapidly extracted from pulmonary arterial blood, while others may pass through unaffected.[12–14] Differences in pulmonary handling of some endogenous and exogenous substances are illustrated in Table 16.2. Exogenous molecules (drugs) are also taken up to varying extents by the lungs. Some pulmonary drug uptake is probably by simple diffusion of the drug into the substance of the lungs. Since the lungs receive the entire cardiac output and are usually exposed to drugs in the venous blood before they reach the systemic circulation, such pulmonary drug uptake may be quite extensive. Almost 25% of a dose of intravenously administered fentanyl may be sequestered in the lungs within 10 minutes of injection.[8] Some drugs also bind to fairly specific receptor sites in the lung and may show competition for these binding sites. Chlorpromazine and imipramine are examples of drugs that bind to specific sites in the lungs. If chlorpromazine is administered to a patient receiving chronic imipramine therapy, some of the tricyclic will be displaced from pulmonary binding sites and released into the systemic circulation.[13]

Table 16.2
Handling of Various Substances by Normal Lung[8, 12–14]

Substances taken up by the lung
- 5-HT (serotonin) ±95%)*
- Prostaglandin E (95%)
- Norepinephrine (30%)
- Chlorpromazine
- Propranolol
- Fentanyl

Substances released by the lung
- Angiotensin II
- Prostaglandin E_2
- Bradykinin

Substances unaffected by the lung
- Dopamine
- Epinephrine
- Prostaglandin A
- Histamine

* Numbers in parentheses are the percentages of first-pass extraction by the lungs.

Following CPB, the ability of the lungs to extract some substances such as serotonin and norepinephrine in enhanced. This may lead to decreased activity of such circulating hormones in the systemic circulation.[12]

Under certain circumstances, the lungs may produce vasoactive substances and release them into the systemic circulation. Most familiar is the conversion of circulating angiotensin I to the powerful vasoconstrictor substance angiotensin II. In response to stimuli such as handling or overdistention, the lungs may also elaborate substances such as prostaglandin E-2 and bradykinin.[13]

The practical implications of the nonrespiratory functions of the lungs during CPB have not been investigated, but theoretically some of the changes in systemic hemodynamics observed during or after CPB could be explained in part by alterations in pulmonary handling of vasoactive substances. The lungs may also serve as a "protected" reservoir for drugs during CPB. Drugs given before CPB may be "stored" in the unperfused lungs, to be released after restoration of pulmonary blood flow. Release of stored fentanyl from the lungs in response to initiation of positive pressure ventilation has been described.[8] In addition, drugs such as fentanyl or propranolol given during CPB may lose some pharmacologic effect when the lungs are reperfused, due to pulmonary uptake.

ALTERATIONS IN PROTEIN BINDING

Many drugs are reversibly bound to plasma proteins, although the extent of binding varies widely. Diazepam and propranolol in plasma are over 95% protein bound, whereas only about 25% of plasma digoxin is bound. The extent of protein binding has great impact on a drug's kinetic behavior.[15] Only unbound drug in the central compartment is free to be distributed into the peripheral compartment. If the degree of binding of a highly bound drug such as propranolol is reduced suddenly, more drug will diffuse into the tissues. The measured plasma concentration (C_1) will fall, since most assay techniques do not differentiate between bound and free drug. However, the concentration at the site of action (C_2) may rise, and the net result would be an increased pharmacologic effect with a lower measured plasma level.

The effects of alterations in protein binding on a drug's elimination depend on the mechanisms for elimination that affect that drug. If elimination is *restrictive*, only free drug is eliminated, and an increase in free drug would enhance clearance. Glomerular filtration is an example of restrictive elimination. Hepatic clearance may be either restrictive or nonrestrictive. Coumadin demonstrates restrictive hepatic elimination, and its metabolism is proportional to the amount of free drug in plasma. Propranolol, on the other hand, demonstrates nonrestrictive hepatic clearance. This means that the hepatocyte will actively extract propranolol from blood, whether protein-bound or not, and thus propranolol elimination is for the most part independant of protein binding.

Plasma protein binding will obviously be altered by the acute decrease in plasma protein concentration that occurs with CPB. However, more important effects on drug-protein interactions during CPB probably occur because of alterations in drug-protein binding properties caused by changes in temperature and alterations in other plasma constituents. Free fatty acids compete for the same sites on proteins that also bind several drugs, including propranolol. Heparin causes an increase in free fatty acid concentration by stimulating the action of lipoprotein lipase. An increase in the free fractions of drugs such as propranolol and diazepam has been found following administration of heparin for cardiac catheterization or CPB, paralleling the rise in plasma fatty acids.[16] The binding of propranolol is so extensive (>95% protein bound) and so sensitive to competition that alterations in propranolol kinetics have been found in patients using "heparin-locks" for venous access.[7]

The interactions of all of the factors that influence drug kinetics following acute alterations in protein binding are complex, but usually are of only limited clinical importance. A significant increase in drug action due to an acute reduction in protein binding is seen with very few drugs. In fact, only the coumadin anticoagulants and the oral hypoglycemic agents have been regularly reported to demonstrate this effect.[15] Even though propranolol is readily displaced from protein binding sites, its volume of distribution is so large that most of the released drug disappears into peripheral storage sites. Also, the difference between an "effective" concentration and a "toxic" concentration (the therapeutic index) is fairly large with propranolol. Alterations in protein binding may have implications during chronic propranolol therapy or research when plasma levels are being measured and correlated with clinical effect. However, there appears to be little chance of an appreciable increase in clinical effect following acute heparinization.

SITE OF ADMINISTRATION OF DRUGS DURING CARDIOPULMONARY BYPASS

Drugs may be given by way of several routes during CPB. The most efficient method would be to inject the drug into the arterial outflow side of the oxygenator circuit. This would deliver the drug directly into the central arterial circulation. However, this route is not favored because of the danger of injecting small air bubbles or even foreign bodies into the systemic circulation. If drugs are being given by anesthesia personnel, it is most convenient for them to inject into the same catheters they have been using throughout the case. These will commonly be central venous catheters placed in the superior vena cava or right atrium. Kamath *et al.*[17] have demonstrated that injection of drugs into a central venous catheter during CPB may result in erratic and unpredictable entry of the drug into the patient's circulation. Figure 16.3 shows some of the results of their studies. Sodium pertechnetate ^{99m}Tc) was injected into various sites and sensed by a detector placed on the arterial outflow line. "Normal" appearance is illustrated by curve "A." After central venous injection at point "I," the tracer appears quickly in the arterial line, followed by a smaller recirculation peak.

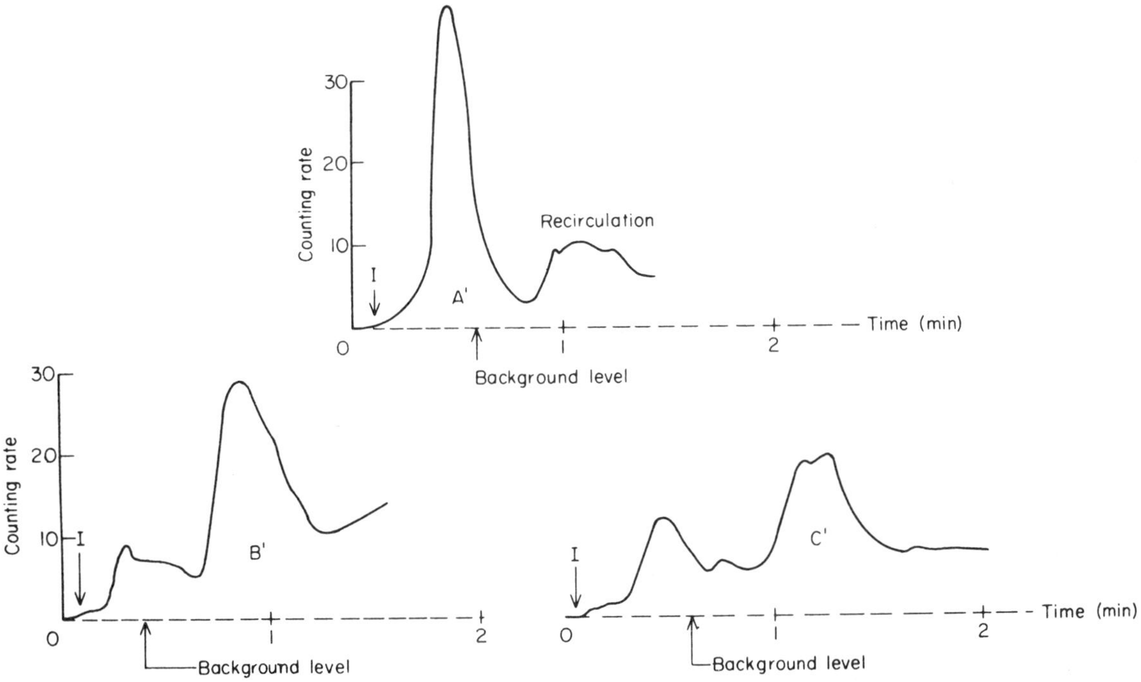

Figure 16.3. Curves demonstrating appearance of a bolus of ^{99m}Tc-injected through a central venous catheter of a patient during CPB at a sensor placed on the arterial outflow cannula. *Curve A'*, normal appearance. *Curves B' and C'*, delayed appearance. (Reproduced with permission from B. S. K. Kamath et al.[17])

However, as shown by "B" and "C," some injections resulted in slow, delayed appearance with tall late peaks that often corresponded to times that the heart was picked up or manipulated by the surgeon. In some trials, tracer appeared abruptly as late as 5 or 6 minutes after injection. These late peaks never occurred if the tracer was injected into the venous inflow side of the oxygenator.

Kamath postulated that some of the tracer injected via a central venous catheter might become sequestered in a relatively isolated low-flow "pocket" at the site of the venous drainage cannulae, to be released either gradually by diffusion or abruptly if the surgeon manipulated the heart.

To ensure prompt and complete delivery into the systemic circulation, therefore, all drugs should be administered via the oxygenator during CPB, and injection into a central venous catheter should be avoided if possible.

ANESTHETIC DRUGS

Narcotics

Very high doses of potent narcotic analgesics are commonly used during anesthesia for open-heart surgery. Morphine sulfate has been used extensively in the last two decades,[18, 19] but in recent years fentanyl citrate has been gaining in popularity.[6, 20, 21] Some of the reasons for this increase in the use of fentanyl include a claimed lower incidence of both serious hypotension and intraoperative hypertension when compared to morphine.[6, 21] However, experiences reported with the two drugs are difficult to compare because of differences in methodologies. Although fentanyl may cause less acute hypotension than morphine, probably due to less marked histamine release, the lower incidence of hypertension may be dose related. The usual reported dose of fentanyl for open-heart surgery is 50 to 100 μg/kg.[6, 21] Since fentanyl is probably about 100 times as potent as morphine, this would correspond to morphine doses of 5 to 10 mg/kg.[20] Morphine is commonly used in doses of 1 to 3 mg/kg for cardiac anesthesia, although doses of up to 8 mg/kg have been reported.[18–20] Therefore, reports that fentanyl can more reliably prevent increases in blood pressure during cardiac surgery may be related to the relatively higher doses used.

The kinetics of both morphine and fentanyl have been studied in detail, and provide excellent examples of the difficulties inherent in clinical pharmacokinetic research. Table 16.3 presents data on fentanyl pharmacokinetics obtained from four recent sources.[8, 22–24] There are obvious differences in model, assay technique, and dose used. The large volume of distribution reported by Murphy is compatible with results from other groups, indicating fentanyl is very avidly taken up by tissues. However, the differences in reported elimination half-lives are striking. It is probably no coincidence that the longest half-life is reported in the study employing patients undergoing cardiac surgery, since elimination would be expected to be slower in a group of patients with serious cardiovascular disease. However, some of the differences are due to variations in mathematical modeling and analysis. Some of the groups employed a two-compartment model similar to that in Figure 16.1, yielding a biexponential decay curve,[8, 22] while others used a three-compartment model requiring three exponential expressions.[23, 24] There were also differences in opinion on such basic issues as whether or not fentanyl concentrations in cerebrospinal fluid (CSF) showed any correlation with plasma concentrations; Murphy et al.[23] found such a correlation but Schleimer et al.[24] did not.

Studies of morphine kinetics show the same variability, often due to simple factors such as the speed of injection or whether or not ventilation was controlled during injection to prevent changes in arterial PCO_2. Morphine is also rapidly taken up by tissues, with a volume of distribution of between 3 and 6 liters/kg.[2, 25] The smaller volumes are often observed with larger doses, probably because the greater degree of hypotension that occurs with large doses limits peripheral distribution.[25] Reported elimination half-lives range from about 1 hour in the dog to 1.5 to 3 hours in human subjects.[2, 25]

Even though the elimination half-life of fentanyl is longer than that of morphine, it is usually considered to have a shorter duration of clinical action. This is explained by the different mechanisms which terminate the

Table 16.3
Examples of Pharmacokinetic Parameters of Fentanyl Reported in the Recent Literature

	Data			
	Ainslie et al.[22]	Murphy et al.[23]	Schleimer et al.[24]	Bovill and Sebel[8]
Assay technique	Trtiated fentanyl	Tritiated fentanyl	Radioimmunoassay	Radioimmunoassay
Model	Dog	Dog	Noncardiac surgery	Cardiac surgery
Dose	12.5 μg/kg	10–100 μg/kg	1 mg/m²	60 μg/kg
Volume of distribution		9.8 liters/kg		
Elimination half-life	89 min	200 min	346 min	423 min
Compartments	2	3	3	2
CFS [fentanyl] correlates with plasma [fentanyl]		Yes	No	

effects of the two drugs. The effect of fentanyl is terminated by redistribution, that of morphine by elimination.[6, 8, 23–25] The difference is illustrated by the composite decay curves shown in Figure 16.4. The volume of distribution of fentanyl is much larger than that of morphine, so that the plasma concentration following bolus administration is lower after the alpha (distribution) phase is complete. The beta (elimination) phase is then very prolonged, mainly due to slow release from peripheral storage sites (slow k_{21}). Plasma levels during the beta phase, however, will be below "effective" levels. As the drug is redistributed away from the vessel-rich organs (including the brain) into peripheral storage depots, the effect of the drug dissipates rapidly.

Morphine, on the other hand, has a much faster k_{21}, so that as drug is eliminated from plasma it is replaced rapidly from tissue depots. Plasma levels approach tissue levels, and the brain-blood gradient is not as large at any given point during the elimination phase as with fentanyl. Brain levels will tend to fall in parallel with total body stores, then, and the drug effect will terminate when plasma and tissue levels are reduced below "effective" concentrations by elimination.

One could predict from this data that fentanyl would show a much more pronounced tendency to accumulate in the body following repeated administration or very high doses, and this is indeed the case. In fact, following the doses commonly used for cardiac anesthesia (50–100 μg/kg), fentanyl cannot be considered a "short-acting" narcotic, and its pharmacologic effect on consciousness and respiratory drive is even more prolonged than

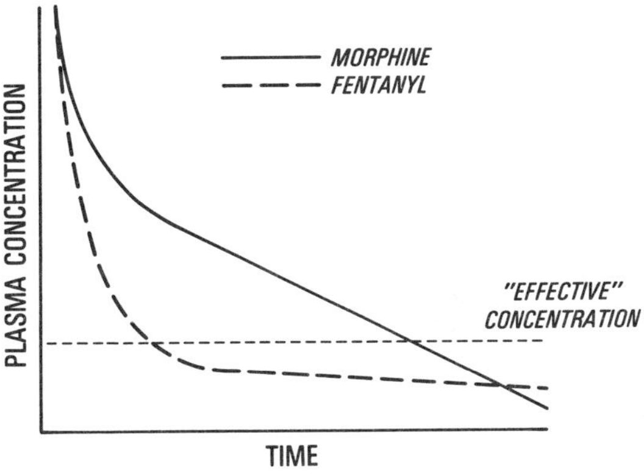

Figure 16.4. Schematic decay curves for plasma concentrations of fentanyl and morphine after intravenous administration. Note more extensive "distribution" of fentanyl, with longer alpha-phase, but slower beta-phase elimination. (Adapted from data of Hug et al.[25] and Schleimer et al.[24])

after large doses of morphine.[6, 8, 23, 24, 26] As more fentanyl is sequestered in peripheral stores, the steady-state beta-phase plasma level will be higher, and redistribution out of the brain will be slowed. Although brain or CSF fentanyl kinetics have not been described during CPB, plasma levels have been found to remain fairly stable, and it is probably not necessary to administer more fentanyl during routine CPB if a full 100 μg/kg dose has been given prior to bypass.[6, 8]

Muscle Relaxants

Although factors such as hypothermia and electrolyte disturbances are known to have significant impact on both the kinetic and dynamic behavior of nondepolarizing neuromuscular blocking drugs such as pancuronium and *d*-tubocurarine (curare),[27] the pharmacology of these drugs during CPB has not been well described. It is common to observe motion of the diaphragm during CPB, however, especially at normothermia. Therefore, during operations involving entry into cardiac chambers, it is rational to give liberal doses of muscle relaxants before cardiotomy to prevent aspiration of air into the pulmonary veins caused by respiratory effort.

Inhalation Anesthetics

Potent volatile inhalation anesthetics (halothane, enflurane) may be administered during CPB by inserting the appropriate vaporizer into the oxygen inflow line to the pump oxygenator. It is rational to use these agents to maintain anesthesia during CPB if they have been used as part of the anesthetic technique prior to bypass. However, they are not inherently particularly effective vasodilators[28] and may have disadvantageous effects on visceral perfusion, in addition to the risks of visceral cellular toxicity.[29] Therefore, there is little reason to use these agents to control perfusion pressure during CPB if the patient has been given effective doses of one of the potent narcotics, and an intravenous vasodilator should be used instead.

If a volatile inhalational agent is used, it should be discontinued at least 15 minutes prior to termination of CPB, as all of these agents in common use today are potent myocardial depressants and may impede the transition to spontaneous circulation.

Digoxin

Studies of the behavior of digoxin during and after CPB have provided good examples of some of the ways that both pharmacokinetics and pharmacodynamics may be perturbed during this period. Digoxin has a very large volume of distribution and a very slow beta elimination phase slope, due primarily to extensive body stores (mostly in skeletal muscle) and slow release from those stores. Elimination is primarily by glomerular filtration, and digoxin clearance usually parallels creatinine clearance over wide ranges of renal function.[2]

Plasma digoxin levels usually fall with the initiation of CPB, probably due mostly to acute dilution.[30–32] However, little actual loss of digoxin from the body occurs during CPB, as elimination is slow and inefficient. With the termination of CPB, plasma digoxin concentrations often rise to equal or even exceed preoperative levels.[30, 31] Referring to Figure 16.1, this may be the result of extensive body stores with a slow k_{21} and relatively efficient k_e. If k_e is reduced, as may happen with digoxin if creatinine clearance falls, C_1 will rise to approach C_2, and a new steady state will be established. As might be expected, this phenomenon is more often seen in older patients than in children, and when bypass times are prolonged.[31, 32]

Whatever the reason, plasma digoxin concentrations in patients on chronic therapy may be expected to be no lower after CPB than before, and may be higher. For this reason, administration of digoxin to patients receiving chronic therapy is not recommended during or immediately following CPB. Digoxin may be restarted 12 to 24 hours after surgery, assuming renal function is normal.

Alterations in digoxin pharmacodynamics also occur during CPB. Morrison and Killip[31] found that plasma digoxin concentrations were higher in patients experiencing postoperative dysrhythmias than those in patients with stable rhythms. However, these dysrhythmias occurred at mean digoxin levels of 1.3 ng/ml, and in almost no case was the digoxin concentration greater than the recognized "toxic" level of 2 ng/ml. Hence, the apparent sensitivity of the heart to digitalis is increased by CBP. This change in dynamics is still unexplained, but there are several factors commonly present following CPB that might contribute, including hypokalemia, hypomagnesemia, and even iatrogenic hypercalcemia from therapeutic administration of calcium salts. Direct myocardial cell damage from surgical manipulation or ischemia may also play a role. From Morrison's data, it would appear that the "toxic" plasma digoxin concentration after CPB is closer to 1 ng/ml than to 2 ng/ml.[31] For this reason, patients who are on stable chronic digoxin therapy should probably have the drug discontinued at least 24 hours before surgery.

The situation is even more complicated with patients who have been started on digoxin therapy within 2 weeks of surgery. Following acute administration of digoxin, myocardial concentrations of the drug are higher relative to peripheral skeletal muscle stores and plasma concentrations than during chronic therapy.[32] Therefore, the "normal" plasma levels expected during chronic therapy will actually reflect higher myocardial levels following acute administration. Dysrhythmias will thus tend to occur at lower measured plasma levels. When therapy with digoxin is to be started within a week or so of surgery, blood levels should be carefully controlled, and possibly should not exceed 1 ng/ml at the time of surgery.[31, 32]

Propranolol

Propranolol pharmacology during CPB offers interesting contrasts to that of digoxin. Propranolol, like digoxin, has a very large apparent volume of distribution (3.9 liters/kg body weight).[2] However, unlike digoxin, it is completely metabolized in the liver, with a beta-phase half-life of 3.9 hours.[2] Hepatic extraction is nonrestrictive and very efficient; two-thirds of an orally administered dose is removed from portal blood in a single pass through the liver.[2, 33] As has been mentioned in a previous section, even though *in vitro* hepatic microsomal metabolism of propranolol is slowed by hypothermia, propranolol elimination during hypothermic CPB may be relatively efficient.

While McAllister et al.[9] found an increase in plasma propranolol concentrations with hypothermic CPB, other authors have usually found a decrease in these levels.[5, 7] Despite this disagreement, most authors agree that postoperative propranolol levels are lower than preoperative.[5, 7, 9] This is paralleled by a similar decrease in pharmacodynamic effect, so that heart rates after CPB are usually higher than rates before CPB, and the response to beta-agonist agents such as isoproterenol or dopamine is well preserved.[4, 5]

In addition, it would appear that only patients receiving propranolol within about 12 hours of surgery will have detectable plasma levels during CPB. Even then, plasma levels may be significant only in those patients receiving doses higher than 160 mg/day. Differences in experiences reported in the literature can be ascribed in part to different methodologies. Hug et al.[5] reported significant prebypass plasma levels (up to 80 ng/ml) in patients receiving up to 350 mg/day, in whom the last dose was given 10 hours before surgery, although by the end of the CPB no level was in excess of 15 ng/ml. Wechsler[4] found much lower prebypass levels (less than 40 ng/ml) in patients in his series, who were given the last dose 4 hours before surgery. However, his patients who were on doses greater than 160 mg/day were tapered to this dose at least 24 hours before surgery. This study also found that patients receiving recent doses of propranolol who required inotropic drug support following CPB had prebypass propranolol levels in excess of 10 mg/ml. He did not measure postbypass levels.

In general it appears that, in contrast to digoxin, propranolol is readily mobilized from body stores when administration is stopped and is eliminated rapidly during CPB. Since propranolol's negative inotropic effects parallel its plasma concentrations, it would be expected that little residual effect would remain at the end of CPB.[3] When inotropic support is required, no adverse pharmacodynamic effects have been reported to make such support more difficult than in patients not receiving propranolol.[4, 5] On the whole, then, continuing propranolol is advantageous in terms of modifying the hemodynamic response to anesthesia and surgery. These beneficial effects may be achieved with little fear of increasing the patient's risk of adverse hemodynamic effects in the postoperative period.

ANTIBIOTICS

The use of prophylactic broad spectrum antibiotics is widely accepted in cardiac surgery; the drugs most often used are the cephalosporins. Cephalothin has been the cephalosporin antibiotic most commonly studied during CPB.[34–37] It has the advanatage of being the cephalosporin most resistant to the action of bacterial beta-lactamase enzymes, and thus is the cephalosporin of choice for treating established penicillin-resistant gram-positive infections.[38] However, when used for prophylaxis it has some disadvantages compared to other cephalosporins.

Cephalothin is rapidly eliminated, even during CPB.[34–36] This may be due in part to the fact that multiple mechanisms are effective in cephalothin elimination, including renal glomerular filtration, tubular secretion, and hepatic metabolism.[38] Austin et al.[35] found that even doses of 2 gm of cephalothin given intravenously prior to CPB in adults failed to maintain adequate serum levels to protect against gram-negative bacteria until the patient reached the postoperative ICU.

In contrast, a drug such as cefazolin has several advantages. First, its V_d is lower than cephalothin's (0.12 liter/kg *vs.* 0.26 liter/kg), indicating that a given serum level could be achieved with a dose half as large as cephalothin.[2] Secondly, its elimination half-life is longer (108 minuts *vs.* 34 minutes for cephalothin), so the intervals between doses can be longer.[2] It is well-absorbed after intramuscular administration and is not as irritating after injection as cephalothin.[38] Its spectrum of activity is broad, and it is effective against gram-negative rods.[36, 38]

Finally, it is eliminated almost solely by glomerular filtration and is poorly excreted during CPB.[2, 38] Akl and Richardson[37] found that a dose of 1 gm of cefazolin given intramuscularly with the preoperative premedication produced adequate, stable blood levels throughout CPB, even when bypass was prolonged for several hours.

Therefore, it can be suggested that intramuscular cefazolin, 1 gm in adults (20 mg/kg in children), is a good choice for antibiotic prophylaxis during CPB. Additional doses need not be given until the postoperative period, even if bypass is prolonged. If cephalothin is used, it may be given intravenously in doses of 2 gm (up to 30 mg/kg in children) at the time of induction of anesthesia, and again at the termination of bypass to ensure adequate blood levels.

ADRENAL CORTICOSTEROIDS

Recommendations in the literature differ about the use of large doses of adrenal glucocorticosteroids during CPB.[39, 40] The described pharmacologic effects of large doses of corticosteroids include peripheral vasodilation with increased microcirculatory flow, stabilization of lysosomal membranes, improved oxygen transport, and increased gluconeogenesis.[40–42] While many of these effects should be beneficial during CPB, few studies have described an objective benefit with the use of pharmacologic doses of steroids. The circulatory and subcellular metabolic effects of up to 30 mg/kg body weight of methylprednisolone, appear to be modest and short lived.[41–43]

The most consistently reported circulatory effects of corticosteroids during CPB are a decrease in apparent systemic vascular resistance and an increase in total flow at the same perfusion pressure, both during spontaneous circulation and CPB.[40–42] Opponents of the use of steroids point out that these changes are not any more significant than those which may be produced with the use of vasodilators such as sodium nitroprusside.[39] However, it is not at all clear that the decreased resistance obtained with nitroprusside is associated with an increase in effective capillary flow. If it could be shown that the decreased resistance caused by corticosteroids was the result of improved microcirculatory flow, the use of such agents would be advantageous. However, the evidence is still incomplete, so the use of corticosteroids must still be considered of unproven benefit.

DIURETICS

Potent diuretic agents such as furosemide are commonly administered during CPB.[44]

Most of the alterations in renal perfusion and function that ocur with CPR are self-limiting and revert to normal postoperatively. There is evidence, however, to suggest that furosemide is capable of ameliorating some of the alterations in intrarenal blood flow associated with CPB. Specifically, furosemide may restore renal cortical blood flow and improve urine flow and possibly creatinine clearance during bypass that lasts longer than 60 minutes.[45, 46] These effects resemble those seen when furosemide is administered to patients with impending acute renal failure following traumatic shock or other similar insults.[47, 48] Since the use of furosemide appears to be associated with an improved outcome in such situations, its use during prolonged CPB or when urine output is unacceptably low is reasonable. There appears to be little advantage to the use of diuretics if bypass time is less than 1 hour, nor is there any particular advantage to the use of other agents such as mannitol.[45, 46]

Vasoconstrictors and Vasodilators

Vasoactive drugs are commonly used to manipulate total systemic vascular resistance (SVR) during CPB.[44] Ideally, SVR should be adjusted to provide adequate perfusion pressure in the central circulation while maintaining a low resistance in vessels supplying vital capillary beds to allow adequate flow. This ideal is very difficult to attain in practice, however. Because of changes in rheology and regional vascular resistances it is difficult to know what an "ideal" perfusion pressure is. Mean arterial pressures (MAP) during CPB of 50–100 torr are usually considered adequate, although much lower pressures are sometimes accepted.[44] Increasing MAP by using a vasoconstrictor such as phenylephrine may not result in better tissue perfusion, even in the coronary vascular bed. While increasing MAP with a vasoconstrictor will usually increase subendocardial blood flow and the endocardial/epicardial flow ratio in normal hearts,[49, 50] this may not be true in areas supplied by collateral vessels. In the dog model, at least, coronary collateral arteries appear to respond to vasoconstrictors as resistance vessels, with increased resistance and decreased flow.[50, 51] This may be because coronary collaterals arise from epicardial vessels and retain the alpha-receptors derived from their parent arteries, whereas normal endocardial and conducting vessels are poorly supplied with alpha-receptors.[50] This coronary vasoconstrictor response seems to be particularly apparent when the vasoconstrictor is given rapidly and is attenuated by a slower infusion rate.[51]

In the peripheral circulation, vasopressors may restrict muscle blood flow. When a group of patients given phenylephrine during CPB was compared to a group at the same MAP achieved by increasing flow rates rather than using the constrictor, the high-flow group had better intramuscular oxygen tensions and showed better rewarming.[52] The use of vasoconstrictors to raise MAP during CPB requires additional study before reasonable indications can be identified. The basis for their use now must remain the individual judgment of the clinician.

Vasodilators such as chlorpromazine and sodium nitroprusside are useful to reduce undesirably high perfusion pressures and increase peripheral flow.[44] The major demonstrable benefit of this redistribution of flow is improved rewarming and temperature maintenance.[53] An actual advantage in terms of improved tissue metabolism has not been proven, however, since the increased flow may not be directed to nutrient capillary beds.[54]

It may be that future work will be directed towards finding ways to influence flow in specific tissues with more selective agents. Possible examples of this approach include the effects of carbon dioxide on cerebral blood flow and those of furosemide on intrarenal perfusion.

References

1. Greenblatt DJ, Koch-Weser J: Clinical pharmacokinetics. N Engl J Med 293:702, 1975.
2. Benet LZ, Sheiner LB: Design and optimization of dosage regimens: Pharmacokinetics data. In *The Pharmacologic Basis of Therapeutics*, Ed. 6, edited by AG Gilman, LS Goodman, and A Gilman. New York, Macmillan, 1980, p. 1675.
3. Boudoulas H, Beaver BM, Kates RE, Lewis RP: Pharmacodynamics of inotropic and chronotropic responses to oral therapy with propranolol. Studies in normal subjects and patients with angina. Chest 73: 146, 1978.
4. Wechsler AS: Assessment of prospectively randomized patients receiving propranolol therapy before

coronary bypass operation. Ann Thorac Surg 30:128, 1980.
5. Hug CC Jr, Kaplan JA, Rigel EP: The effect of cardiopulmonary bypass on plasma propranolol concentrations and response to isoproterenol. Abstracts of Scientific Papers, ASA Annual Meeting, 1977, p. 501.
6. Lunn JK, Stanley TH, Eisele J, Webster L, Woodward A: High dose fentanyl anesthesia for coronary artery surgery: Plasma fentanyl concentrations and influence of nitrous oxide on cardiovascular responses. Anesth Analg 58: 390, 1979.
7. Wood M, Shand DG, Wood AJJ: Propranolol binding in plasma during cardiopulmonary bypass. Anesthesiology 51:512, 1979.
8. Bovill JG, Sebel PS: Pharmacokinetics of high-dose fentanyl. A study in patients undergoing cardiac surgery. Br J Anaesth 52:795, 1980.
9. McAllister RG Jr, Bourne DW, Tan TG, Erickson JL, Wachtel CC, Todd EP: Effects of hypothermia on propranolol kinetics. Clin Pharmacol Ther 25:1, 1979.
10. McAllister RG Jr, Tan TG, Todd EP: Effect of hypothermia on the metabolism of propranolol, quinidine and verapamil. Clin Pharmacol Ther 23:121, 1978.
11. Milnor WR: Pulsatile blood flow. N Engl J Med 287: 27, 1972.
12. Gillis CN: Metabolism of vasoactive hormones by lung. Anesthesiology 39:626, 1973.
13. Comroe JH Jr: Nonrespiratory functions of the lungs and pulmonary circulation. In *Physiology of Respiration*, Ed. 2, Chap 23. Chicago, Year Book Medical Publishers, 1974, p. 285.
14. Nunn JF: *Applied Respiratory Physiology*, Ed. 2. Boston, Butterworth, 1977, p. 21.
15. Koch-Weser J, Sellers EM: Binding of drugs to serum albumin. N Engl J Med 294:311, 1976.
16. Wood AJJ, Robertson D, Robertson RM, Wilkinson GR, Wood M: Elevated plasma free drug concentrations of propranolol and diazepam during cardiac catheterization. Circulation 62:1119, 1980.
17. Kamath BSK, Thomson DM, Johnston B: Administration of drugs during cardiopulmonary bypass. An analysis of the fate of the bolus injected through different routes using radio-active technetium. Anaesthesia 35:908, 1980.
18. Hasbrouck JD: Morphine anesthesia for open-heart surgery. Ann Thorac Surg 10:364, 1970.
19. Arens JF, Benbow BP, Ochsner JL, Theard R: Morphine anesthesia for aortocoronary bypass procedures. Anesth Analg 51:901, 1972.
20. Stoelting RK, Gibbs PS, Creasser CW, Peterson C: Hemodynamic and ventilatory responses to fentanyl, fentanyl-droperidol, and nitrous oxide in patients with acquired valvular heart disease. Anesthesiology 42:319, 1975.
21. Stanley TH, Webster LR: Anesthetic requirements and cardiovascular effects of fentanyl-oxygen and fentanyl-diazepam-oxygen anesthesia in man. Anesth Analg 57:411, 1978.
22. Ainslie SG, Eisele JH Jr, Corkill G: Fentanyl concentrations in brain and serum during respiratory acid-base changes in the dog. Anesthesiology 51:293, 1979.
23. Murphy MR, Olson WA, Hug CC Jr: Pharmacokinetics of ^{3}H-fentanyl in the dog anesthetized with enflurane. Anesthesiology 50:13, 1979.
24. Schleimer R, Benjamini E, Eisele J, Henderson G: Pharmacokinetics of fentanyl as determined by radioimmunoassay. Clin Pharmacol Ther 23:188, 1978.
25. Hug CC Jr, Murphy MR, Rigel EP, Olson WA: Pharmacokinetics of morphine injected intravenously into the anesthetized dog. Anesthesiology 54: 38, 1981.
26. Hug CC Jr, Murphy MR: Fentanyl disposition in cerebrospinal fluid and plasma and its relationship to ventilatory depression in the dog. Anesthesiology 50:342, 1979.
27. Ham J: Factors affecting administration of nondepolarizing neuromuscular blocking agents. In *Refresher Courses in Anesthesiology*, Vol. 8, edited by SG Hershey. Philadelphia, J. B. Lippincott Co., 1980, p. 61.
28. Eger EI, II, Smith NT, Stoelting RK, Cullen DJ, Kadis LB, Whitcher CE: Cardiovascular effects of halothane in man. Anesthesiology 32:396, 1970.
29. Ngai SH: Current concepts in anesthesiology: Effects of anesthetics on various organs. N Engl J Med 302: 564, 1980.
30. Coltart DJ, Chamberlain DA, Howard MR, Kettlewell MG, Mercer JL, Smith TW: Effect of cardiopulmonary bypass on plasma digoxin concentrations. Br Heart J 33:334, 1971.
31. Morrison J, Killip T: Serum digitalis and arrhythmia in patients undergoing cardiopulmonary bypass. Circulation 47:341, 1973.
32. Krasula RW, Hastreiter AR, Levitsky S, Yanagi R, Soyka LF: Serum, atrial and urinary digoxin levels during cardiopulmonary bypass in children. Circulation 49:1047, 1974.
33. Kornhauser DM, Wood AJJ, Vestal RE, Wilkinson GR, Branch RA, Shand DG: Biological determinants of propranolol disposition in man. Clin Pharmacol Ther 23:165, 1978.
34. Williams DJ, Steele TW: Cephalothin prophylaxis assay during cardiopulmonary bypass. J Thorac Cardiovasc Surg 71:207, 1976.
35. Austin TW, Coles JC, McKechnie P, Sandoval W, Doctor A: Cephalothin prophylaxis and valve replacement. Ann Thorac Surg 23:333, 1977.
36. Kini PM, Fernandez J, Causay RS, Lemole GM: Double-blind comparison of cefazolin and cephalothin in open-heart surgery. J Thorac Cardiovasc Surg 76:506, 1978.
37. Akl BF, Richardson G: Serum cefazolin levels during cardiopulmonary bypass. Ann Thorac Surg 29:109, 1979.
38. Mandell GL, Sande MA: Antimicrobial agents. Penicillins and cephalosporins. In *The Pharmacologic Basis of Therapeutics*, Ed. 6, edited by AG Gilman, LS Goodman, A Gilman. New York, Macmillian, 1980, p. 1126.
39. Yates AK: Maintenance of adequate hemodynamics during open-heart procedures and in the postoperative period. Anesthesia for open heart surgery. Int Anesthesiol Clin 14(3): 1, 1976.
40. Santoli FM, Pensa PM, Azzolina G: Anesthesia in open-heart surgery for correction of congenital heart diseases in children over one year of age. Anesthesia

for open heart surgery. Int. Anesthesial Clin 14(3): 165, 1976.

41. Dietzman RH, Lunseth JB, Goott B, Berger EC: The use of methylprednisolone during cardiopulmonary bypass. A review of 427 cases. J Thorac Cardiovasc Surg 69:870, 1975.
42. Niazi Z, Flodin P, Joyce L, Smith J, Mauer H, Lillehei RC: Effects of glucocorticosteroids in patients undergoing coronary artery bypass surgery. Chest 76: 262, 1979.
43. Thompson MA, Broadbent MP: Methylprednisolone prior to cardiopulmonary bypass. Anaesthesia 35:345, 1980.
44. Finlayson DC, Kaplan JA: Cardiopulmonary bypass. In *Cardiac Anesthesia*, edited by J. A. Kaplan. New York, Grune & Stratton, 1979, p. 393.
45. Engelman RM, Gouge TH, Smith SJ, Stahl WM, Gombos EA, Boyd AD: The effect of diuretics on renal hemodynamics during cardiopulmonary bypass. J Surg Res 16:268, 1974.
46. Nuutinen LS, Kairaluoma M, Tuononen S, Larmi TKI: The effect of furosemide on renal function in open heart surgery. J Cardiovasc Surg (Torino) 19: 471, 1978.
47. Brown RS: Renal dysfunction in the surgical patient. Maintenance of the high output state with furosemide. Crit Care Med 7:63, 1979.
48. Bastron RD: Pathophysiology of acute renal failure. In *ASA Referesher Courses in Anesthesiology*, Vol 8, edited by S. G. Hershey. Philadelphia, J. B. Lippincott Co., 1980, p. 1.
49. Symmonds JB, Kleinman LH, Wechsler AS: Effects of methoxamine on the coronary circulation during cardiopulmonary bypass. J Thorac Cardiovasc Surg 75:577, 1977.
50. Sink JD, Hill RC, Chitwood WR Jr, Abriss R, Wechsler AS: Effects of phenylephrine on transmural distribution of myocardial blood flow in regions supplied by normal and collateral arteries during cardiopulmonary bypass. J Thorac Cardiovasc Surg 78: 236, 1979.
51. Williams DO, Most AS: Responsiveness of the coronary circulation to brief *vs.* sustained alpha-adrenergic stimulation. Circulation 63:11, 1980.
52. Stanley TH, Jackson J: The influence of blood flow and arterial blood pressure during cardiopulmonary bypass on deltoid muscle gas tensions and body temperature after bypass. Can Anaesth Soc J 26:277, 1979.
53. Noback CR, Tinker JR: Hypothermia after cardiopulmonary bypass in man: Amelioration by nitroprusside-induced vasodilation during rewarming. Anesthesiology 53:277, 1980.
54. Evans PJD, Ruygrok P, Seelye ER, Harris EA: Does sodium nitroprusside improve tissue oxygenation during cardiopulmonary bypass? Br J Anaesth 49: 799, 1977.

CHAPTER 17

POTASSIUM KINETICS DURING CARDIOPULMONARY BYPASS

EDWARD P. TODD, M.D., PH.D.

It is well documented[3, 8, 11] that during both surface cooling for deep hypothermic arrest and during cardiopulmonary bypass with moderate hypothermia, potassium concentration decreases. Characteristically, it progressively decreases and remains low during bypass, then increases somewhat during the warming process before cessation of bypass, and then declines again in the early postbypass period.[21]

The significance[15, 20, 26] of hypokalemia during cardiac surgery is clear. Shanahan et al.[17] demonstrated that they could decrease the incidence of ventricular arrhythmia from 44% to 18% and the incidence of ventricular fibrillation from 16% to 0% with potassium supplementation in patients on cardiopulmonary bypass. It was also noted that despite supplementation with potassium in the improved group of patients, serum potassium levels fell and were routinely below normal during cardiopulmonary bypass and in the immediate postoperative period.

The purpose of the chapter presented here will be to review the factors which can cause alterations in potassium concentration during cardiopulmonary bypass in order to clarify their respective roles. The factors which must be considered include urinary losses, hemodilution, alterations in acid-base balance, glucose metabolism, and catecholamine mechanisms.

URINARY LOSSES

Urine volume during and after hemodilution perfusion for cardiac surgery varies widely. Similarily, external potassium losses also are variable. Isotope techniques,[3] utilized to evaluate external potassium losses after surgery, have demonstrated large individual variations between patients ranging from 120 to 266 mEq of potassium in the first 24 hours after surgery. Patrick and Sivapragasam[12] have shown that 5 hours after cardiopulmonary bypass, potassium losses correlate with urinary volumes and therefore, potassium replacement can be planned on the basis of the urine volumes of the previous hours.

During cardiopulmonary bypass, however, potassium losses[12] do not correlate with urinary volumes. As part of the stress response to cardiopulmonary bypass, vasopressin secretion[13] is increased, urinary sodium concentration increases, and urinary potassium concentration actually decreases. Thus, external losses decrease at the same time serum potassium concentration decreases. Studies such as these and others[4] have led to the conclusion that neither urinary losses or dilution of serum potassium by the pump prime are adequate to explain the fall in potassium. The data suggest potassium must move from the circulation to an interstitial space not in equilibrium with the circulating blood or into the intracellular space.

HEMODILUTION

Initially, it was thought that hemodilution might be a major factor in the production of cardiopulmonary bypass-induced hypokalemia. This seemed logical enough, as pump primes without potassium will dilute potassium, but it was noted that the potassium level continued to fall even after mixing was complete. It was also demonstrated[9] that when one uses a hyperkalemic prime, or a prime containing 4 mEq of potassium,[21] the potassium concentration progressively decreases during cardiopulmonary bypass. Thus, the decrease can in no way be correlated with the hemodilutional effect.

ACID-BASE BALANCE

Initial investigators proposed respiratory alkalosis as a factor. They theorized[1] that metabolic alkalosis would be buffered by an exchange of extracellular potassium for intracellular hydrogen, thus producing a decrease in serum potassium. This mechanism can contribute to hypokalemia in patients who are hyperventilated or given exogenous base in excess so that their pH increases. This mechanism, however, does not explain the standard hypokalemia which occurs during bypass, as hypokalemia has been shown to occur despite careful control of PCO_2 between 35 and 45 mm Hg and development of metabolic acidosis requiring sodium bicarbonate during bypass.

GLUCOSE METABOLISM

Numerous studies have pointed out that, with the institution of cardiopulmonary bypass with moderate hypothermia, glucose levels increase.[16] The increase in glucose level is partially related to the intravenous administration of glucose in fluids given during the anesthetic or that glucose contained in the pump priming volume. When these factors are controlled, however, glucose still increases, except in the fasted, glucose-depleted patient undergoing bypass without additional added glucose.[6] The observations have caused some investigators to propose that glycogenolysis in the liver and the direct inhibition of glucose uptake by muscle is the major cause for the elevation in glucose which occurs during cardiopulmonary bypass. One might initially speculate that glucose, then, would be a major factor in the production of the alterations in potassium. It is known that glucose moves into the cell under the influence of insulin, and with transport, potassium also moves intracellularly. In studies from our laboratories[21] and others,[9,16] however, it is now well known that insulin secretion is inhibited during cardiopulmonary bypass, and that the hyperinsulinemic response to a glucose load is markedly inhibited. It is thought that two factors are involved in the inhibition of insulin. First, hypothermia[5] produces a definite suppression of beta-cell secretory activity to produce a primary decrease in insulin secretion. In addition, the stress response[9] to cardiopulmonary bypass and hypothermia produce elevated catecholamines, which also inhibit insulin secretion. It is now known that glucose metabolism does not return to normal until approximately six hours after cardiopulmonary bypass.[16] Thus, glucose metabolism seems to play little, if any, role in the redistribution of potassium during cardiopulmonary bypass.

CATECHOLAMINES

It is now well documented[1,14,18] that catecholamine secretion, including both epinephrine and norepinephrine, is increased during cardiopulmonary bypass in response to the surgical stress. This response occurs in patients in which either pulsatile or nonpulsatile flow are utilized.

The possible significance of catecholamine mechanisms in potassium kinetics was first suggested from studies from our laboratory which clearly indicated an important role for the normally circulating catecholamines, epinephrine, and norepinephrine in normal potassium homeostasis. In these studies carried out in dogs,[19] it was first shown that continuous infusion of 2 μg/kg/minute of epinephrine (Fig. 17.1) and later norepinephrine[25] produces an initial transient increase in potassium concentration which was followed by a progressive decrease below control level. The increase in potassium was shown to be due to the release of potassium from the liver.[27] When lesser doses of epinephrine were infused,[24] the initial increase in potassium was significantly reduced, but the secondary decrease in potassium was similar for all doses. These data suggested that the decrease in potassium might be the more physiologic response. Studies using single injections of epinephrine[23] added credence to this assumption as the increase in potassium was

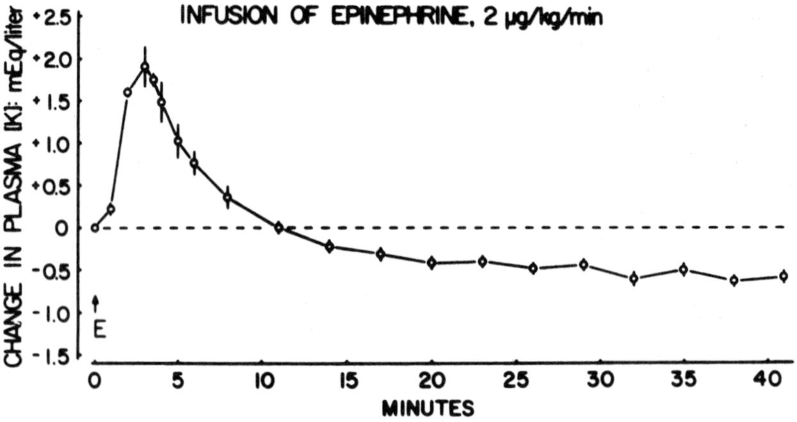

Figure 17.1. The changes in arterial plasma [K+] (mean ± SE) produced by the continuous infusion of 2.0 µg/kg/minute epinephrine in 12 dogs for 41 minutes.

transient, lasting only 1–3 minutes, but the decrease persisted for an hour or more after a single dose.

Studies were then carried out to determine which adrenergic receptors were responsible for the alterations in potassium. It was demonstrated that the initial increase in potassium was a complex response which required both alpha and beta receptor stimulation[27] to duplicate the effect of epinephrine, but the increase in potassium was inhibited by phenoxybenzamine, the alpha-adrenergic blocking agent.

The decrease in potassium was more easily classified. Isoproterenol, the beta adrenergic stimulator,[27] produced essentially a pure decrease in potassium concentration. Propranolol, the beta-adrenergic blocking agent (Fig. 17.2), totally inhibited the decrease in potassium, such that epinephrine infusion produced only an increase in potassium after propranolol pretreatment. These observations led to the conclusion that plasma potassium concentration can be significantly reduced by the intrinsic catecholamines epinephrine and norepinephrine and that the reduction in potassium, which appeared to be the more physiologic response, was produced by beta adrenergic mechanisms and thus inhibited by propranolol, the beta adrenergic blocking agent.

Initially, it was thought that the decrease in potassium might be an indirect effect related to glycogenolysis and glucose moving from the liver to the periphery rather than a direct effect of epinephrine on muscle. Therefore, a study[27] was designed to test this hypothesis. Epinephrine in a dose of 0.2 µg/kg/minute was infused into the femoral artery of a dog. Blood samples for potassium concentration were obtained from the ipsilateral femoral vein, contralateral femoral vein, and systemic artery simultaneously. It was reasoned that any direct effects would cause potassium to change in the ipsilateral vein first. Indirect effects, though, would be apparent in both the ipsilateral and contralateral veins simultaneously, as they would become apparent after recirculation. The data clearly indicated that potassium concentration fell in the ipsilateral vein first; thus, it was demonstrated that the effect of epinephrine on the decrease of potassium was a direct effect. Potassium left the circulation and entered a space not in equilibrium with the circulation, presumably, the intracellular space, such as the muscle distally in the distribution of the femoral artery being perfused.[9]

Other studies[27] were then carried out to determine whether the hypokalemia could be reversed in addition to being inhibited by propranolol. In this study, epinephrine (2 µg/kg/minute) was infused continuously. The potassium was significantly below control level by 11 minutes and stayed down until propranolol was infused. Despite the continuing infusion of epinephrine, potassium rose to control level over the ensuing 30 minutes,

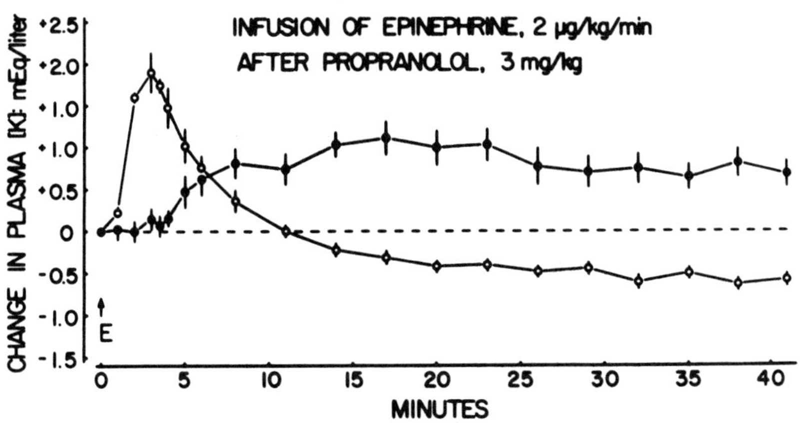

Figure 17.2. The changes in arterial plasma [K+] (mean ± SE) produced by the continuous infusion of 2.0 gm/kg/minute epinephrine for 41 minutes in 9 dogs pretreated with the beta blocking agent propranolol (*half-filled circles*) and in the control group receiving no previous treatment (*open circles*).

indicating that propranolol could reverse the hypokalemia produced by beta-adrenergic mechanisms in addition to inhibiting it. These background studies then established the characteristics of the alterations in potassium produced by the catecholamines.

PROPRANOLOL

Studies were then undertaken to determine whether beta-adrenergic mechanisms are significant factors in the production of the hypokalemia which occurs with hypothermia and cardiopulmonary bypass.

To test the effects of hypothermia, dogs[20] were cooled in a water bath to 25°C. Seven animals served as controls; six animals received propranolol, the beta-adrenergic antagonist, 30 minutes prior to and during cooling; and six animals were given propranolol after they had cooled to 25°C.

The magnitude of the decrease in potassium during the cooling process is indicated in Figure 17.3. In the control animals, plasma potassium concentration progressively decreased to −0.97 ± 0.15 mEq/liter below control at the end of the 30 minute period at 25°C. Potassium decreased in the animals pretreated with propranolol to only −0.34 ± 0.08 mEq/liter below control. The differences in potassium between the control and propranolol-pretreated animals during cooling and while at 25°C were significant to a *p* value less than 0.001. In the six animals given propranolol at 25°C, potassium rose to a level which was almost identical to the value noted in the animals pretreated with propranolol and statistically significantly higher than that of the control animals. No statistically significant differences in insulin, glucose, or urinary losses of potassium were observed between the groups.

The data[20] indicate that propranolol significantly inhibited the decrease in potassium and also reversed the potassium decrease when the propranolol was given later, after the dogs were cooled to 24°C and potassium had fallen. These data indicate that beta-adrenergic mechanisms are important in the production of hypokalemia during hypothermia. The effects of propranolol on hypothermia-induced hypokalemia are so similar to the effects produced by propranolol in the alterations in potassium produced by epinephrine that one must suspect that the increase in catecholamines produced by the hypothermic stress response is a major factor in the production of potassium changes during hypothermia.

In this study ventricular arrhythmia occurred in 5 of 7 control animals but in only one of six pretreated with propranolol ($p < 0.05$). It is tempting to speculate that the increase in potassium in the propranolol-treated animals decreased arrhythmia. Other investigators[17] have shown that adding ex-

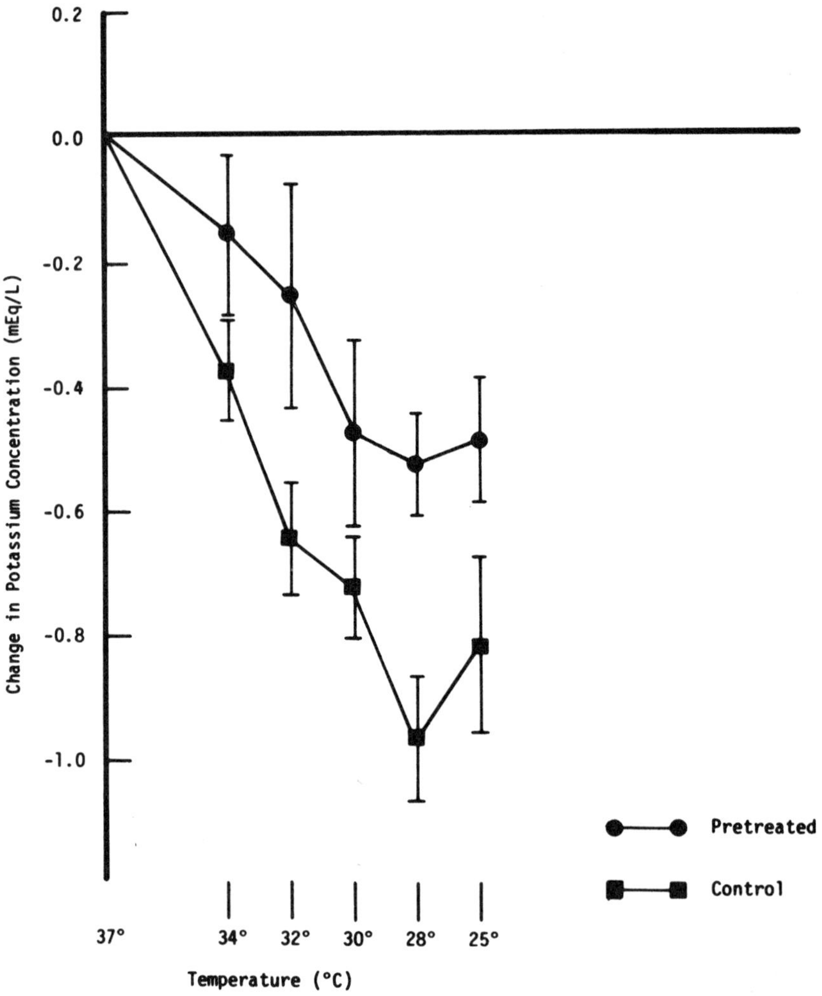

Figure 17.3. The changes in arterial plasma [K+] (mean ± SE) produced by hypothermia to 25°C. Six animals received propranolol (*closed circles*), and seven animals served as controls (*closed squares*).

ogenous potassium certainly significantly decreases arrhythmia, but our conclusions here had to be tempered by the realization that propranolol may have other salutary antiarrhythmia effects besides its effect on potassium.

The studies discussed above were limited to the effect of hypothermia and, further, were purely animal studies, but were a good basis for subsequent clinical studies. Clinical studies were then undertaken. Patients undergoing coronary artery bypass surgery who were on no diuretic therapy were selected for the study. Six were on no preoperative propranolol and 13 were chronically medicated with propranolol daily up to the day of surgery. Blood samples were obtained for determinations of arterial blood gases, insulin, and glucose, before and after cardiopulmonary bypass. The priming solution was Ringer's lactate solution containing 4 mEq/liter of potassium. Patients were routinely cooled to 28°C. Urine was collected for determination of potassium losses. No significant differences in urine volumes, urinary potassium losses, or PCO_2 were observed between the two groups of patients.

Glucose (Fig. 17.4) rose in both groups of

patients. The increase was somewhat greater in the patients on propranolol, and the level stayed higher throughout the period of the study. The differences in glucose can be explained on the basis of similar differences between the patients in the amount of exogenous glucose which they received rather than any intrinsic metabolic effect of propranolol pretreatment.

During cardiopulmonary bypass, insulin levels (Fig. 17.5) reduced in both groups despite high glucose levels. During warming, insulin levels increased dramatically, but the increase was somewhat less in the propranolol-pretreated patients despite the fact that glucose levels were slightly higher in that group of patients. The increase in insulin continued during the first hour after bypass.

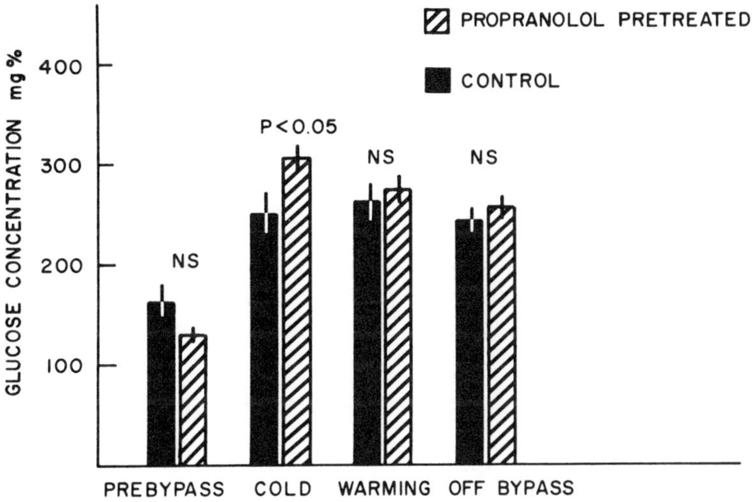

Figure 17.4. Changes in glucose during four phases of cardiopulmonary bypass. Control patients on no propranolol. Others on propranolol up to the day of surgery.

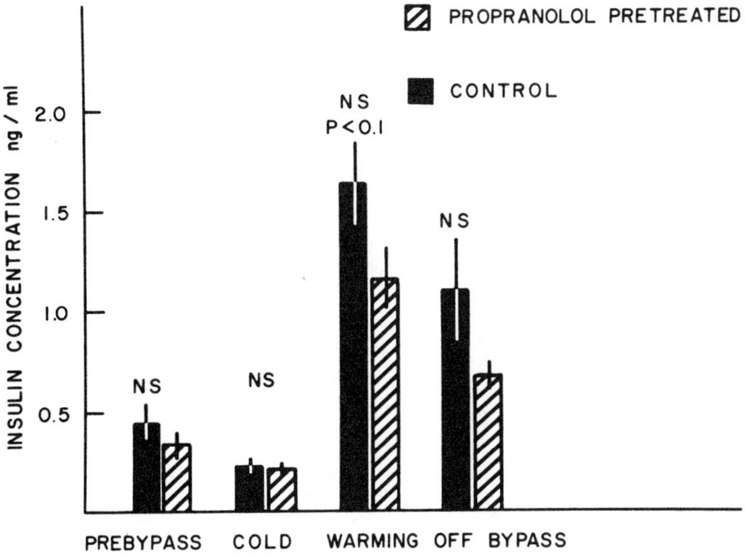

Figure 17.5. The changes in insulin during four phases of cardiopulmonary bypass. Control patients on no propranolol. Others on propranolol up to the day of surgery.

The differences in insulin response were not statistically significant.

During cardiopulmonary bypass, potassium decreases (Fig. 17.6) in both groups of patients with institution of bypass, but the decrease was statistically significantly less in the patients who were pretreated with propranolol. The differences became even greater during the warming process, with the potassium increasing slightly in the patients on propranolol but staying low in the patients who did not receive propranolol. After the patients were off cardiopulmonary bypass, the potassium levels became more similar, although the levels in the propranolol-pretreated patients were consistently higher. These data indicate that beta-adrenergic blockade with propranolol significantly inhibits the decrease in potassium which occurs during cardiopulmonary bypass with moderate hypothermia and suggests that beta-adrenergic mechanisms are significant factors in the production of hypokalemia during cardiopulmonary bypass.

These studies indicate that beta-adrenergic mechanisms are significant factors in normal potassium homeostasis and, therefore, patients pretreated with propranolol might be more sensitive to potassium during cardiopulmonary bypass, as one of the mechanisms for clearing potassium was significantly inhibited. Preliminary studies[22] have been undertaken to test this hypothesis. Two groups of patients were studied. Group I consisted of patients on more than 120 mg/day of propranolol up to the day of surgery, and Group II consisted of patients on no preoperative propranolol. During cardiopulmonary bypass all received cardioplegic solutions, with a total potassium dose of from 15 to 45 mEq. Differences in total dose between groups were nonsignificant. During cardiopulmonary bypass, potassium decreased in Group II despite the addition of potassium. In the patients on chronic propranolol therapy, potassium rose dramatically during surgery and reached levels 3 mEq above control and remained elevated after the patients were off bypass. In the propranolol-pretreated patients, potassium concentration frequently rose above 7 mEq/liter but stayed at normal levels in the patients on propranolol. It is apparent that while on bypass at 28°C, during the warming process and after the patients were off bypass, that potassium concentration was significantly elevated in the patients on chronic propranolol therapy. These observations indicate that potassium cardioplegia for myocardial preservation or potassium supplementation during surgery may pro-

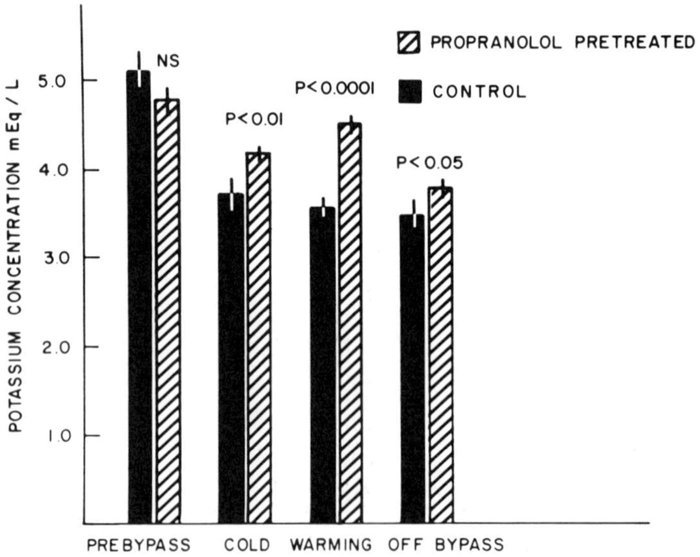

Figure 17.6. The changes in potassium during four phases of cardiopulmonary bypass. Control patients on no propranolol. Others on propranolol up to the day of surgery.

duce elevations in plasma potassium concentration which are potentially dangerous in patients on chronic propranolol therapy.

PRACTICAL CONSIDERATIONS

The significance of cardiac arrhythmia[15, 17] and the association with hypokalemia during cardiac surgery are clearly documented. The arrhythmia problem is compounded in patients on digitalis preparations because hypokalemia potentiates digitalis toxicity. Characteristically, several approaches have been used to minimize the problem with hypokalemia during and immediately after cardiac surgery. They are as follows:

1. Stop digitalis and diuretics 24 to 48 hours before surgery.
2. Replace any potassium deficits preoperatively.
3. Add potassium liberally during bypass based on potassium determinations every 15–30 minutes during surgery.
4. Replace potassium hourly in the postoperative period to maintain serum potassium greater than 4.0 mEq/liter.

Potassium replacement during and after cardiopulmonary bypass can be administered using various regimens. The approach at our institution has been to prime the pump with Ringer's lactate containing 4.0 mEq/liter of potassium. Potassium determinations are made every 30 minutes during bypass, while the patients are hypothermic, every 15 minutes while the patients are being warmed, every 2 hours after bypass as long as potassium is below 4 mEq/liter and then every 4 hours for the remainder of the first 24 hours after surgery. Potassium replacement is given according to the regimen in Table 17.1.

In patients on bypass the potassium is given over a 1- to 5-minute period. Supplementation is then given every 15 to 30 minutes when the routine potassiums are obtained. Postoperatively, the calculated potassium dose, from Table 17.1, is given each hour for 2 hours, then the serum potassium concentration is repeated before any additional potassium is given. Each replacement dose is given slowly over an hour to avoid transient hyperkalemia. Using this approach, hypokalemia-induced arrhythmias are seldom observed.

Table 17.1
Potassium Replacement for Hypokalemia*

1. If serum potassium is less than 3.7 mEq/liter, 1/4 mEq/kg is given for patients who weigh less than 40 kg. Patients who weigh over 40 kg routinely receive 10 mEq.
2. If potassium is between 3.7 and 4.0 mEq/liter, then recommended dose is one-half the dose calculated in no. 1 above.

* Frequency and rate of administration are discussed in text.

Table 17.2
Management of Hyperkalemia

1. Liberal administration of calcium chloride to maintain ionized calcium between 2.2 and 2.5 mEq/liter to minimize the negative effect of hyperkalemia on cardiac function.
2. Correct any acidosis.
3. Establish a vigorous diuresis with diuretics.
4. Give glucose (50 gm) and insulin (20–25 units) to force potassium intracellularly.
5. Kayexalate (Winthrop Laboratories, New York, New York) enema every 1–2 hr.
6. Hemodialysis.

In the past, hyperkalemia was quite unusual, occurring only in patients with renal failure or in patients receiving injudicious potassium replacement. In the last few years, however, elevated potassium concentration has been seen frequently in patients on high dose propranolol who require myocardial revascularization and where potassium-containing cardioplegic solutions are used for myocardial preservation. The body of this report explains the reasons for these changes. The significance is obvious, as hyperkalemia[2] can produce a decrease in myocardial contractility which may be critical in patients with poor basic cardiac function.

Our approach to hyperkalemia is indicated in Table 17.2. This approach has been uniformly successful, except in patients with cardiogenic shock and renal failure postoperatively. Dialysis is seldom necessary but can be done either on bypass or postoperatively, as necessary, with good success.

References

1. Barnard MS, Saunders SJ, Eales L, Barnard CN: Hypokalemia during extracorporeal circulation. Lancet 1:240, 1966.

2. Hammarsten JF, Ginn HE, Smith WO: Normal and abnormal potassium and magnesium metabolism. In *Clinical Metabolism of Body Water and Electrolytes*, Chap. 21. W. B. Saunders, Philadelphia and London, 1963, pp. 569.
3. Breckenridge IM, Deverall PB, Kirklin JW, Digerness SB: Potassium intake and balance after open intracardiac operations. J Thorac Cardiovasc Surg 63:305, 1972.
4. Clark RE, Beasley WE III, Sode J, Mills M: The lack of influence of hemodilution perfusion on alterations in total body potassium. J Thorac Cardiovasc Surg 65:112, 1973.
5. Curry DL, Curry KP: Hypothermia and insulin secretion. Endocrinology 87:750, 1970.
6. Hill DG, Sönksen PH, Braimbridge MV: Levels of plasma insulin and glucose after open-heart surgery. J Thorac Cardiovasc Surg 67:712, 1974.
7. Landymore RW, Murphy DA, Kinley CE, Parrott JC, Moffitt EA, Longley WJ, Quirbic AA: Does pulsatile flow influence the incidence of postoperative hypertension? Ann Thorac Surg 28:261, 1979.
8. Mandal AK, Callaghan JC, Dolan AM, Sterns LP: Potassium and cardiac surgery. Ann Thorac Surg 7: 428, 1969.
9. Moffitt EA, Sessler AD, Molnar GD, McGoon DC: Normothermia *versus* hypothermia for whole body perfusion. Effects on myocardial and body metabolism. Anesth Analg 50:505, 1971.
10. Obel IWP, Marchand P, Du Plessis L: Biochemical changes associated with the use of haemodilution with 5% dextrose in water and mannitol for open-heart surgery. Thorax 22:180, 1967.
11. Paton BC, Rosenkrantz JG, Blount SG Jr: Clinical and physiological results of perfusion with diluted blood. Circulation 29(Suppl 1):29:63, 1964.
12. Patrick J, Sivapragasam S: The prediction of postoperative potassium excretion after cardiopulmonary bypass. J Thorac Cardiovasc Surg 73:559, 1977.
13. Philbin DM, Coggins CH, Emerson CW, Levine FH, Buckley MJ: Plasma vasopressin levels and urinary sodium excretion during cardiopulmonary bypass. Comparison of halothane and morphine anesthesia. J Thorac Cardiovasc Surg 77:582, 1979.
14. Replogle R, Levy M, DeWall RA, Lillehei RC: Catecholamine and serotonin response to cardiopulmonary bypass. J Thorac Cardiovasc Surg 44:638, 1962.
15. Selmonosky CA, Flege JB Jr: The effect of small doses of potassium on postoperative ventricular arrhythmias. J Thorac Cardiovasc Surg 53:349, 1967.
16. Stremmel W, Schlosser V, Koehnlein HE: Effect of open-heart surgery with hemodilution perfusion upon insulin secretion. J Thorac Cardiovasc Surg 64: 263, 1972.
17. Shanahan EA, Anderson ST, Morris KN: Effect of modified preoperative, intraoperative, and postoperative potassium supplementation on the incidence of postoperative ventricular arrhythmias. J Thorac Cardiovasc Surg 57:413, 1969.
18. Tan C-K, Glisson SN, El-Etr AA, Ramakrishnaiah KB: Levels of circulating norepinephrine and epinephrine before, during, and after cardiopulmonary bypass in man. J Thorac Cardiovasc Surg 71:928, 1976.
19. Todd EP: Studies on the kalemotropic effects of epinephrine. Baylor College of Medicine, Baylor University, Houston, Texas. 1969.
20. Todd EP, Campbell HC, Utley JR, Miller RE, McAllister RG Jr, Wachtel CC, Collins JC, Erickson JL: Effect of β-adrenergic blockade on hypothermia-induced hypokalemia. Surgical Forum 28:275, 1977.
21. Todd EP, McAllister RG Jr, Campbell HC, Miller RE, Utley JR, Zeok JV, Erickson JL, Wachtel CC: Effect of propranolol on hypokalemia induced by cardiopulmonary bypass. Circulation 56(Suppl 2):60, 1977.
22. Todd EP, McAllister RG, Miller RE: Potential potassium toxicity with routine cardioplegia. Unpublished observations.
23. Todd EP, Vick RL: A re-evaluation of the effects of single rapid injections of epinephrine on plasma [K]. Proc West Pharmacol Soc 12:114, 1969.
24. Todd EP, Vick RL, Bonner RM, Luedke DW: The influence of the rate of infusion on the kalemotropic effect of epinephrine. Arch Int Physiol Biochim 77: 33, 1969.
25. Todd EP, Vick RL: Kalemotropic effect of epinephrine: Analysis with adrenergic agonists and antagonists. Am J Physiol 220:1964, 1971.
26. Todd EP, Vick RL: The influence of plasma potassium concentration on hydrocarbon-epinephrine arrhythmia. Proc West Pharmacol Soc 11:112, 1968.
27. Vick RL, Todd EP, Luedke DW: Epinephrine induced hypokalemia: Relation to liver and skeletal muscle. J Pharmacol Exp Ther 181:139, 1972.
28. Vick RL, Todd EP: The effects of autonomic blocking agents on plasma [K]. Proc West Pharmacol Soc 12: 124, 1969.

INDEX